SICKNESS, RECOVERY AND DEATH

Sickness, Recovery and Death:

A History and Forecast of Ill Health

James C. Riley

Professor of History

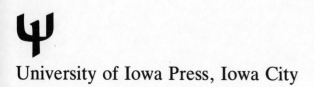

University of Iowa Press, Iowa City

For Sharyn
and for Mike Aronoff, Ann Carmichael,
Della Cook and Gene Weinburg

Contents

List of Tables

List of Figures

Preface

> The menace of disease is one of the
> components of health.
>
> Georges Canquilhem

Today as in the past most episodes of ill health do not end in death. The most common outcome is something called recovery. An individual who falls ill or is injured convalesces and resumes ordinary activity. This book takes a step toward a history of sickness and its outcomes, more especially the outcome called recovery. The narrative extends across time from the mid-seventeenth century into the future, and across space from Western Europe and Britain to the United States. Between the seventeenth century and the twentieth, the risks posed by illness and injury changed. In the earlier period most sicknesses were resolved quickly although still more often in recovery than in death. Life involved a series of confrontations with ill health, confrontations of which the 'menace of disease' mentioned in the epigraph to this chapter represents only one type. During the nineteenth century, protracted ill health began to take over. Aged people became more numerous, but among the young and the old sicknesses were resolved less and less often in death. In the twentieth century health has been dominated by two new and stunning achievements of humankind. First, death has been pushed by and large into the realm of the old. Whereas in the seventeenth-century West about half of the population died before reaching adulthood, today more than 90 per cent survive past age 50 and more than 75 per cent past age 65. Second, the likelihood that any given episode of ill health will be resolved in death, or at least in death in the near future, has been curtailed.

Did the prototypical story of health over the life course also change character, from a narrative of short lives dominated by ill health to a narrative of long and healthy lives? That is the question this book seeks to answer. At first glance it is a simple question, and its answer is obvious. Surely we are now healthier. Who among us would trade places with someone living in the seventeenth century without dreading the vastly greater health risks of that era? But the answer is not altogether simple. More especially, it is not simple once we stop telling the story of health from the record of deaths rather than recoveries. To see the more complex implications of this question, consider the issues of health, ill health, and the timing of death within a spatial framework. How many years might a group of people born at the same time live, given what we know about the human life span? How many of those years are now lived, and how many have been lived in different periods of human history? Among years lived, how many have been lived in health rather than ill health? How have the ill health episodes survived influenced later health and the timing of death? How does distant and more recent experience with ill health influence the forecasts we should make about future life and health?

In search of answers this book offers a number of dialogues, in which an historian relates some things known about past human experience to knowledge and curiosity in other specializations: biology, medicine, public health, gerontology, epidemiology and demography. The narrative is organized around a theory called insult accumulation, which is summarized in Chapter 2. Insult accumulation is a theory about how sicknesses survived influence later health. This theory is an important organizing principle because it provides a way to consider evidence about recoveries and deaths and because it emphasizes the value of an historical record that includes individual and aggregate-level health experience over the life course. History is ordinarily thought of as a relation of individual experiences. Here, however, it is rarely the individual and more often the historical period and the group of people born around the same time that assume the leading roles.

In the nineteenth century, more so apparently than in the eighteenth or the twentieth, people in Western Europe and the United States worried about whether they might be mistaken for dead. To the customary cautions, which called for careful scrutiny to determine death and advised against too hasty burial, they added new practices, outfitting coffins with strings reaching above ground to bells. I have no idea how often people taken for dead regained vitality. A few accounts circulated, and some of them may have been grounded in fact. Nevertheless, the living will not often have been taken for dead. The sick, however, may often take themselves for being well, and the well may often present themselves as sick. The issue of a threshold was settled in a certain way in the sources consulted for this book. Its settlement was usually matter-of-fact.

The people who made distinctions between health and sickness in the creation of these records apparently considered their decisions matters of common sense.

That is not to say that threshold, definition, and categorization are in fact simple matters of common sense. That they are not is obvious. So, too, is it obvious that the records used to compile this history will fail to satisfy those of us who want subtle distinctions, much less those who want to distinguish an objectively verifiable gauge of 'real' ill health. On the one hand, readers interested in emotional as well as physical health, or in the health experiences of women and children, may be disappointed. Most of the record yet regained deals with physical disorders plus gross mental illness—insanity (whatever that may mean). And most of it deals with adult males. These focuses will be taken over and in more recent circumstances, when emotional health and the health of women and children might be discussed in greater detail, the physical health of men will continue to draw most of our attention. On the other hand, readers interested in determining the level of ill health that prevailed at a given place and time will also find their preoccupation shifted behind a feasible goal. Whereas it is reasonable to infer the trend of ill health over time, it is much more difficult to decide whether the level reported for one time and place can be stated in the same terms as that given for another time and place. Thresholds, definitions and categories may change even when ill health is reported in the same terms.

This is an exploration. Many historical records remain to be consulted; many problems of theory, method and characterization remain to be solved. An attempt at a general history is nevertheless worth while. It may provoke people who would not otherwise look for evidence or attack problems to do so. It may help organize the exploration, lending it a body of propositions and inferences open to testing and, in many cases no doubt, to rejection. But the most important contributions this book may make are, I hope, these two. First, this book is intended to assert the importance of historical experience and historical exploration in fields in which researchers turn too quickly to animal models, computer simulations and prospective studies. Questions about life-long health experience and the influence of prior health on future health need not depend, for satisfactory answers, only on laboratory and clinical studies. Second, this book focuses on quantities. Sickness cannot be understood merely by measuring its incidence or prevalence, or merely by describing its characteristics; quantitative and qualitative dimensions

both require consideration. The focus of this book is a consequence
of the sources consulted and the need to establish quantitative issues
in a clear way rather than of a sense of where the answers ultimately lie.

Acknowledgments

It is a joy to acknowledge some of my collaborators in researching and writing this book. The Dean of Faculties at Indiana University, Anya Royce, sponsored the first step by initiating a program of multidisciplinary faculty development. Five of us organized a seminar called 'Morbidity', and spent a year exploring some of the dimensions of sickness. I've dedicated this book to my colleagues in that seminar, and to my wife, Sharyn. The Netherlands Institute for Advanced Study in the Humanities and Social Sciences provided time off from the usual responsibilities of academic life and a congenial group of people in whose company I spent the year 1985–86. The John Simon Guggenheim Memorial Foundation allowed me to continue to work on this project, and to compose this book, during the year 1986–87. Additional financial assistance has been provided by BRSG S07-RR07031 awarded by the Biomedical Research Support Grant Program, Division of Research Resources, National Institutes of Health, and by Indiana University.

A book like this falls outside everyone's field. In hopes of limiting the number of large mistakes I might make, I enlisted the help of readers who agreed to lend their expertise in several fields. For the good advice that they offered, advice that I usually took, I thank George Alter, James H. Cassedy, Alfred W. Crosby, Wilbur G. Downs, Myron Gutmann, Eric Jones, K. David Patterson, M. Jeanne Peterson, Steven Stowe, and Eugene D. Weinberg. Allyn Roberts suggested a number of ways in which the text might be made easier to follow. I claim responsibility for the flaws that remain.

A book like this also depends on cooperation from librarians and archivists. The people who helped me locate useful material have been too numerous to mention by name. I want, however, to identify some who have earned my gratitude for their contributions to this book and to other projects carried out at Indiana University in the past thirteen years. Miriam Bonham, Tom Glastras, Jeffrey Graf, Betty Jarboe, Fred Musto, Pat Riesenman, Rhonda Stone, Gloria Westfall and Alice Wickizer are not the only librarians in the reference, interlibrary loan, and government publications departments at Indiana, but they are the people I've gotten to know best by calling on them repeatedly. The firm AMEV, formerly a life insurance company known as 'the Utrecht', allowed me to use items from their extensive library. Mr G. Haughton and Mr George Swetman of the Independent Order of Odd Fellows Manchester Unity allowed me to consult material from their library and answered questions about the Order. Mr Douglas Carr, High Secretary of the Independent Order of Rechabites, provided access to the Rechabite library.

Although I have already mentioned George Alter as reader of an earlier draft, my debt to him is grander than that. George fostered my interest in sickness and its history by developing an interest of his own in this field and by teaching me how he would approach its questions and problems.

I wish to thank the following for permission to reproduce material from their publications:

Academic Press, Inc., for a figure initially published in *Advances in Biological and Medical Physics*, vol. 4 (1956) in an essay by Hardin B. Jones.

Editions Société d'Histoire et d'Archéologie de Genève and Professor Alfred Perrenoud for a figure from Perrenoud's *La population de Genève du seizième au début du dix-neuvième siècle: Etude démographique* (1979).

The *Milbank Memorial Fund Quarterly/Health and Society* for four figures initially published in an essay by Lois M. Verbrugge, which appeared in vol. 62, no. 3.

W.H. Freeman and Company for a figure from *Vitality and Aging* by James F. Fries and Lawrence M. Crapo, Copyright 1981.

James C. Riley

Bloomington
November 1987

This book has been awarded the 1988 Ernst Meyer Prize, given by the Association Internationale pour l'Étude de l'Économie de l'Assurance, Geneva. This prize is given annually by the Geneva Association for 'university research work which makes a significant and original contribution to the study of risk and insurance economics'.

Introduction

How fascinating the drama of death as acted out by the royalty of early modern Europe and the favored people able to ape the behavior of kings. On that stage everyone seemed to die an anticipated death. The lead player took to the deathbed on some hidden signal, called in intimates and children, reminisced, offered advice, wrote or dictated memoirs, set a courageous example, and then died. To all appearances it was an era of open and almost benign death. Even Louis XV of France, whose misfortune it was to die at age 64 in 1774 of an acute childhood disease, smallpox, died slowly enough to participate in a more than ordinarily elaborate version of the ritual. But what a curious and unlikely image. To be sure, the old may have died in a lingering manner, old kings and old beggars alike, each on his or her own stage. But the typical death of the early modern era was neither benign nor lingering. It was a death in anguish, anguish compounded by the joint operation of two forces: the diseases that killed were mostly painful ailments quickly resolved by death or recovery; and the therapies that combatted those diseases offered additional pain without apparent efficacy. It was a death experienced more often than not by infants and children rather than by the aged. From the demographer we learn about the prototypical death scene: an infant falls ill and, before acquiring any other means to express suffering than a cry, dies after a few days.

Except for infants, death was also an event likely to be recorded, leading to a situation in which, for many of the people who lived in Europe or North America in the seventeenth, eighteenth or nineteenth centuries, it is possible to recover a name, a date of christening and a date of death or burial, but little else. So many lives, so many histories, recorded only as entrances and exits. These characteristics of the record have been allowed to shape our understanding of the history of sickness. Sickness was, we infer, disease or sometimes injury remarkable by the occasions in which it was resolved by death. And because disease, especially epidemic disease, and death were so commonplace at every stage within the human life course, the supposition that these historical societies were distinguished by their ill health becomes inescapable. Sickness, the transient event preceding death, hardly needs notice in its own right.

1

In the final analysis all this is true. Death was the dominant event, the more so because it was so often premature, because so often it occurred before old age. But it was not so overwhelming in importance that we can afford to neglect the transient event that preceded it or, more especially, the series of transient episodes in the life course that did not end in death. Death was preceded by sickness or injury. But sickness did not usually end in death. Even in the seventeenth and early eighteenth century, when lethal epidemics were common and the crude death rate exceeded 30 people per 1000 a year (in contrast to about 9 per 1000 per year in the same regions of the world today), most ailments ended in recovery. The sufferer resumed his or her ordinary activities.

The customary manner of understanding sickness, whether in the seventeenth century or the twentieth, begins with the concept of disease or condition. People are sick when they have smallpox, coronary heart disease, a cold, AIDS, or another malady. At some point in the development of an ailment the sufferer recognizes the existence of malady and its symptoms, and may ask for diagnosis and treatment from a medical practitioner. Once given, the diagnosis establishes the reality of the malady; the disease is real when its nature has been deciphered by a third party. For all the value of this approach at the individual level when the overriding issue is to identify an efficacious therapy, it is not a model that is always easily applied to historical investigation or even to the present. Most sicknesses experienced in the past went undiagnosed and unrecognized in this formal sense. Those most likely to be diagnosed were the sicknesses most likely to be resolved in death, an unrepresentative group, since the risk of fatality varied substantially from disease to disease and from person to person. What is more, the individuals who gave diagnoses – identities for diseases – were often unqualified to do so within any system that can now be reconstructed.

It matters that the people charged with assigning cause of death in eighteenth-century Sweden were clergymen who had known the victim, in England the searchers of the dead – women, often widows – who supplemented meager incomes by taking this official position, and in Milan licensed physicians. The significance lies at two levels. First, diagnoses by lay persons referred to short lists of possible causes and to means of determination that have been lost but seem in any event to have been casual or vague. Only the physicians shared a system of identification that can now be reconstructed and that can therefore serve as the basis for attempts to transfer historical identifications into terms now in use. Inevitably the effort is less than fully satisfying, if only because the textbook of pathology has expanded so much and come to depend on features of diagnosis alien to licensed physicians, much less clerics and searchers, in the early modern era. The second level of significance consists of the possibility of diagnostic error even when an expert verdict has been given within a known system. Although the results are biased by the likelihood that difficult cases will be chosen for reconsideration, present-day post-mortem examinations find rates of diagnostic error as high as 50 per cent and continue to report a small but significant percentage of cases in which no diagnosis can confidently be made. What is more, many people die of multiple or overlapping pathologies, so that it is difficult to distinguish an overriding cause of death or to distribute responsibility for death among the causes identified.

The weaknesses of the diagnostic model are not sufficient to undermine confidence in the desire to learn about sickness in the past or present, nor are the strengths of this model – its argument toward disease identification and its capacity to use the rich accumulated body of medical knowledge about diseases – sufficient to satisfy curiosity. Too many dimensions of the historical phenomenon of sickness escape notice when the diagnostic model is applied by itself. It is not essential to rely only on the historical sources ordinarily consulted to answer questions about disease identity: medical commentaries and registers of death by cause. Other approaches and other sources complement these and bring into light aspects of sickness experience heretofore poorly known or not known at all.

Sickness has three dimensions. It is, first, a passage out of 'wellness'. (Even the language makes it difficult to describe health in structural terms, for it offers no ready oppositional terms. Ill health is not the complement of health; wellness is an awkward term of uncertain meaning; disease has no simple counterpart.) For the moment the key feature is the event: to fall sick is at least to create the possibility of historical notice. It is something worth remarking. Second, sickness is an event with a temporal dimension. Even when its duration is too brief to warrant measurement – such as the stroke that kills suddenly or the sharp but unidentified pain that quickly fades – some time passes between the point at which the individual could still claim good health and the outcome of the episode. Often sickness lingers for hours, days, weeks, years, even decades. Third, sickness is a matter of intensity. Not everyone takes the same opinion about whether an apparently identical degree of distress should constitute sickness. Even when the judgment is shifted to a third party, such as the physician who identifies a disease and determines whether therapy is required, opinions will vary (although much less so than in a world in which all judgments rest with the individual). Historians, social scientists, and philosophers often write about this third dimension of sickness by comparing its degrees to the strata of physical objects. The iceberg metaphor is sometimes employed and a distinction made between visible and invisible sickness. A subtle range of distinctions is provided by the model of the onion, with its rings that stand for degrees of ill health but are not always concentric.[1] Sometimes they overlap and in overlapping suggest the ultimate ambiguity of the point at which the event of sickness begins. Each of these dimensions has its own complexities. For example, will the individual who experiences an unambiguous passage into sickness allow himself or herself to be scrutinized by anyone who may record the event? In simple present-day terms, will this person consult a physician or report an illness to anyone else?

Like the diagnostic model, the temporal model can tell only part of the story about sickness. Together the two models complement one another, so that one can foresee a history and a story of current and future events that incorporate both models to probe the experience of sickness. That time has not yet arrived. At this moment it is important to examine the characteristics of the temporal dimension of sickness, to pose questions that have a reasonable prospect of being answered, and to begin to fashion the part of the history of sickness that can be told from sources recording events, durations, and degree. The temporal approach, which is often quantitative, should later be amalgamated with the diagnostic approach, which is sensitive to qualitative issues. The characteristics of this amalgamated model cannot all be foreseen, but it will emphasize patient and case histories and it will also require new methods for the simultaneous and collaborative treatment of quantitative and qualitative information.

The temporal model, too, requires a specialized vocabulary and the assignment of special meanings to familiar words. It also requires a methodology. In the vocabulary the key word is sickness, which is defined here as a degree of ill health that compromises the individual's ability to perform ordinary activities. For most of the historical period in which sickness can be discussed in this form – from the seventeenth century to the present – ordinary activities consisted of work and the passage from wellness to sickness occurred when, in a third party's judgment, an individual became incapable of work. It was the incapacity to earn the wages of work that gave rise to the recognition of sickness in this form as an event. The passage was recorded because workers organized insurance funds to compensate themselves for some of the income lost to sickness. They paid premiums, thereby creating a financial record of their time at risk to sickness, and they drew benefits, creating a record of sickness events. Thus the insurance records, like familiar diagnostic sources, identify events of the numerator. Unlike familiar sources, they also distinguish the duration of the events and the size and temporal dimensions of the denominator, allowing sickness rates to be computed. This is what distinguishes them from hospital and physician records from which it is seldom possible to gauge the size of the population at risk.

In the methodology of a history of sickness the key concept is risk. Who is at risk to sickness, and what are the dimensions of the risk? The methodology draws heavily on demography and epidemiology, especially in turning attention away from the experience of the individual toward that of the group and in adopting means to discuss leading features of risk and their evolution over time.

In the matter of death the historical trend is clear. In Europe and North America in the late twentieth century fewer people die at every stage of life before old age; the trend consists of fewer 'premature' deaths and, on average, more years lived in each life. One manifestation of this trend is increasing life expectancies. It is customary to suppose that the era of premature death and the era of transition toward death in old age were characterized by ill health. Somehow the short life expectancy of times past seems testimony of ill health among survivors as well as among victims of illness and injury. That assumption will be contested here but not in an effort to show that, in the era of premature death, people were seldom sick. That, after all, cannot be shown. Instead, it will be contested in order to see more clearly the intricacies of ill health in the early modern era and since, especially to see that identifying the terminal sicknesses of those who died will not reveal the state of health of those who lived.

Inevitably the question will arise whether the sickness rate has increased or diminished in the long run. This is a question that must be asked but also one that cannot yet be answered with assurance. Sickness is more difficult to specify than death, and its specifications have changed over time. For example, the concept of sickness has expanded. In the twentieth century it includes psychological disorders not recognized one or two hundred years ago, a longer list of physical disorders, and probably also an inclination to take symptoms that are not incapacitating more seriously. Definitions may also vary from one culture to another, which means not only across well-demarcated cultural frontiers but also across time within the same region and among subgroups in the same culture. No simple way exists to quantify these definitional and conceptual shifts and thereby to hold constant the standard by which events or episodes may be admitted to the numerator. However, trends can be discerned when the sickness experience of a group is followed over time and when the specification of sickness has been held constant. The trends themselves can be compared. A certain image arises from the history of these various trends, and that is the way in which the history of sickness can now be told. It is not yet a history in which levels of ill health in a seventeenth-century workforce can be usefully compared on the same scale to those obtained through twentieth-century health surveys. A comparison can nevertheless be made. While it is important to know whether work time lost because of sickness in the seventeenth century may have been distinguished in a way similar to the twentieth-century discrimination of sickness from health among working people, it is also important to know how much time was lost from work in the two eras even if different judgments may have been made about the threshold between capacity and incapacity.

Although the issue of trend in health status is important, and the tentative answer about trend to be given here may seem to be the most provocative part of the study, the most significant issue lies elsewhere. It concerns not population-level experience as understood through sickness rates, but population-level experience as understood through an aggregation of individual life histories of sickness and health. After its end, each life can be seen in a telescoped manner as an assemblage of health experiences. If the life has been reasonably long, then its health history is a record of some diseases and injuries survived and, ultimately, of at least one not survived. In the diagnostic model, the most important aim is to identify the cause or causes operating at the time of death. Individual diseases and injuries assume importance when they figure prominently as causes of death. In the temporal model, in contrast, the aim is to follow health experience over the life course.

In an ideal world, one in which the historian, like a laboratory scientist, could design the sources from which information would be gathered, health experience might be followed at the individual level from birth to death. Reliable and precise data would be obtained about all episodes of health and ill health, those of which the individual was aware and those not, those clinical and those subclinical in manifestation, as well as information about genetic characteristics, environmental hazards, and many other variables. The experiment would be designed to answer questions about the degree to which the experience of ill health earlier in life influenced later health and the timing of death. Since the historical process must be retrospective, the actual record will lack many of these ideal features and conclusions will often be flawed. Individual life histories of health experience, which are the basic data of the insurance records, speak nevertheless to questions about the long-term effect of ill health. Are individuals who suffer more sickness earlier in life prone to more sickness later in life or to earlier deaths? How are groups of people born at the same time and raised in the same epidemiologic regime and ecological domain affected by the health experiences they share and accumulate? How do the remote causes of death – earlier illness and injury episodes incompletely repaired, reallocations of resources toward repair, and the assaults of disease and violence on the elements of vitality (such as the immune system) – affect health? These, too, are questions that need to be carefully framed before they can be answered adequately. But these questions can be addressed from historical sources. It is not necessary to follow the experience of people now alive in prospective epidemiologic studies, to rely on animal models, or to turn to computer-aided simulations, though each of these sources complements the historical record and assists the search for answers.

Toward the end of the twentieth century it is appropriate to turn away from the diagnostic model and toward a combined and, eventually, an integrated model of diagnoses and life histories. Remote causes of death – events that occurred years, even decades, in the past but which condition health in the present – have never been more important in human experience with morbidity and mortality. Today in the developed countries the prototypical death occurs through the operation of chronic and degenerative disease in an aged individual suffering several ailments at once. Some of the ailments can be traced to distant events that are known, in the way, for example, that lung cancer can be related in many individuals to a history of cigarette smoking. Some are traced to distant events that are less readily specified, such as the acquisition of habits of diet and exercise that fail to serve longevity in an optimal way. Some are related to specific health events or to repeated ill health that diminishes vitality. And some ailments are recent and exogenous in origin.

The passage from a regime of premature death usually caused by acute diseases to a regime of death in old age from mostly degenerative diseases is a history worth reconstructing. It is also a history that bears directly on the health experience of today and tomorrow and that, therefore, forms itself into patterns that can be projected forward in time. Historians have usually been loath to forecast future events, knowing all too well the unlikelihood of finding reliable forecasts in a mere forward projection of historical patterns. I have not elected to toss caution aside but instead to project a range of future experience. The basis for these projections will be given by a combination of the assumptions about morbidity and mortality that are the most warranted, according to the evidence assembled here, and by recent morbidity and mortality experience. The forecast will be gloomy, not because I believe the future must contain an increasing burden of sickness but because signs of the alleviation of that burden are rare. To have a different future we should behave differently now and thus change the assumptions about mortality and morbidity that today appear most justified.

1 The Boundary of Survival

The last enemy that shall be conquered
is death.

I Corinthians 15:26

THE SPACE OF LIFE

Life leaves us in suspense, not about the eventuality of death but about its timing and causes. Like many other organisms, the human species faces a boundary on survival, a maximum or potential life span quantifiable on a graph. It is difficult to imagine a situation in which all of the space up to this boundary might be filled, in which, that is, everyone would survive to the limit of the human potential. The difficulty arises from our familiarity with the history of death. This history shows that some people will die in every stage of life, and that illnesses and injuries likely to cause death will accumulate, especially in old age. Eliminating each of the causes reported on death certificates would not extend the human life span indefinitely, but, at least in theory, such an achievement would allow all members of the species to live to the boundary.

The location of the boundary – the maximum age to which members of the species might live – is a matter of speculation rather than knowledge. Although people have long been curious about it, and the life spans of exceptionally old individuals have often been reported, little reliable information is available. The true birthdates of historical figures reputed to have lived exceptionally long lives are seldom known, and those individuals rarely appear in corroborative records. The boundary should be fixed at an age above 100, for it can readily be shown that people have lived longer than 100 years. Above 110, however, it becomes difficult to find reliable examples, despite the millions of people who die each year and who now die in societies in which birthdates and corroborative evidence are available.[1] A few people survive to higher ages, but the significance of their survival is difficult to evaluate.

9

The assumption that the life span of the human species should be identified from the longest life yet reliably recorded is itself a speculative one. It is an assumption that in turn guides the idea that many species have maximum life spans. Fragmentary evidence about animal and insect life spans suggests that other organisms, whether similar to humans or not, also confront boundaries to survival but that the upper limits can be achieved only when these species are protected from predators, parasites, and other exogenous threats to survival. Animals in the wild rarely live as long as animals in controlled environments, such as the zoo or the laboratory. Hence the life span of animals in a given species has usually been estimated from the longest life of a member of the species observed in captivity. For example, a lemur once lived to age 39, and the life span of the genus *Lemur* has been estimated at 40. Rockstein and Lieberman constructed a life table for male house flies, showing that one in the population of 4627 lived 59 days but that, at the end of 16 days, the population had been reduced by half.[2] The analogy from humans to animals or insects can then be reapplied to humans. If the maximum life span is manipulatable, if it can be altered in ways that enhance the likelihood of survival, and perhaps in ways that allow enough individuals to live beyond 110 or some higher age to show that the maximum life span for humans is greater, what, then, are the boundaries of manipulation? But such discussion threatens at once to become metaphysical. I wish only to suggest that it is reasonable and plausible to conceive of a longer human life span than will be acknowledged here. That is reasonable and plausible because one argument to be developed in this book – an argument about the remote causes of death – demonstrates that the conditions necessary to discover the human life span have not been established. Compared to the lemur kept in a zoo or the house flies raised in a laboratory, or to any animal or insect living in a controlled environment, humankind has not yet managed its own environment to a point at which we can be confident that the maximum life span has been achieved. Humans have shown that they can create the protected environment that allows a lemur to live 39 years, but they have not elected to subject themselves to the same degree of control.

Nor is it necessary to know the upper boundary in order to proceed. It is not the boundary that needs to be known but two other quantities that fall short of it. One of these, known too awkwardly as the *maximum average life span*, can be called the *modal age of death*. It is the appoximate age at which deaths cluster among long-lived members of a given generation. If all births are considered, that age would, until recently, have been between birth and the first birthday. Up to the twentieth century more people died in the first year of life than at any other age. But if infancy and childhood are excluded, the modal age of death will be higher and will identify a point before very old age at which the probability of dying in adulthood peaks. That point has changed over time. The other quantity is the *life expectancy* – the average span that individuals can expect to live in a given place and time.

Although potential life span has often been and remains a matter of speculation, these two other quantities have been objects of legal and scientific investigation. The psalmist suggests a life span of three score and ten years, meaning apparently to approximate a limited version of the modal age of death rather than the potential span, which biblical testimony fixed at much higher ages, or life expectancy, which assuredly fell short of 70 years. This limited version represented an approximate life span of adults. A similar version of the modal age was implied in computations of the Roman jurist Ulpian, who sketched what appears to have been a table of life expectancy at some ages. Ulpian implied that the modal age would be 65 years or slightly higher, a juridical version of the span. Early in the eighteenth century the mathematician Abraham de Moivre, interested in the probabilistic as well as the juridical side of the problem, revised Ulpian's figure to 86 years. De Moivre possessed some evidence about actual life spans because he had studied the survival of people on whose lives annuities had been purchased and who had, therefore, been under scrutiny from the time they entered observation, in childhood or early adulthood, until their deaths. He argued not that no one lived longer than 86 but that years lived at higher ages would have little effect on the juridical and financial decisions revolving around life span because they would be so few.[3] In those terms de Moivre's figure remains appropriate today. At the end of the twentieth century a larger proportion of the population lives to an age above 86, but as yet the number of years lived at higher ages remains a small part of the total.

Recent discussion has often accepted age 85 as a reasonable approximation of the 'complete' maximum average life span or, in the terms preferred here, the highest modal age of death likely to be achieved by humans.[4] That is, it seems reasonable to hope that, by bringing all the means now available to bear on increasing the number of years lived, we might enable birth cohorts to die at a modal age of about 85. The contrast with past experience would lie in the age from which modal age at death was measured – not adulthood but birth. In other words, this view suggests that life expectancy might be extended to the modal age of death. Other observers continue to focus on the modal age of death among adults, and suggest that a higher age can be achieved.

Because no convention exists for establishing the modal age of death, it is a figure whose definition has shifted, a value estimated by a process standing about midway between calculations from experience and approximation. Life expectancy, in contrast, is a figure obtained by computations following a strict set of conventions. One devised in the seventeenth century used historical evidence to follow a cohort as its members died. For example, the Dutch jurist and mathematician Johannes Hudde, interested in estimating the cost of different loan formats, consulted documents in 1671 detailing experience in a life annuity loan organized between 1586 and 1590. The life annuity contracts had been sold far enough in the past so that nearly everyone on whose survival an annuity had been purchased had died. Since the advent of the census, in the eighteenth century, it has been more common to take a cross section of the population within an interval of time and to estimate mortality at each age from that experience.

The experience is usually organized in a life table, such as the abridged (rather than complete, or age-by-age) US life table for 1979–81 given in Table 1.1. The life table begins with a radix (or base) population, often 100 000, and applies the current probability of dying at each age to determine decrements from the radix, or how many survivors will remain at each higher age. This basic information appears in the l_x column, so that, for example, Table 1.1 shows that 91 526 out of 100 000 people can be expected to survive to age 50. The decrements – deaths – at each age, given in the d_x column, make it possible to state the probability of death between any two ages, called the q_x function. Other columns report the number of complete years lived between any two ages (L_x), the total number of years lived at all subsequent ages (T_x), and the life expectancy (e_x). For US males and females together, life expectancy at birth in 1979–81 amounted to 73.88 years, which is all the years lived at all ages from 0–1 up by the initial population, or 7 387 758 divided by 100 000.

Consider the meaning of these columns by looking at what Table 1.1 says about each function at the highest ages included, where the numbers involved are small. Among 100 000 births this table indi-

TABLE 1.1 *Detail from the US life table for 1979–81*

Age	Number living of 100 000 born alive	Proportion dying	Number dying	Years lived at each age	Sum of years lived at each age and later ages	Life expectancy
	l_x	q_x	d_x	L_x	T_x	e_x
0	100 000	0.01260	1260	98 973	7 387 758	73.88
1	98 740	0.00093	92	98 694	7 288 785	73.82
2	98 648	0.00065	64	98 617	7 190 091	72.89
3	98 584	0.00050	49	98 560	7 091 474	71.93
4	98 535	0.00040	40	98 515	6 992 914	70.97
5	98 495	0.00037	36	98 477	6 894 399	70.00
10	98 347	0.00020	19	98 338	6 402 327	65.10
15	98 196	0.00069	67	98 163	5 910 885	60.19
20	97 741	0.00120	118	97 682	5 420 937	55.46
25	97 110	0.00132	128	97 046	4 933 778	50.81
30	96 477	0.00133	127	96 414	4 449 812	46.12
35	95 808	0.00159	153	95 731	3 969 060	41.43
40	94 926	0.00232	220	94 817	3 492 100	36.79
45	93 599	0.00366	343	93 427	3 020 551	32.27
50	91 526	0.00589	540	91 256	2 557 359	27.94
55	88 348	0.00902	797	87 950	2 107 175	23.85
60	83 726	0.01368	1145	83 153	1 676 326	20.02
65	77 107	0.02059	1587	76 314	1 273 347	16.51
70	68 248	0.03052	2083	67 206	909 003	13.32
75	56 799	0.04507	2560	55 520	595 390	10.48
80	43 180	0.06882	2972	41 694	344 612	7.98
85	27 960	0.10725	2999	26 461	166 556	5.96
90	14 154	0.15868	2246	13 031	62 666	4.43
95	5 043	0.22976	1159	4 463	16 840	3.34
100	1 150	0.29120	335	983	3 137	2.73
105	179	0.33539	60	150	428	2.38
109	33	0.35988	12	27	73	2.20

SOURCE US, National Center for Health Statistics: United States Life Tables, *U.S. Decennial Life Tables for 1979–81* (Washington, 1985), pp. 6–7.

cates that 33 individuals entered age 109–110. The probability of dying within that year of age (q_x) had risen to 0.36 out of a possible 1.0, and 12 individuals died (d_x) before reaching age 110. The 33 who entered age 109 lived a total of 27 years (the L_x value), and the 21 survivors lived an additional 46 years after age 109–110. The quantities of years lived combine to provide the T_x value (i.e., 27 + 46 = 73), and that amount divided by the number of individuals entering age 109 (33 people) gives the life expectancy at age 109 (e_{109}): 2.2 years.

It is important to notice that this is a period rather than a cohort table. Its values for each age group are derived from experience during 1979–81 rather than from following a cohort as it ages, as Hudde could do. A period table sacrifices the more precise values that would be obtained by following a cohort through life to the need for current information. Table 1.1 also assumes that the population is neither growing nor shrinking.

Although the custom is to focus attention on life expectancy, especially life expectancy at birth, other features of the life table are of more interest here. The l_x values, which recount the proportion of the initial population living to each higher age, sketch a survival curve for this population, taking males and females together. They help provide both a visual image with which to consider survival and its boundaries and a quantitative image. The visual image appears in Figure 1.1, a survival curve for the complete US population according to the mortality risks that prevailed in the period 1979–81.

The quantitative image consists of a proportion between the years that might be lived, assuming that everyone born alive achieved a given life span, and the years actually lived. In Table 1.1 this space takes the form of a rectangle whose boundaries are fashioned by the radix (100 000) and the limit of the life table, which ends at age 110, a figure approximating but not quite attaining the potential human life span. But it is more realistic to consider this space in terms of the modal age of death, which should be estimated at some point between 85 and 100. If age 85 is taken as a reasonable limit, then the space consists of 8.5 million years that might have been lived per 100 000 people. If 100 is the reasonable limit, then the space consists of 10 million years that might have been lived. Whether one figure is preferred to the other has some implications for the importance that might be attached to preserving life between ages 85 and 100 and for health programs. These are weighty matters, but they are not yet at issue here.

If the space – and therefore the denominator – is given as 8.5 million years, the numerator will consist of the sum of years actually lived to age 85, a value obtained from the T_x column of the life table after subtracting years lived at ages higher than 85 from the total value in the row for age 0, which refers to the first year of life: $T_0 - T_{85}$, or 7 387 758 − 166 556 = 7 221 202. The proportion of years

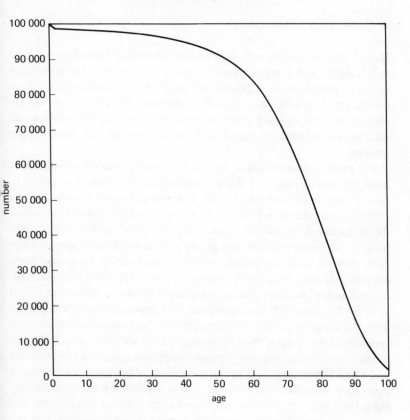

FIGURE 1.1 *Survival curve of the US population, 1979–81*

SOURCES See Table 1. 1.

lived to years available will be 85 per cent. If the space is given as 10 million years, the numerator will be years actually lived to age 100, or 7 384 621, giving a proportion of 73.8 per cent. Depending on how the limit has been set, the quantitative image suggests that between 74 and 85 per cent of the available space has been filled, even though the complete US population in 1979–81 had achieved neither the highest life expectancy at birth of any world society nor a homogeneous distribution of life span by sex, race, income, and other characteristics.

A CONQUEST OF SPACE

If we think of human survival in terms of one or the other of these two images, and if we review the history of survival, the story that emerges resembles a conquest of space. It is a dramatic story of movement between two radically different survival curves, or between two sharply divergent proportions, if still a story told in an undramatic manner of visual and quantitative rather than human images.

For most of human history only a few people reached old age. Not until the last decades of the nineteenth century was it possible to detect a persistent increase in life expectancy. Before that the history of life expectancy is a history of variation and fluctuation, in which the expectation varied from place to place and fluctuated from time to time. In some periods and places – William Shakespeare's England, around 1600, for example – life expectancy at birth may have approached late nineteenth-century levels, some 40 years, only to decline again.[5] In other places and periods this value fell so low that it is difficult, given the characteristics of human reproduction, which limit the range of possibilities, to conceive mathematically of how the segment of the species then living could have sustained itself. On the whole, survival fashioned a particular pattern consisting of variations and fluctuations around a gradual increase. The number of humans estimated to have lived grew in a way resembling the manner depicted in Table 1.2. Presented as population totals at given times, the increase is impressive: the habitable earth has been peopled. But the pertinent way to think about these values is in terms of the annual rate of change. Until the latter part of the eighteenth century the annual rate of growth remained modest, even though periods of regression were usually crowded out by an underlying tendency of the population to increase. These numbers and rates of change are informative. But they reveal less than we can learn from considering human history in terms of the survival curve and from considering space not as habitable land but as years that might be lived at each stage of life.

For early humankind the evidence about longevity is sparse and difficult to interpret. What is known about longevity in prehistory is known from skeletal remains, often mere fragments. A specialized branch of science, paleopathology, seeks to interpret this record, dating remains, estimating age at death, examining remains for signs of the cause of death and for morbid conditions present but not

TABLE 1.2   *World population, 4.5 million years ago to 1985*

	Population (in millions)	Growth rate per annum
4.5 million years ago	0.1	
		0.00000046
1 million years ago	0.5	
		0.00000191
500 000 years ago	1.3	
		0.000003
10 000 years ago	6	
		0.000425
400 BC	153	
		0.001245
1 AD	252	
		0.000004
1000	253	
		0.001201
1500	461	
		0.002059
1750	771	
		0.004771
1850	1241	
		0.005517
1900	1634	
		0.008782
1950	2530	
		0.018465
1985	4800	

SOURCES   Kenneth M. Weiss, 'On the Number of Members of the Genus Homo Who Have Ever Lived, and Some Evolutionary Implications', *Human Biology*, 56, no. 4 (Dec. 1984), p. 642; Jean-Noël Biraben, 'Essai sur l'évolution du nombre des hommes', *Population*, 34, no. 1 (Jan.–Feb. 1979), pp. 15–16; and *The World Almanac* (New York, 1987), p. 544. See also Ansley J. Coale, 'The History of Human Population', *Scientific American*, 231, no. 3 (Sept. 1974), 41–51; Colin McEvedy and Richard Jones, *Atlas of World Population History* (New York, 1978), esp. pp. 14 and 342; and Fekri A. Hassan, *Demographic Archaeology* (New York, 1981), pp. 193–208.

necessarily responsible for death. The unknowns are significant. Infant and child skeletal remains have seldom survived the 8000 to 10 000 years since the beginning of the transition from hunter-gatherer, or paleolithic, to settled agricultural, or neolithic, societies because their bone tissues were too soft. Many paleopathologists believe that survival experience before age 15 can be estimated for paleolithic humans from the remains of people living in similar circumstances, but more recently, such as American Indians, or from the experience of twentieth-century hunter-gatherers such as the !Kung San. While teeth and bones record some signs of trauma and disease – wounds and tuberculosis, for example – they provide little or no information about many other possible causes of death. Even if it is plausible to suppose that many infectious diseases and parasites identified later were absent or rare in paleolithic societies because human populations were too small and sparsely distributed to support them, skeletal remains fail to reveal signs of some maladies that may have been present. Building a life table from the skeletal record requires a further assumption that the population from which skeletons are drawn was stationary – neither changing in size nor influenced by migration – and that the individuals dying at each age represent essential characteristics of the living. These assumptions must be made in order to proceed, but they can rarely be supported, much less verified. The remains of only a few people are recovered at any site or in any region; paleolithic and neolithic life tables must be based on populations so small that the margin of possible error is quite large.[6]

Any one of these problems might undermine confidence in the findings, except for the general agreement that independent surveys reach regarding the location and shape of the survival curve. Although the experts disagree on whether the neolithic transition from hunting-gathering to settled agriculture caused life expectancy to improve or deteriorate, their disagreement revolves around a narrow band within the survival rectangle. More probably, as sedentarism increased, so did fertility, but the new social structure brought a deterioration in mortality, morbidity, and life expectancy. Only in the long run did responsive strategies or adaptations regain earlier levels of life expectancy.[7] Figure 1.2 provides a selection of late paleolithic and neolithic survival curves, enough to show their proximity and rough agreement and to reveal how little of the space of life had yet been overtaken. The two Dickson Mounds curves (Late Woodland mixed and Middle Mississippian) in Figure 1.2 represent one view of the transition, a view holding that life expectancy deteriorated with the neolithic revolution.[8] The opposite view is represented by the contrast between the Maghreb-type paleolithic curve, which is described as the most favorable portrayal of late paleolithic mortality, and the Alsónémedi neolithic curve.[9]

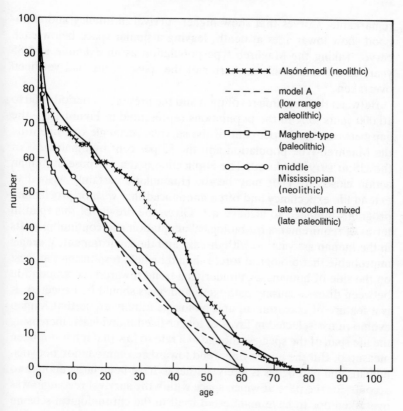

FIGURE 1.2   *Survival curves for some paleolithic and neolithic populations*

SOURCES   Gy. Acsádi and J. Nemeskéri, *History of Human Life Span and Mortality*, trans. by K. Balás (Budapest, 1970), pp. 160, 205, 266–7, 282–3; Alan H. Goodman *et al.*, 'Health Changes at Dickson Mounds, Illinois (AD 950–1300)', in Mark Nathan Cohen and George J. Armelagos, eds, *Paleopathology at the Origins of Agriculture* (New York, 1984), pp. 272–6; and Fekri A. Hassan, *Demographic Archaeology* (New York, 1981), p. 116.

In the quantitative image each paleolithic and neolithic curve sketches its own picture. The differences are worth noting if the purpose is to follow what each curve suggests about risks to life at each stage (and if we are willing to accept assumptions and estimates about the two weakest areas of the evidence: mortality in infancy and childhood and the age at death of older individuals in the record). But, in the overall picture, it is the resemblances that are more remarkable. Curves that show higher survival in infancy and childhood show lower ages at death, leaving a similar space below each curve. Taking the Maghreb-type population as an example and 85 years as the limit, only a quarter of the space of life had yet been overtaken.[10]

Between the neolithic revolution and the present – a period 1000 to 10 000 years long in the populations represented in Figure 1.2 – the gap between the 25 per cent of the survival rectangle overtaken by the Maghreb-type population and the 85 per cent by inhabitants of the US in 1979–81 closed. The implication is that purposeful human action closed it. That may be so. Humankind certainly wished to extend life expectancy and often announced that wish or proclaimed programs intended to achieve it.[11] Given the brevity of this span in terms of requirements for biological adaptation and continuing shifts in the human association with disease and the environment, it seems improbable that biological forces should be held responsible, at least on the side of humans. An underlying trend toward accommodation between disease-causing pathogens and hosts should be expected. It is a feature of coexistence, and biologists usually argue that human evolution has selected in favor of longer-lived individuals, increasing the life span of the species, though at a rate so low that it has not been measured. But the underlying trend toward accommodation between humans and pathogens is likely neither to have been large enough to account for the pace at which space within the survival rectangle was overtaken nor to have manifested itself in the chronological scheme suggested by Figure 1.3. The scheme is one of increasing returns, which seems to imply learned behavior, albeit behavior that for a long time was learned slowly.

The inference of learned behavior is stronger still when survival curves are compared for populations differing in social characteristics. Slaves in the Roman era had shorter life expectancies than free individuals, and individuals with greater wealth – a feature determined by artifacts excavated with the skeleton – seem to have lived longer.[12] In the aggregate, though not in every individual case, the differentiation is a sign of control over some causes of death, and it raises the question of what was controlled.

Figure 1.3 brings the two images together by sketching survival curves for some populations from the Maghreb-type of the late paleolithic era to the US in 1979–81, and by indicating the proportion of space overtaken by each.[13] Except for the mid-nineteenth-century curve, each population deals with the two sexes together, and each proportion relates years lived at each age to the assumption that the

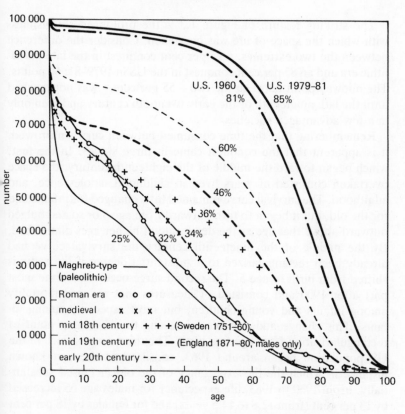

FIGURE 1.3 *Survival curves for selected populations*

SOURCES See Figures 1.1 and 1.2 and Acśadi and Nemeskéri, *Human Life Span*, pp. 70–1, 220–1, 289–90 and 308–9; Great Britain, House of Commons, Sessional Papers 1884–85, *Supplement to the 45th Annual Report of the Registrar-General of Births, Deaths, and Marriages in England*, v. 17, 365, vii–viii; Gustav Sundbärg, *Bevölkerungsstatistik Schwedens, 1750–1900* (Stockholm, 1907), pp. 131–2; US, Bureau of the Census, *United States Life Tables 1910* (Washington, 1916), pp. 16–17; and US, National Center for Health Statistics, *Vital Statistics of the United States: 1960*, Department of Health, Education, and Welfare (Washington, 1963), II, pt. a, section 2, pp. 7 and 9.

modal age of death is, and has been, 85 years. Although this assumption is incorrect – we have seen that the modal age has increased – it is useful as a basis for comparing overall survival experience over time and as an alternative to comparisons based on life expectancy at certain ages.

The striking feature of Figure 1.3 is the prolonged sluggishness with which the space of life was overtaken. Consider the difference between the two extremes, a 25 per cent conquest in the late paleolithic era and an 85 per cent conquest in the US in 1979–81: 60 points. The midway point between the two – 55 per cent – was not reached until the late nineteenth or the early twentieth century and then only in a few advantaged societies.

Remembering that the time consumed between curves narrowed, it is apparent that the conquest came in three surges. In the first, which began toward the middle of the eighteenth century, the space overtaken consisted of years lived in childhood, adolescence, and adulthood. The survival curve remained little changed for infants and for the old, but it began to turn outward from age 5 or so and bulged outward above that age as the death rate at higher ages diminished. By the middle of the nineteenth century the survival curve had already been rectangularized to a substantial degree if the radix is shifted from birth to age 5. The second surge occurred for the most part after 1900 and consisted of measures that reduced mortality among infants and young children, but most especially among infants. This change added space by raising the beginning point of rectangularization from age 5 to birth. The third surge, which in the US population began around 1963, consisted of the first known instance in which the life expectancy of the old increased substantially. From 1960 to 1983, life expectancy for males age 65 increased by 13 per cent (from 12.8 to 14.5 years) and for females by 18 per cent (from 15.8 to 18.6 years). Since 1983 there has been little change in the US. It is premature to claim that the third stage has closed but not to observe that a series of rapid and concentrated increases in life expectancy has moved through the life cycle. To repeat itself, the series will have to begin again, and begin at a point at which there is much less space available to be overtaken in each stage of life. Even large decreases in the death rates of the present-day US population would add comparatively little to life expectancy at birth or any higher age.

HAZARD

If the first feature of particular interest in Table 1.1 is the survival curve derived from the l_x column, the second is the mortality risk given in the q_x column. The q_x figures allow the plotting of a curve that portrays the distribution of the risk of death by age. For the US

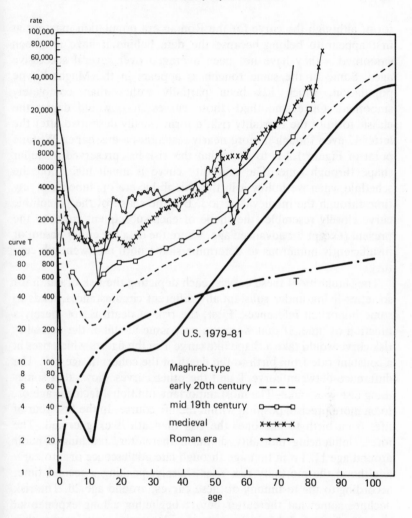

FIGURE 1.4 *Age-specific mortality risk in selected populations
(per 100 000)*

SOURCES See Figure 1.3.

population in 1979–81, the risk of dying declined from 1260 per
100 000 in the first year of life – 0.0126 – to 0.0002 in the tenth year,
and then rose to 0.35988 at age 109–110.

Figure 1.4 sketches mortality curves for the populations whose
survival curves have already been considered. As a figure it requires
some patience to interpret. Each of the curves presents a similar

form, although the curve for the Roman era population may not at
first appear to belong because the data behind it have not been
smoothed – they have not been averaged over several successive
ages. Some of the same roughness appears in the Maghreb-type
population, which has been partially rather than completely
smoothed. Once smoothed, those curves, too, would depict the
classic form of the mortality risk, a form usually described after the
letter U even though it more nearly resembles a misshapen W. One
point of Figure 1.4 is to show that this risk has preserved a similar
shape through time. The mortality curve is much higher on the
schedule when we follow it in the paleolithic era or, indeed, at any
time through the medieval period. But the shape of the paleolithic
curve closely resembles the shape of each subsequent curve to the
present (except for advanced age, where the data are either absent or
insufficiently numerous to determine shape until the twentieth century).

The similarity of these curves, each depicting the risk of death for
societies living under substantially different circumstances, leads to
some important inferences. First, the risk of death is not merely a
function of time. If that were the only issue at stake, the mortality
risk curve would take a shape like curve T in the figure, which rises at
a constant rate from birth to the death of the cohort at age 110. The
difference between curve T and the other curves shows that something else is at stake. The most important additional factor is age or,
to be more precise, position within the life course. In the first year of
life, from birth to age one, the risk of death is exaggerated. The
forces influencing mortality diminish thereafter, reaching a nadir
around age 11. From that age through late adolescence or into early
adulthood the mortality risk rises sharply, peaking a second time,
according to the testimony of these curves, around age 20. The risk
declines somewhat thereafter before beginning a long exponential
increase. (Figure 1.4 appears on a semi-log scale, which means that
straight lines on it represent a stable *rate* of increase rather than the
linear or stable *amount* of increase from age to age that guides the
hypothetical curve T.) The nature of the force called aging is much
less well understood than are the specific hazards – diseases and
injuries – that cause death.

The second inference is that changes in the profile of diseases and
injuries causing death and in the skill with which humankind has
controlled specific diseases and injuries have caused the mortality
curve to shift on the graph, mostly by moving downward. Late in the

twentieth century the risk of death is lower at each age than it has ever previously been, which is another way of noticing that the potential for life represented by the human life span – portrayed above as a rectangle – has been overtaken to an increasing degree. But the underlying structure of the mortality risk has remained unchanged in the passage through mortality regimes.

Other factors than age exert some influence over mortality risk. The curves in Figure 1.4, with one exception, deal with populations combining males and females. But members of the two sexes seem seldom to have experienced an equivalent risk. In the Roman-era populations represented in the figure, male life expectancy at birth exceeded female by 30.4 years to 22.9 years. A similar relationship appears in prehistorical populations and in many other but not all populations of classical antiquity.[14] By the seventeenth century in Europe, however, females could expect to live longer than males and, lower life expectancies at some ages in some nineteenth-century populations notwithstanding, that advantage has been retained to the present. It now appears to be increasing. Although considerable attention has been given to this issue, demographers have found it difficult to provide convincing explanations for the superior life expectancy of one sex or for the crossover. Social or environmental factors are suspected of having been generally disadvantageous to females in prehistoric times and classical antiquity. There are, however, reasons to suppose that biological traits favor female survival from conception forward, at least for certain ages. But the force of the two factors remains obscure, perhaps chiefly because the available historical evidence is seldom adequate to specify the scale of socio-environmental factors.

Among other matters requiring consideration, the standard of living – a general term referring to nutrition, housing, and other circumstances of material life – is acknowledged to play a role in the location of the mortality risk on the schedule. In theory, standard of living might also influence the shape of the mortality curve. For example, deficient or unbalanced nutrition early in life is known to retard growth and is believed to affect the timing of death. Two populations that fed their infants and children quite differently might, therefore, be expected to produce adult mortality curves with different shapes. Figure 1.4 does not rule out that possibility. It represents only a few examples of experience, and represents those on a scale lacking the detail required to detect nutrition effects of the kind hypothesized.

The profile of diseases and injuries causing death – the mortality regime – also influences the mortality risk. Most specific historical populations can be associated with a short list of leading causes of death. In the paleolithic era infant deaths are usually attributed to nutritional disease, malnutrition, and violence (a broad category covering injuries and accidents). Among juveniles and adults the leading causes were violence, childbirth, wear and tear on the organism, and the cumulative effects of earlier injuries and diseases. Infectious diseases took over the leading role in the neolithic era and retained that role in Europe and the US into the nineteenth century. But the regime of infectious diseases causing death underwent many radical shifts during that long period. Toward the end of that era air-borne infections, especially those assisted by crowding, such as tuberculosis, played the largest role. In earlier times that part had been taken sometimes by infections associated with filth, sometimes by those associated with insect vectors, and sometimes by diseases transmitted by other means. Toward the end of the nineteenth century chronic and degenerative diseases replaced infections. In the US heart disease has remained the leading cause of deaths since the beginning of the twentieth century. Accidents and injuries also regained prominence. The skeletal record shows that the risk of fracture declined as sedentarism replaced hunting and gathering, but a comparison of cause of death information from the last three centuries shows an increase in the proportion of deaths caused by injuries.[15]

In theory shifting mortality regimes might be expected not only to raise or lower the mortality curve on its schedule but also to influence its shape. For example, two populations in each of which infants and children faced quite distinctive disease profiles might be expected to display adult mortality curves with different shapes. That would occur if one disease regime caused lasting damage among survivors or extracted from the population individuals especially susceptible to infection. Figure 1.4 also does not rule out these possibilities. At this level of generalization it merely establishes age as the leading cause of variations in mortality risk in any given population. And it raises two other possibilities. First, although economic and mortality regimes have differed substantially over time and the differences have pushed mortality curves up or down the schedule, the differences may be less imposing than the similarities. That is, another territory of factors not yet identified may exert more influence than the standard of living or the mortality regime. A second possibility consists of substitution. Although economic and mortality regimes may themselves change, the characteristics of each regime may be less influential than the larger body of hazards of which these have been only a part.[16]

THE SPACE OF HEALTH

Each population is an assemblage of events and episodes of health and ill health, similar to the manner in which each life is a sequence of events and episodes. The period life table, so useful a device for calculating life expectancy and comparing the survival experience of different populations, can be extended by adding to it the risk of sickness as measured among the different ages of a population in the same period. Instead of the life expectation arrived at by dividing years lived by the entering population, or the population surviving at each age, the amended table will provide a sickness expectation or a health expectation. Given the threshold specified for a division between health and ill health at each age, the table will reveal how many years of ill health or health may be forecast, or how many ill-health events can be expected to occur within the remaining lifetime. The health expectation will always fall short of the life expectation, for any quantity of ill health time must be subtracted from the total of survival time. At issue is the size of the shortfall, and its trend.

In developed countries humankind has conquered the space of life, or nearly so. Members of each cohort who formerly died in infancy or, in any event, before old age, now survive to old age. Do they survive in good health? Does a year added to life expectancy represent something approaching a year added to health expectancy, too? The answer will depend on what we learn about the risk of ill health, its history, and its prospects. Relying now on our imagination, it is not difficult to conceive of a second territory that humankind might conquer, this one composed of the space of health. While it may not be realistic to think about eliminating ill health, it is realistic to think about diminishing its proportions. First, however, it is necessary to learn about those proportions and their history.

CONCLUSION

Death is not the subject of this book – obviously. In one chapter we have swept from the paleolithic era to the present. But death and its history have important empirical and theoretical properties and implications. Their study helps identify certain boundaries, such as the human life span, and certain parameters, such as those sketched by paleolithic and recent mortality curves. The study of death and its causes furnishes a variety of mathematical tools appropriate for the study of health and ill health. Even if health and sickness lack the clear definition of life and death, they can nevertheless be approached via the same means of analysis. If, therefore, we wonder about the number of survivors at each age in a population, we may also wonder about the number of sick and healthy among those survivors. If we wonder about the probability of death at each age according to sex, standard of living, and other factors, we may also wonder about the risk of sickness at each age according to the same set of variables. If we wonder about life expectancy in a given place and period, we may wonder also about health expectancy: the portion of life remaining that will be spent in good or ill health. Finally, if we wonder about death as an outcome of illness and injury and thus see sickness as a mediator between health and death, we may wonder about those episodes of sickness that do not end in death. They are still more commonplace than death. And they serve the roles of similarity and substitution. The causes of sickness, like the causes of death, change from one economic or mortality regime to another. But sickness itself remains a feature of every regime.

2 Sickness, Aging and Death

> The uniform nature of the age-dependent
> deteriorations that occur in human beings
> dictates that any significant prolongation
> of life-span . . . will require a uniform
> prolongation of general health
> maintenance.[1]

Death is almost always attributed to disease or injury. The likelihood that a given episode will result in death is a function of three things. First, each disease or injury taken by itself poses a certain risk. These risks range from a negligible likelihood of death – such as is associated with minor ailments and injuries and ailments as well as disabilities that are major but bear little or no fatality risk – to a nearly complete likelihood – such as is associated with virulent diseases appearing in a virgin soil population, a group previously unexposed to them. Second, the vulnerability of the human organism increases with age during most of the life cycle. Third, some experiences – disease and injury insults that are imperfectly repaired, some lifestyle and dietary practices, and excessive radiation exposure are examples – have deferred effects. The organism's 'memory' of these prior insults influences the timing of death. This chapter will explore a particular realm of the theory of death, a realm in which the leading issues deal not with immediate causes but with features of experience that affect the timing of death and contribute indirect or incremental steps toward death.

When historians have considered death as an event rather than an idea, they have been interested chiefly in immediate causes. This interest has been important for the biological sciences, for it produced the record of human experience with death summarized in the first chapter, a record that informs biological thinking about the way in which death and the timing of death may be approached as events open to understanding, explanation, and manipulation. But the biological scientist recognized something new in the historical record: immediate causes diminish in importance as the human organism ages. Among people who die young, as most of humankind did until

29

the early eighteenth century, immediate causes are of special concern. They dominate the profile of all causes and deprive the society of the largest blocks of the space of life, blocks composed of years not survived from infancy or childhood into old age. But among people who die old, as for the most part people in Europe and the United States now do, immediate causes are less important. They have been supplanted by multiple pathologies, by the ways in which aging itself depletes vitality, and by the memory of prior health experience that the individual, the cohort, or the population has accumulated.

In reviewing evidence and theory from the biological sciences about aging and insult accumulation, this chapter will clarify ways in which aging influences the risks of mortality and morbidity, and lay foundations for considering health experience over the life course. The objective is to consider the timing of death and the risk of ill health as functions of prior health experience, thus to see the usefulness of historical sources relating sickness experience over the life course. The essential point remains the observation that health experience is a continuing narrative in the life course of the individual, the cohort, and the population.

AGING

The viability or vigor of the human organism decreases and its vulnerability increases with age in ways that are apparent from clinical examination and post-mortem analysis, and from laboratory experiments with animals that, reasoning selectively from analogy, provide insights into human experience. The process, called aging or senescence, is usually associated with the part of the life cycle following somatic growth. In humans it is now sometimes held to begin at conception or birth, or upon reaching physical maturity, age 18, but the more common view is that it begins after age 30. It becomes manifest between ages 40 and 50. Although the processes of deterioration begin to prevail in a noticeable way in most individuals between ages 40 and 50, they do not for some time thereafter play a determinant role. Only at or above the modal age of death, between about ages 85 and 110, is death not necessarily linked to disease. At that extreme the probability of dying from *any* disease or injury is so great that, while death may be attributed to one or several diseases or injuries, its underlying cause is senescence. The aging hazard is defined as a property of the organism in general, so that it includes neither the risks of disease and injury nor those associated with hereditary features peculiar to some but not all members of the species.

While it is easy to find grounds to suspect that aging is a distinct process, it is difficult to demonstrate its existence in an unambiguous way or to isolate its quantitative properties. The most common argument for the existence of an aging process is based on an interpretation of the survival curve. As explained by the biologist Alex Comfort, 'a progressively increasing *force of mortality* and decreasing expectation of life in a population . . . is evidence of the senescence of its individual members [if significant variation in the exposure rate can be excluded]'.[2] In other words, a stable mortality rate implies that deaths should be attributed to causes unrelated to senescence. Such a situation is approximated by the experience of paleolithic humankind as appeared in Figure 1.3. Few individuals survived to ages at which senescence might play a role, and most died earlier in life from diseases and injuries that might have caused death at any age. (It is for the moment merely incidental that the causes shifted somewhat with age, relating more to nutrition early in life and to activity among juveniles and adults.) In contrast, a mortality rate that increases with age, such as appears in Figure 1.3 for the US population of 1979–81, implies senescence. In it most individuals survive to advanced age but 'after a certain age' they 'die from causes that would not have killed them in youth'.[3] Diminishing vigor and increasing vulnerability are not merely related to age but are related in such a way that aging exerts a regularly increasing influence on survival. Individuals age at slower or faster rates, but a regular rate of increase appears when large groups are surveyed. The regular rate of increase in the death rate is called the Gompertz function after the nineteenth-century mathematician, Benjamin Gompertz, who devised a formula to express the correspondence.[4] Stable functions of this kind have also been found in the healing time and mortality rates associated with some specific insults, such as burns, in mortality from some individual diseases, and in a linear rather than an exponential form in some physiological functions, such as the basal metabolic rate, which measures oxygen consumption at rest.[5]

The properties of the mortality risk curve that are said to reveal the existence of aging show up more clearly on the logarithmic scale of Figure 2.1, which reproduces a figure comparing the empirical data that Gompertz consulted from eighteenth-century England with some death rate curves from the first half of the twentieth century.

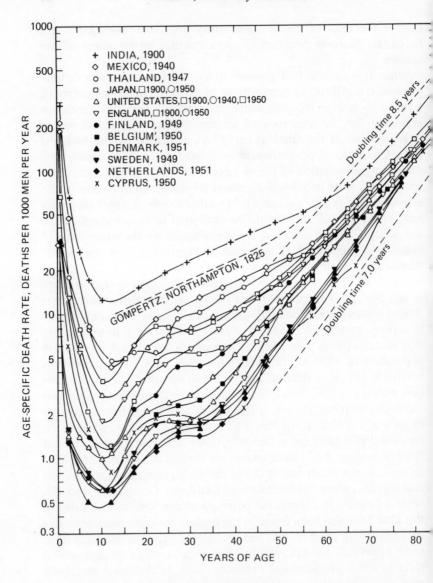

FIGURE 2.1 *Age-specific mortality risk and the Gompertz function*

SOURCE   Hardin B. Jones, 'A Special Consideration of the Aging Process, Disease, and Life Expectancy', in John H. Lawrence and Cornelius A. Tobias, (eds), *Advances in Biological and Medical Physics* (New York, 1956), IV, 284.

On the logarithmic scale a stable rate of increase in the death rate appears as a straight line, a feature approximated by each curve in this figure but approximated better by the curves based on large rather than small populations (e.g., Thailand 1947 and Cyprus 1950). The figure was initially constructed to illustrate the Gompertz function and to show that the doubling rate should be expected to vary from one population to another (in this instance between 7 and 8.5 years would pass before the death rate doubled). That is, the gradient of the function differs from population to population, but all populations exhibit periods during the life course when a regular rate of increase in the death rate appears for some years during adulthood.

Figure 2.1 also indicates that the location of the Gompertz function (or straight line) within the life course not only varies from one population to another but also varies within an historical pattern. Excepting Gompertz's Northampton curve, based on the experience of insured lives from eighteenth-century England, all the death rate curves in Figure 2.1 refer to the first half of the twentieth century. But they refer to populations with quite different levels of mortality and life expectation, some of which can be characterized as 'favored' and others as 'unfavored'. Comparing Gompertz functions in these terms, it appears that the location of the function underwent a peregrination. In unfavored populations, including the insured lives of eighteenth-century England, a first Gompertz function appeared in early adulthood but gave way in mature adulthood to a second function in which the death rate was higher and took less time to double. As age-specific mortality risk shifted downward over time, the first Gompertz function peregrinated, beginning and ending at a later age. It appeared around age 30 in unfavored populations (including nineteenth-century Sweden and England, not shown here) and disappeared around age 50, while in favored populations it appeared around age 45 and persisted for longer and longer periods. In the US during the period 1979–81 (Figure 1.4) the straight line occurred between ages 45 and 90, and was then replaced by a slower rate of increase in the death rate.[6]

The slower rate of increase at high ages can be explained as the result of changes in the characteristics of survivors, changes related to the amount of variety, which is called heterogeneity. Heterogeneity is an important issue in describing the composition of populations. Each cohort is born with a certain range of vitality and vulnerability among its members. The range is unobserved, but evidence about it can be collected from mortality and morbidity data. Although some deaths and sicknesses have completely random causes, most are associated to some degree with characteristics of the individual and, in the aggregate, of the cohort. At birth the cohort's heterogeneity extends from individuals condemned to early death because of genetic or congenital abnormalities to individuals who for most of their lives will resist or avoid major threats to health and survival. More or less by definition the part of the cohort that dies at each age, whose deaths are the basis for deriving the q_x function of the life table, is a select population. Over time, deaths diminish heterogeneity by removing susceptible individuals, but illnesses, injuries, and other experiences introduce fresh heterogeneity by leaving memories that influence future susceptibility to disease and death. The balance of heterogeneity remains unobserved. Most authorities expect it to diminish as the cohort ages. Clearly the range between the most and the least susceptible member of the cohort narrows, but the average or median value of heterogeneity in the cohort may increase. Late in life there is a transition from heterogeneity toward homogeneity, a transition that occurs at a point at which the cohort's survival comes to be dominated by *less* susceptible individuals.[7] The increase in the age at which this transition has occurred – its peregrination – is a sign that the heterogeneity necessary to maintain the Gompertz function is preserved for a longer part of the life cycle in favored than unfavored populations. In other words, higher risk people are living longer.

The rising age of this transition is another illustration of how the survival rectangle has been overtaken. It indicates that the overtaking is an effect of changes in survival within the limits of a life span specific to the human species. It also indicates that, below the transition, overtaking the space of the rectangle occurs by adding to the longevity of more susceptible members of the cohort. That is, the changes that have occurred in longevity and life expectancy have had little to do with the rate of aging. They are effects of changes in the rate of survival.

Many authorities nevertheless believe that the rate of aging can be manipulated and that it can be controlled in ways that add to the sum of years of vigor and health rather than merely to the sum of years lived.[8] Animal experiments and, more recently, work in cell biology appear to confirm the theoretical possibility of adding time to the human life span, extending it beyond the limit so far postulated, about age 110, to a higher figure. But the most promising of the methods so far demonstrated on laboratory animals, which focus on dietary restriction rather than chemotherapy, have limited potential for application to humans and ambiguous implications. Experiments conducted by C.M. McCay in the 1930s, and since replicated and expanded, show that the life span of rats can be increased by severely restricting caloric intake while maintaining a balance of vitamins and minerals. Rats fed 50 per cent fewer calories lived nearly twice as long, and those fed 25 per cent fewer calories lived about a third longer. The longer-lived rats appear to have had years added to the part of the life span marked by vigor rather than to old age. They were able to reproduce longer and, when the restricted regime had been begun before physical development was complete, it deferred maturity. Further experiments considering the effect of dietary restriction on susceptibility to disease have shown mixed results, in general an increase in bacterial and parasite infections but a decrease in some tumors.

Even though similar findings have been shown for other laboratory animals, including mice, guinea pigs, fish, and fruit flies, interpretation of the results is unclear. Who knows what the vitamin and mineral requirements of these organisms may be, and who can say that the diets given in a controlled manner represent optimal diets? One possible interpretation is that dietary restriction restored the experimental animals to the life spans they would have had had they eaten in the laboratory the diets of the wild to which their species had adapted through natural selection, and that the control groups, which were fed *ad libitum*, lived shorter spans because of overeating. In that case the results might be interpreted more as evidence about the negative effects of overeating than the positive effects of undereating.[9]

Another reason for skepticism lies in the antiquity of this idea of long life through diet, as of other elements of Hippocratic advice about health maintenance. An association between dietary restriction and extended longevity appears repeatedly in medical literature. For example, George Cheyne, a physician practicing in Bath, England, early in the eighteenth century, cited reputedly long lives of ascetic eastern Christians subsisting on 'very little Food' as evidence of an association, and developed the idea by repeating dietary advice from long-lived individuals.[10] He also described the components of an appropriate diet.

Testimony about superior longevity and dietary reasons for it fails to stand up to critical scrutiny or to produce populations of extreme aged people composed to a great degree of individuals who have practiced such diets. The historical evidence, which tends to be vague about dietary composition, suggests that restriction is not an adequate means to extend the potential life span or at least that appropriate forms of dietary restriction have not yet been found. Roy Walford, a pathologist interested in the field of life span extension, cites the example of a Venetian nobleman, Luigi Cornaro, who converted from dissipation and excess to temperance and dietary restraint around age 37, and lived until 1565 or 1566, when he was age 98 or 104, or something in between.[11] Cornaro 'discovered' how to live longer by taking up ideas of the classical Greek physician Galen about dietary regulation. Cornaro spread those ideas in a series of books written in the 1550s – including *Compendio della vita sobria* – which were republished and translated in numerous editions into the twentieth century. Yet it is at least as easy to cite examples of people who practiced lifelong dissipation and still lived long lives. And there is the difficulty of identifying long life spans of people directly influenced by Cornaro or Galen. The historical record includes abundant examples of involuntary undernutrition and some diets resembling those that laboratory animals were fed – nutritious diets restricted in calories that are linked in laboratory populations to longer life spans. But historians seem to associate all population-level dietary restriction with excessive mortality.

There are other directions from which the aging rate might be influenced. Animal experiments suggest that lowering metabolic rate might extend the life span. Fruit flies and fish live longer when their body temperature is lowered, suggesting a mammal model in which hibernation or torpor – for example, a small reduction of body temperature during sleep – might reduce the aging rate. Other sectors of research focus on body chemistry and cells, examining how additions or deletions of hormones influence animal aging and mortality, on means to repair cell damage associated with age, and on the immune system. The immune response matures around age $2\frac{1}{2}$ and begins to deteriorate after adolescence, a point at which the autoimmune response increases. The two dysfunctions, immune response deterioration and autoimmune response increase, which may be related in their development, play a major role in the onset of and development of some leading degenerative diseases, including many cancers and autoimmune diseases. In this way aging is tied directly to some of the leading diseases causing death in adulthood and old age, but the association is not unique to aging. Prior health experience, diet, radiation, and other exogenous factors also influence the age of onset and the risk of cancers. In an interesting combination of results, rats and mice fed restricted diets show a higher immune response later into life. That is, disease frequency appears to be open to manipulation by several means working jointly.

But it remains unclear whether the single or joint operation of these or any other techniques would extend the potential life span or influence the proportion of people living to that potential. Many biologists are hopeful about a breakthrough in means to slow the aging rate, but none of the paths yet explored has been shown to be effective in humans. The optimism rests more on the absence of compelling reasons to believe that the potential life span cannot be extended than on the availability of effective or plausible means of extension. To some extent at least it rests also on continuing difficulty in distinguishing between interventions that increase the likelihood of survival to more or less 110 years and those that extend the life span in the desired manner, by adding years of vigor and good health.[12]

Although it is usually suggested that the potential human life span has either remained unchanged or increased very slightly since the paleolithic era, biological research also raises the possibility that the aging rate has instead quickened and the life span thus contracted. In one form of this idea, it is suggested that toxic substances such as chemicals and radiation have been added to the diet and the environment more rapidly than the body has learned how to compensate for them. And, in a variant on that idea, Richard Cutler thinks that health and life span may be dependent on 'the degree to which repair and protective processes have evolved to protect an organism against its own endogenous production of toxic by-products.'[13]

The biological inquiry into genetic and biochemical control of the aging rate and of health maintenance in turn influences the questions that may be posed of historical data. Records about health and illness over the life course assume more importance when the questions posed deal with ways in which life experiences influence the timing of death, the more so when the historical record furnishes opportunities to examine cohorts whose life course is complete and whose experience with health, diet, and other macro-level variables can be reconstructed. Retrospective post-mortem investigations assume new importance, especially with regard to people who died more recently, when human remains can contribute answers to the micro-level questions posed by the biologist as well as the macro-level counterparts of these questions formulated by the historian.

Distinguishing Aging from Vulnerability

The most compelling evidence for the existence of a distinct aging component within mortality risk is provided by the regularity in the rate of increase of the mortality rate in mature adulthood. But the Gompertz function is not the product of aging operating by itself. It has two sources. The increase is, in the first place, a consequence of survival time, of continuing exposure to disease and injury hazards, and of the accumulating effects of earlier insults. Second, it is an effect of aging. The unsolved problem is to determine the force of the senescence risk and to distinguish intrinsic changes associated with aging from other sources of vulnerability that accumulate with age but are not intrinsic.[14]

An eighteenth-century observer like de Moivre, who estimated a juridical version of the modal age of death as 86, might have set the gradient of the senescence risk in quite another way than would an actuary or a biologist familiar with recent experience. In de Moivre's day hazards unassociated with senescence ensured that most individuals would die before being able to reproduce, but those same hazards took a high toll of individuals surviving past 30, or to between 40 and 50, when the senescence risk is now held to intervene in an observable way.[15] Recent gains in longevity, especially in the longevity of people age 65 and over, imply a later and lower senescence risk than appeared to exist in de Moivre's day or even as recently as the mid-twentieth century. Nor have the limits of survivorship after 65 been reached. Most authorities predict further gains in life expectancy at higher ages. Since senescence is believed to be a characteristic property of the human organism as formidable (albeit theoretically) in paleolithic as in modern times and one not yet influenced by medical measures or other forms of intervention, these continuing gains reflect controls over other categories of risk.[16] All the gains in life expectancy observed so far may be attributed to some combination of public health, medical, standard of living, or environmental control measures, and none to measures that slow or suspend the intrinsic process of aging. Returning to the metaphor from Chapter 1, humankind has not put itself into a zoo or a laboratory, but it has made considerable progress in controlling threats in the wild.

To appreciate this historical trend is to find reasons to reduce the portion of the risk expressed by the Gompertz function that should be assigned to aging and to increase the part that should be assigned to vulnerability. The problem of distribution has a second dimension, consisting of passage along the continuum of age. A distribution of the two components suitable for age 50, for example, will not be suitable for age 75. It is clear that the part to be assigned to aging is weak when the Gompertz function appears, around ages 45–50 in nineteenth- and twentieth-century populations, and much stronger when it disappears, at 75 or higher. The stability of the function implies a regular rate of increase from the beginning to the end of the effect. But the level of either portion remains unobserved at either end. It seems reasonable to suggest that aging plays so little role in the mortality risk at ages 45–50 that its part for those ages could be set at or close to zero. If the value at the other extreme could be fixed, portions of risk could be estimated for each intervening age by backcasting from the distribution fixed for the higher age to zero at ages 45–50. But, in populations heretofore observed, the Gompertz function – the stable rate of increase in the death rate – has disappeared at ages earlier than it is plausible to suppose that aging is the only or even necessarily the dominant factor over vulnerability.

The effort to partition the vulnerability and senescence components – or terms – remains worthwhile, but it requires more sensitivity to historical and prospective experience. In the hands of biologists this effort has concentrated on showing the significance of aging as a term in the equation of health and mortality risks in adulthood and among the elderly. The net effect of casting the issue within a history of survivorship is to enhance the part of vulnerability over that of aging. That is, the vulnerability term is larger than it has been taken to be, and the evidence of that consists of large and continuing changes in the mortality rate at those ages to which the Gompertz function applies, and at higher ages also. To stress vulnerability in turn places more emphasis on the components of vulnerability.

VULNERABILITY

The hazards and processes that collaborate with aging to cause death have been treated above as the 'vulnerability term' in an equation in which the risk of death has only two terms: aging and vulnerability. There is no easy distinction between the two, in language or practice. Aging is styled an intrinsic or endogenous process, and most factors contributing to vulnerability are considered extrinsic or exogenous. But some elements of vulnerability are intrinsic to begin with, and some are 'endogenized'. The complexity of the risk of death can be reduced somewhat by adopting a simplifying assumption, which is that all deaths are preceded by sickness, even if the sickness is instantaneous. Here sickness has been defined to include illnesses and injuries in such a way that being struck by lightning and dying immediately can register on both the morbidity and the mortality scales. Thus all deaths, even those that might be attributed solely to chance and might therefore be detached from any reasonable effort to link the death to features peculiar to the individual, the cohort, or the population, are considered.

Another step toward bringing the complexity of the mortality risk within manageable bounds lies in breaking the vulnerability term into leading components, three of which are proposed here. *First*, genetic and congenital abnormalities and propensities influence many members of a cohort in ways that determine later morbidity and mortality. This part of the vulnerability term is largely complete at birth, and the cohort bears a pattern that will subsequently change, chiefly through selective mortality among members whose genetic programing causes or contributes to death. There will be few fresh increments to genetic vulnerability as the cohort ages. *Second*, every cohort faces a range of illness and injury risks, a range that is influenced somewhat by the characteristics of the cohort but that is chiefly a function of time and place. A cohort born in sixteenth-century England faced a barrage of infectious diseases, including plague, but one born in late twentieth-century England can be expected to contract many fewer infections, to survive childhood in larger proportion, and, correspondingly, to acquire immunity to fewer diseases by means of clinical or subclinical episodes. The effects of time periods – period effects – are, by definition, extrinsic or exogenous. Both their occurrence and their nonoccurrence influence the cohort. They cause deaths, and these contribute further to changes in the composition of the cohort. The members who die are a select population (or rather a set of select populations), and, increasingly, the members who do not die become a select population in their own right. The period effects also contribute to sicknesses that end in recovery, or in which death is at least deferred. In this way they are held to be endogenized, and to form part of the *third* segment of the vulnerability term, a segment representing collectively all previous illness and injury experience that has some bearing on subsequent health and the timing of death. The third segment can be styled the 'insult history', and its operation 'insult accumulation', a phrase already familiar.

Each of the three segments is difficult to observe, but the ways in which health services have been organized in the US and Europe make it more likely that evidence will have been gathered about the second segment than the first or third. This is so because of something called the medical model, an abstract construction represented in practical ways by health personnel and institutions that are responsive to health problems identified by the individual. People who practice the medical model – patients and physicians – want to categorize ill health, usually by specifying a physical or mental disorder that is recognized in lay or professional circles and about which information has been acquired concerning treatment. In the best case, recognition leads to the identification of a program of therapy and to recovery. Most of us expect or hope for recovery from the health services we use, so that the beneficiaries of health services – patients – contribute to the reign of the medical model just as surely as do deliverers of health services, such as physicians and hospitals.

But this medical model is not the only way in which health problems might be identified, and many authorities have come to be persuaded that it is not the model most appropriate for current and future needs. They argue that it is suited best to an era in which ill health was usually exogenously determined and consisted for the most part of discrete bouts of sickness attributable to infection. The model helped conquer infections, although more via public health reform than strictly medical means. Success is documented by an epidemiologic revolution in which causes of death shifted from infections to degenerative diseases and people lived longer.[17] In the new circumstances, so the argument goes, the medical model is no longer appropriate because most ill-health episodes, and especially most episodes likely to cause death, discomfort, or pain are not susceptible to identification or treatment in the same way as infections. A different pattern of diseases calls for a different model.[18] Although various ideas have been expressed about the characteristics the revised model should have, there is some agreement that it should be concerned with identifying propensities toward illness and that its conception of therapy should be much broader than the chemotherapeutic and surgical orientations of present-day medicine. The debate is fascinating, but it is not itself the issue here. If health services and the expectations that providers and recipients of those services have were different, more might be known about the first and third segments of the vulnerability term – genetic anomalies and previous sicknesses. It is comparatively easy to find information about the incidence of death by disease and, at least in the twentieth century, the incidence (or prevalence) of diseases deemed important enough to be made 'notifiable' – to enter the list of diseases about which data are regularly collected. It is much more difficult to find quantitative information about the first and third segments. The three segments are unequal in their impact on mortality and morbidity, but not enough information is available to apportion them accurately.

Genetic Vulnerability

Major structural defects – congenital malformations – presently occur in about 20 per cent of fertilized ova. Most of these ova die before becoming viable fetuses so that congenital malformations occur in about 2 per cent of newborns. Of these defects about 25 per cent are related to genetic causes and about 10 per cent to environmental sources (infections, drugs, and irradiation) during fetal development. Causes of the remaining 65 per cent of congenital defects remain unknown. Before the twentieth century most individuals with life-threatening malformations – about 1 per cent in each birth cohort – failed to survive to adulthood and thus failed to reproduce. In the long run the failure to reproduce had functioned as a form of natural selection. At least in theory it had limited the incidence of malformations to a trend stable fraction of birth cohorts and to a fraction composed chiefly of malformations caused by mutation.

During the twentieth century some major malformations – affecting about 0.5 per cent of the birth cohort – became treatable. Comparing early twentieth-century life tables to recent life tables, individuals with these problems gained more in life expectancy at birth than did the overall population. Increased survival within this group does not appear to have influenced the rate at which malformations occur, but it has influenced the composition of each birth cohort and thus the population. In terms of mortality selection, as discussed above, survival prolongs the period in which the cohort is marked strongly in its susceptibility to sickness by heterogeneity. That is, as this part of the population has lived more years, it has carried with it a higher risk of sickness. Of the remaining portion of the cohort with congenital malformations – 1.5 per cent – most malformations consist of anomalies that pose no particular health risk to the people who bear them and the remainder of those for which no treatment is yet available.[19]

A much larger part of any cohort is born with malformations that remain undetected at birth but appear later in life, especially in the form of renal and cardiac anomalies, or with propensities to disease that may be known or suspected on the basis of parental experience. Several degenerative diseases, including some of the leading causes of death in late-twentieth-century populations (heart diseases, neoplasms, and diabetes) have been linked to heritable propensities (as have also a number of diseases seldom associated with fatality, such as schizophrenia and allergies). But it is difficult to distinguish the origins of these propensities because the genetic characteristics passed on by parents to children are usually melded with environmental characteristics, habits, and attitudes that become part of the child's lifestyle. The case of longevity 'endowments' provides a good example of this problem. Long-lived parents, especially long-lived mothers, pass to their children an endowment toward long lives and, correspondingly, short-lived parents pass on the opposite endowment.[20] Experiments with laboratory animals in which some environmental factors, such as exposure to infection, are controlled, show that these endowments curtail the maximum life span. The experiments appear to confirm genetic differentiation in all mammals. But in humans the environmental traits that also contribute to longer or shorter life spans have not been successfully measured, and the evidence is insufficient to distinguish the value of genetic from environmental effects. Although genetic propensities are recognized and include some important diseases such as diabetes, Alzheimer's disease, and Parkinsonism, most authorities maintain that most of these diseases and most cases of disease in which the propensity plays some role occur chiefly because of exposure or lifestyle rather than genetic endowment.[21] People known to have a given genetic propensity often fail to develop a given disease, and people without any evidence of such a propensity often develop the disease.

This review of information about genetic vulnerability leads us to expect that each birth cohort is programed to repeat some diseases that occurred among its parents, but that the programing is probabilistic rather than determinant. The programing works in two ways. Parents pass along propensities toward disease, consisting mostly of propensities they have at birth but also of some they acquire before reproducing. And parents may also pass along dispropensities, such as genetically programed resistance. Historical populations that developed some genetic resistance to infectious diseases conveyed some of that resistance to their children.[22] In the very long run this kind of endowment gradually decreased the incidence of disease or at least the incidence of disease as manifested by fatalities. Except in a few specific diseases, such as syphilis and tuberculosis, the effect has been too small to measure accurately on the scale of human time.

From the survey of mortality in Chapter 1, it is evident that the risk of death from infectious disease remained quite high from the neolithic revolution into the eighteenth century, especially for infants. The death rate fluctuated from period to period, but the very long-run trend was stable. In that high mortality regime people who died early in life included individuals preselected for death by their congenital malformations, and perhaps also some with less genetic resistance to common diseases, especially infections. People within one cohort surviving to each successive age constituted a somewhat fitter group – if we define fitness as the absence of malformations and propensities plus the presence of genetic resistance. But cohort after cohort produced a trend stable mortality rate. Over time the disease profile shifted, and the value of inborn qualities changed. Each cohort was slightly better prepared to resist the profile of diseases its parents had known than the profile it would face. But most deaths in the early modern era can be attributed to infectious diseases, which seem to have offered much smaller chances for resistance or dispropensity than the leading causes of death in low mortality regimes. Survivors were unable to pass along dispropensities of marked value.

In the low mortality regime that has emerged since the eighteenth century, infectious diseases have taken a smaller toll and smaller parts of a cohort have died in infancy and childhood. Lower mortality rates in early life mean that more individuals survive to ages at which genetic propensities toward degenerative disease appear. The genetic composition of successive cohorts has not changed, at least not in these terms, but the genetic composition of the population has changed.

This feature of the history of survivorship provides a second reason to suspect that the incidence of sickness may have increased when the death rate decreased. The first reason arose in discussion of Figure 2.1 (p. 32), from which it appears that, in the shift from a high to a low mortality regime, heterogeneity was preserved for a longer part of the life cycle of successive cohorts. People at higher risk to mortality lived longer than formerly. The second reason arises from the observation that passage from the high to the low mortality regime changed the genetic composition of the population. The change was probably small. Certainly it was if attention falls only on congenital malformations and net changes in heritable resistance. But it may have been large, if genetic propensities toward degenerative diseases constitute a major part of the reason for degenerative diseases in middle and old age. At any given age in adulthood, the low mortality regime cohort will manifest more episodes of degenerative disease because more of its members survive to ages at which degenerative diseases occur. And it will present more episodes of diseases of all types because degenerative diseases dominate the disease profile in adulthood. But natural selection will change genetic endowment only to the extent that it affects reproduction. Genetic differences after about age 40, when fertility is low, should have little effect on the genetic endowment of the next generation.

What is not clear is whether the increase in sickness will be in proportion to the increase in survivorship, or something greater than that. That is, aggregate sickness will have increased, but the effect of a changing genetic composition of the population may not have increased the age-specific sickness rate. The outcome is unclear because of the lack of information about the relationship among genetic endowment, infectious disease, and degenerative disease. If the 'new survivors' – people who live longer in the low mortality regime but would have died at an earlier point in the high mortality regime – had faced genetically influenced, higher risks of *infectious and degenerative* diseases, then the passage from one mortality regime to the next probably increased the age-specific rate of sickness.[23] But if the genetic propensities and dispropensities toward infectious and degenerative diseases were separate or in balance, then this passage may have brought no change in the sickness rate at each age or even a decrease in it.

The net effect of these observations is to suggest that the fitness of the population – its genetic susceptibility to sickness – changed little from generation to generation in the high mortality regime. It also appears to change little from generation to generation in the low mortality regime. But, in the passage from one to the other, there may have been a substantial shift. The reduction of mortality changed the composition of the population, preserving its genetic heterogeneity longer. In successive cohorts more people survived to higher ages, but they survived with health statuses compromised by genetic malformations and propensities. The new survivors have less healthy lives.

Vulnerability to Random Illness and Injury

It is not uncommon to hear or read of people who claim never to have been sick a day in their lives. But the memory of ill-health episodes is faulty. It is so faulty that late-twentieth-century interviewers conducting health surveys have settled on a reference period no longer than fourteen days: respondents are asked to recall ill-health episodes over the two weeks prior to the interview. The short reference period has been adopted because of the discovery that people recall a diminishing percentage of episodes in times more distant from the present and overlook some altogether.

Although it is widely believed that individual medical histories are an important element in health experience, diagnosis, and treatment, the kinds of histories taken seldom provide more than negative evidence about the claim that some lives are free of illness and injury. The histories record episodes remembered or treated. They are not intended to measure either the prevalence of ill health within a life or the complete incidence of sickness, which would consist of the sum of recorded and unrecorded episodes. Quite probably there is no complete health history for any pre-twentieth-century figure, no single instance in which a person's ill-health experiences were recorded in full over a long life. The closest approximation seems likely to consist of diaries that include comments on health. The Reverend Ralph Josselin kept such a diary from the autumn of 1643, not long after Josselin became vicar of Earls Colne in Essex, until July 1683, shortly before his death.[24] It illustrates the incompleteness and unrepresentativeness of individual-level records. Josselin recorded his own ailments with care, but reported those suffered by his wife Jane and other family members less completely. Even this unusual daily or weekly record of his own illnesses and injuries omits Josselin's childhood, youth, and early adulthood – from 1616 until autumn 1643 – and may contain gaps. Even in this form the historical record is so incomplete that it is impossible to decide how seriously claims of sick-free lives should be taken. I believe they can be dismissed as so improbable as not to require notice when our concern lies with population-level health.

For most people the narrative of health over the life course is a narrative of movement into and out of a status recognized as sickness. Some of the sicknesses experienced fall into the category of fresh insults. These consist of illnesses and injuries that are usually called random events, meaning not that their occurrence is entirely random but that the individual's health history and genetic endowment plays no evident role in contraction. For the moment it is enough to recognize that this segment of vulnerability dominates the medical model of ill health, our imaginations, and our histories. It will be the subject of Chapters 3 and 4.

Insult Accumulation

Surviving the high mortality risks of fetal development and birth brings for most individuals a series of ill-health episodes. Each episode bears a certain risk of death. But most episodes are not resolved in death. Most are resolved in something called recovery. The individual resumes ordinary activities, but each episode constitutes an insult to the organism, one that produces a certain amount of damage. The organism strives to repair the damage or to adapt to it and both of these capacities are linked to age. Senescence can be seen as a diminished capacity to repair or adapt. For most of the human life span most episodes are adequately repaired, but some leave lasting damage. Unrepaired damages accumulate, adding to the likelihood that future exposure to pathogens or environmental hazards will produce a clinical level of disease and to the likelihood that future episodes of ill health will result in death. This category of vulnerability consists of the deferred and cumulative effects of prior insults. The history of an individual's health is a history of the accumulation and shedding of insult effects. Like so many other features of sickness, the two processes remain unobserved. It is known that some illnesses and injuries leave lasting damage and suspected that others may do so. It is also known that some damage is permanent, while some is long lasting but ultimately reparable. What is unobserved is the mix between the two, and the overall mix among ill-health episodes that cause permanent, long lasting, or merely temporary damage.

The hazards represented by prior insults can be divided into two categories. One consists of recognized ill-health events, which we call illnesses and injuries. The other consists of events that we do not perceive at the time as illness or injury but that influence later health. The theory about how each type of insult influences later health can be explained by considering the case of illness and injury.

In a general way the history of a theory of insult accumulation is so thoroughly embedded in medical intuition and memory that it is no longer possible to trace its origins. Patients observed and experienced associations and sometimes committed them to knowledge in the form of folkloric sayings. Physicians learned to recognize associations and disassociations between illnesses and committed these to memory as aphorisms. Galenic tradition identified three forms of old age: premature, marked by constitutional infirmities or those traceable to diseases contracted in youth; ordinary, an insidious aging; and late, in which vitality was preserved (tautologically) by the absence of earlier diseases or dissipation.[25] The concept that health experience influences current and future health became embedded in the medical consciousness of practitioners and patients. But the representation of the idea was vague, or the notion was linked squarely to external influences rather than to the internalized effect of prior illness.[26] Nevertheless, this idea promoted a new, complex attitude toward illness and injury. To the notion that ill health should be avoided for the sake of the immediate risks each episode posed to life and comfort, insult accumulation added the idea of incremental hazard: future health is conditioned, and in some ways determined, by prior health.

The idea of insult accumulation acquired an extended theoretical form in a 1955 essay by the medical physicist Hardin B. Jones.[27] Jones examined mortality patterns in mid-twentieth-century populations with high and low death rates and in some historical populations in which birth cohorts could be followed through all or a large part of the life course. Some populations seemed to age more slowly than others. Life expectancy increased both because more people survived the diseases of early life and because favored cohorts experienced less mortality at each later stage of life. Individuals attaining age 70 in favored populations possessed a greater endowment of future life expectancy than counterparts aged 70 in unfavored populations. Jones decided that a formal distinction could be made between physiologic and chronologic age at the population level, not merely at the individual level. Although people aged 70 in favored and unfavored populations have the same chronologic age, those in the favored population have a lower physiologic age.[28]

To explain the different rates of aging, Jones suggested that physiologic age is a function of prior disease experience. Diseases in infancy and childhood seemed to have the greatest impact on later physiologic age, but diseases experienced in adulthood also seemed to play a role.[29] 'Every disease episode does some damage to physiologic function', Jones wrote. 'Diseases tend to facilitate the growth of disease states' at all ages, including adulthood.[30] Favored cohorts –

those that have experienced less disease – enjoy longer life spans and greater vigor at every subsequent stage of life.

Although Jones described the model of physiologic versus chrono-logic age chiefly in terms of mortality risk, it is clear that he had a broader conception in mind, and it is clear that more recent biologi-cal and medical versions extend the territory of the model even further. In principle the theory of insult accumulation encompasses all physical and psychological experiences that have lasting health consequences as well as insult experiences in three areas: diseases, injuries, and risk factors. In practice, the list of insults deemed significant is limited by incomplete or ambiguous information about the health effects of many experiences, and by the variability of effects from individual to individual and perhaps also from period to period. Before considering some examples, it is useful to reflect on the difficulty of identifying causes that operate at a distance and effects that are delayed and occur after intervals during which other factors intervene. In the broader model of health risk, insults remain *necessary* causes. But their degree of *sufficiency* as causes declines from the high levels held to occur with infections, in which a clinical level of ill health is chiefly a function of the volume of pathogens, to a lower level. The operation of cause is not doubted in the instance of insults, but its degree is usually unmeasured.[31]

Diseases.

The physical and psychological effects of disease are understood to an uneven degree. At one extreme, many diseases, especially virulent infections, are known to cause cellular and tissue lesions, blatant signs of illness. At the other extreme, many diseases cause no apparent physical damage. In between the two, clinically manifest instances of disease, and perhaps subclinical episodes too, impose stress on the sufferer, contributing to attitudes concerning pain, health practices, lifestyle, mental health, and in other ways to psycho-logical well-being. In the realm of external damage, some insults are repaired, and the repair process more or less coincides with recovery. The sickness episode is often held to end when visible signs of damage disappear. Internal damage is more difficult to track, and occurs in a number of diseases, including virulent infections common in historical populations, such as streptococcal infections and typhoid fever, that may cause lasting or permanent damage or, in the case of streptococcal infections that convert to rheumatic fever, cause subclinical anomalies that subsequently regain a clinical level of importance. In rheumatic fever, for example, the infection usually occurs in childhood. The disease damages heart valves, but the individual recovers and adapts. The damage has little immediate effect after recovery but regains importance later in life and may later cause heart failure. Yet another category of disease accumulation takes the form of uncured ailments. The sufferer of persistent skin diseases, rheumatism, tuberculosis or diabetes adapts to the disease but finds future health compromised and influenced by the continuing presence of disease.

Injuries.
These too have a range of effects extending from minor damage repaired with no apparent lasting effects to serious disabilities that permanently compromise health, lifestyle, and behavior. Minor injuries – cuts, scratches, burns – are probably the most common of all ailments and leave the least significant traces. But this category includes wounds and structural damage suffered at work, at play, in events of violence such as assaults, small group incidents like automobile accidents, and organized, large-scale episodes such as war. It is, in the twentieth century, a category of growing importance. The proportion of fatal and serious injuries within all sickness episodes has grown in absolute and relative terms compared to the eighteenth or nineteenth century.[32] The medical capacity to repair or substitute for functional impairments, to limit side effects of injury such as infection, and to assist the body's adaptation may have improved more rapidly in the twentieth century than any other realm of medicine. The risk of injury has increased over the last century or so, but the increase in the risk of fatality has been more modest than the increase in the risk of injury. The portion of the population with injury insults has grown, even though the average effect of each injury on activity or the quality of life may have diminished.

Risk Factors.
Epidemiologists have relearned something known to physicians since Hippocrates: health is influenced, and sometimes determined, not merely by disease and injury but also by behavior, lifestyle, and environment. Classical Greek physicians considered these factors as non-naturals – influences external to the body that contribute to health and disease – and that concept of health risks remained strong into the nineteenth century.[33] Physicians who wrote about the means of preserving or restoring health advised of the dangers of unhealthy

behavior, specifically of diets abusive to health in the short or long run; of climatic, weather, and other environmental threats; and of the role of rest, exercise, regularity of habit, moderation, and emotional balance. In that medical model the individual was held responsible for health maintenance, although the physician would assist in the inevitable event in which the narrow and ambiguously identified path had not been followed.

In modern science the non-naturals have been redefined, emerging not in the limited sense that the concept of non-naturals acquired in the nineteenth century – hygiene – but as factors that cause or heighten the risk of illness while remaining extrinsic or, at least, something apart from microorganisms. The path of health mainte-nance has also been defined more broadly – it includes more categor-ies of behavior and lifestyle than those specific among the non-naturals – and it defines those categories with less ambiguity. And it has become disease-specific. Most risk factors are related to individ-ual diseases, and the epidemiologist considers it useful to assess the degree of risk added by each factor. The process relies on a shift from individual- to population-level experience and on the statistical analysis of associations between behavior and disease. These tech-niques point to a long list of risk factors, a list led by cigarette smoking, alcohol abuse, diet, atmospheric pollution, radiation, and stress. Each item stands for a variety of associations not yet fully understood. A common feature of risk factors is their probabilistic nature at the level of the individual but deterministic nature at the population level. Risk factors may or may not promote or produce disease in an individual but, in a population, given levels or degrees of abuse can confidently be associated with given levels of effect.[34] Another feature of risk factors is the capacity of this concept to accommodate a broader variety of psychological insults. Even if stress and other signs or manifestations of psychological ill health short of insanity cannot always be identified in historical sources, present-day theories suggest ways to supply missing information. In this way the record of Ralph and Jane Josselin's sicknesses, which includes some explicit references to depression, might be elaborated further by supplying episodes now linked to unusual stress, such as childbirth, job changes, travel, marriage and marital discord. If such events can be supplied at the individual level they can also be supplied at the aggregate level by consulting average population experience and historical events. It is unreasonable to expect a wholly quantitative record of physical and emotional health; this is an illustration of the need for an amalgamation of the diagnostic and temporal models and of qualitative and quantitative information.

As an example of risk factors, consider the case of cigarette smoking, which has been associated statistically with a wide range of mostly degenerative diseases, among them lung cancer. Cigarette smoking adds to the likelihood of lung cancer by causing lesions in the lungs, but the latent period is a long one. An analysis of lung cancer among white males estimated the average time between tumor initiation and death at 20.3 years. The amount of damage and thus the risk is a function of the quantity of cigarettes smoked and the pace of smoking – measured as 'pack years' – and perhaps also of characteristics of the cigarettes smoked. At a modal pace of smoking, damage also peaks after about twenty years, in a complicated process by which the smoker repairs some of the cellular lesions but adds new damage by continuing to smoke.[35] Former smokers shed some damage because affected cells die off at a faster pace than unaffected cells, and the organism repairs previous insults by adapting to the death of damaged cells. The damage caused by cigarette smoking is lasting but not necessarily permanent; it is variable from individual to individual and on other grounds.

Like diseases and injuries, risk factors have histories and the profile of risks faced by a population changes over time. For example, environmental pollution is often thought of as a recent phenomenon, a byproduct of industrial modernization. Only certain forms of pollution are recent. Some toxic chemicals, such as polychlorinated biphenyls or PCBs, have entered the soil and the air as a byproduct of manufacturing processes introduced in the twentieth century. But toxicity in the environment and human contributions to toxicity are as old as humanity.[36]

Taken as a whole, risk factors constitute another category of injuries. The distinguishing features of this category are the delay between cause and effect or, at least, perceived effect, and the indirectness of cause and effect. The delay – the latent interval – makes it more difficult to measure the degree of effect or to provide compelling testimony that the effect is real in any individual case. Like the physician of the past who professed despair because patients refused to accept sensible advice about the non-naturals, the epidemiologist-physician of the present may despair at the reluctance of patients to accept advice about the probabilistic effect of risk-prone behavior and of risks encountered involuntarily.

Over the life course every individual accumulates insults and, given the range of illnesses, injuries, and risk factors that might be experienced, each individual acquires a unique insult memory. The same is true of cohorts. Each cohort acquires a specific memory as its members confront and either die from or survive disease hazards, as each obtains certain kinds of medical care, and as each faces non-disease hazards taking peculiar combinations. Even when Jones considered these factors of exposure and assistance impressionistically – at the level of high and low risks and good and bad care – he recognized that the experience of each cohort would be unique. Nevertheless, the experiences of cohorts born at nearly the same time would be so similar that he elected to compare cohorts distant from one another in time and space. (At least that seemed to be so during the period that Jones studied, about the last 125 years. Over the longer term it is less likely to have been true because earlier cohorts often experienced rapidly changing disease hazards, with the differences producing substantial variations in life expectancy at birth.)[37]

Across a cohort the timing of death would be a function of the accumulation of past impairments. Medical measures appear in this part of the theory as interventions that shorten or mitigate disease episodes. To a clinician it is obvious that diseases are not of equal importance in the damage they leave. Jones did not maintain a doctrine of equal importance, but he dealt with this aspect by assuming an equation between morbidity and mortality. The mortality of members of the cohort who died would faithfully reflect the average severity of diseases experienced in the cohort and therefore the average development of its vulnerability. In effect, Jones assumed that the case fatality rate of illness and injury episodes would adequately measure insult accumulation, and he assumed further that the most important aspect of accumulation lay in increments toward death rather than toward future ill health.

From his vantage in the 1950s, Jones predicted that the incidence of disease in adulthood would decline sharply in less favored populations as each new cohort suffered fewer diseases at every stage of life, and would decline to the degree that medical measures slowed the rate at which diseases still experienced added insult increments. His hopes for the future included further increases in life expectancy, further reductions in morbidity, and further gains in physiologic age. These are important predictions, and it is worthwhile to pause for a moment to distinguish between conclusions warranted by the evidence available in the 1950s and the assumptions not warranted by that evidence. Jones compared survival curves to infer the difference between chronologic and physiologic age, and he considered some implications of radiation experiments on animal models. At that time medical physicists suspected that radiation exposure influenced the aging rate and, using animal models, investigated both the effects of excessive radiation from such sources as nuclear explosions and the level and effects of radiation encountered in the ordinary environment. The experiments showed theoretical properties similar to illness and injury episodes, in that some damage was incremental, some damage became manifest only later or again later, while repeated episodes added to the risk of additional impairment. The experiments also provided practical information about the effects of excessive radiation and its peculiar health sequence: illness, recovery, and deferred illness that often caused death.

Jones did not report demographic or medical models based on radiation experiments nor, more important, did he report evidence about morbidity in humans or laboratory animals. Instead he drew inferences from a series of implicit and intuitive assumptions. The mortality rate of a population or cohort reflects morbidity experience. A high mortality rate signals a high morbidity rate, and vice versa. It is appropriate to substitute 'disease' for 'mortality' in a phrase such as 'physiologic age is a function of prior mortality experience'. The high *mortality* rate of unfavored populations – those with low physiologic ages – is itself evidence of a high *morbidity* rate and a more rapid rise in the vulnerability term. Longer life spans reveal increased vigor and lower physiologic than chronologic age. In short, Jones estimated the vitality of the surviving population by observing the vulnerability of those who died. He assumed a parallel relationship between mortality and morbidity. And he assumed that the trend of declining mortality risks, which he observed by comparing survival curves, was itself proof of a declining morbidity risk. Furthermore, Jones explicitly rejected the idea of selection, holding that survivors are not selected on grounds of fitness except in the case of infants with severe physical disabilities who die but who make up a tiny part of any cohort.

Modifications to Insult Accumulation Theory

Some of Jones's assumptions have retained the confidence of later researchers, and some have been modified. The most recent version of the initial proposition, which was a statement about the properties of mortality risk during adulthood and the similarity of human experience to that of many animal models, has been provided by T.B.L. Kirkwood and R. Holliday. In the basic form of the problem, stated by Gompertz and restated most effectively by George A. Sacher, two terms – the rate of aging and vulnerability – comprise the mortality risk.[38] Kirkwood and Holliday add a third term representing somatic maintenance and repair.[39] Although this term is presented as a distinct element in the equation, it seems to incorporate properties previously assigned to both aging and vulnerability. It is not yet clear how the addition of this term influences opportunities for testing the equation with animal or human models.

Other modifications derive from closer scrutiny of evidence considered by Jones. Whereas Jones stressed the greater importance of insult accumulation during development, especially up to age 18, Bernard Strehler's modification suggests the continuing, and in some instances growing, importance of accumulation through adulthood. Looking at survival curves, Strehler noticed that the rate of increase in the death rate – the Gompertz function – is stable in favored and unfavored populations but also that its value has been somewhat lower in unfavored than favored populations.[40] In unfavored populations a high mortality rate in infancy and childhood is followed by higher mortality rates in adulthood but a lower rate of increase (i.e., in the terms of Figure 2.1, a more gradual incline). In high mortality regimes the high death rate before age 30 winnows the population, leaving survivors whose longevity is prolonged. The lower rate of increase in the adult death rate appears in all unfavored populations studied, and therefore in a variety of disease- and injury-risk profiles. Unfavored populations resemble one another in their higher death rates but differ from one another in the causes of those higher rates. This characteristic suggests that winnowing in the development stage of life influences the way insult accumulation effects in the postdevelopment stage will accrue.

Strehler's modification also accommodates evidence from postmortem analysis, which shows that the number of lesions unassociated with the cause of death rises with age.[41] And it allows for the influence of risk factors more satisfactorily than does Jones's initial formulation. Risk factors operate at all stages of life, but many injury risks cluster by age. As will be shown in more detail below, one of the most intensive points of clustering occurs in adolescence and early adulthood, a period in which injury exposure resembles the hazards of early childhood exposure to infectious disease. It is this injury exposure that gives the mortality risk curve its interior peak and the form of a misshapen W.[42]

Jones initially proposed that mortality within a cohort does not involve a process of selection except in the case of infants with severe physical disabilities who survive infancy. Survivors present the same characteristics and the same distribution of characteristics as those who have died. He later altered this position by suggesting that children who survive diseases in infancy become a special population more likely to develop other diseases.[43] The comparison between unfavored and favored populations is instructive once more. It suggests that the process of differentiation occurs not only in infancy and childhood but continues throughout life. Members of a cohort shift position from relatively disease-free backgrounds to relatively disease-ridden backgrounds as additional disease and injury hazards are encountered. The issue is not only mortality but also morbidity experience.

Jones' intuitive sense that the morbidity experience of survivors could be inferred from mortality experience will not withstand scrutiny.[44] Disease experience is reflected in mortality rates, but the manner of its reflection changes over time and during the life cycle of a cohort. Every cohort and every member of a cohort is not subject to the same array of insults. A cohort quickly divides itself into numerous segments, each representing clusters of people who share the same or very similar disease-and-recovery experiences. The pertinent issue is whether the process of selection can be separated into constituent parts. In the simplest possibility, cohorts might be found regularly to divide themselves into three categories: members who have died, members who lived but accumulated insults at a notably higher rate, and members who lived but accumulated insults at a notably lower rate. At the other extreme, survival might constitute a process of selection and differentiation with a stunning number of permutations in which the ultimately unique experience of each survivor represented significantly different histories of insult accumulation. The operation of a latent interval further complicates the problem of identifying and measuring causation. In any event, accumulation has its own history in each cohort, and that history can be told as a process of division and selection.

Finally, Jones cast the issue of insult accumulation not in terms of the timing of death but in terms of the differential between chronologic and physiologic age, that is, in terms of vigor rather than vulnerability. If it were plausible to assume a trend stable relationship between mortality and morbidity risks, then vigor and vulnerability might simply be two sides of the same coin. But if the relationship is unstable – if, for example, the morbidity risk is more susceptible to manipulation than the mortality risk, or if it is less susceptible – then the role of insult accumulation will differ between the two outcomes. In one morbidity/mortality complex a higher index of insult accumulation may augment the risk of sickness without increasing the risk of death at any given age. That is, anything other than a parallel and proportional relationship between morbidity and mortality will upset Jones's version of the theory. From discussion above it is already apparent that this relationship will not always be parallel. We will later encounter reasons to wonder whether or not the relationship between these two risks is usually stable and proportional.[45]

Modifications to Jones's theory produce a more realistic but also a more complex theory of insult accumulation. The new theory expands the range of insults, demands information about the degree and term of influence exercised by individual types of insult, and considers insult accumulation at every stage of life rather than chiefly in childhood. The modifications substitute an assumption of life-long selection for an assumption that selection is insignificant or else important only in the early years of the experience of a given cohort. But the most important effect of the modifications is to recast the underlying question. Jones wondered how to account for stability in the mortality risk during a period of adulthood in which populations with quite different disease and medical histories nevertheless manifested a statistical regularity – the Gompertz function. His answer was to suggest that health events early in life condition the average experience of the cohort, a conditioning that shows up statistically when population (rather than cohort) experience is compared because events differ little from one birth cohort to the next. In Jones's formulation the important issue was the timing of death. The important hypothesis held that more sickness early in life coincides with lower physiologic age and earlier death. In the recast version, three fresh issues emerged. How do survivors differ from those who die? How do those who survive (or die) in the same cohort differ from one another? How much do sicknesses experienced earlier in life influence health experience later in life?

CONCLUSION

Death is a sequel of illness and injury, but the relationship between the two is complex. The comparison of survival curves across vastly different populations suggests that the relationship between morbid experience and death should be addressed in the first place by means of a division between intrinsic and extrinsic sources of risk, and in the second place by a division of the life course into three stages. In the first stage, lasting from early fetal development until middle age – now about age 45 – mortality and morbidity seem to be conditioned chiefly by extrinsic risks. Some members of every cohort carry intrinsic risks at birth in the form of serious structural malformations, and many more bear propensities to disease or stress that may be inherited. These characteristics exert limited influence on health experience at the population level until later in the life course. Nevertheless, the mortality risk, which is all that has yet been considered here, exhibits certain regularities suggesting that underlying biological properties are influential. It is not surprising that mortality is regularly higher among infants (0–1) than among children. The peak in mortality risk at which life opens, and the correspondingly predictable peak at which it closes for any cohort, implies an intervening low point. But it is surprising that the low point seems itself to exhibit an age-related regularity. Figure 1.4 (p. 23) suggests that the mortality risk reaches this lowest point at about age 11, even though Figure 1.4 deals with populations facing radically different disease and injury profiles, and radically different profiles of medical assistance. Another regularity appears in the misshapen portion of the W-shaped mortality curve. An initially rapid increase in the mortality risk from the low point around age 11 to a second peak around age 20 gives way to a leveling off or a temporary decline in risk. This portion of the curve deserves closer scrutiny, but the recurrence once more of a certain form – the misshapen W – suggests that underlying biological properties condition the influence of extrinsic risks.

The second stage of the life course also exhibits an underlying biological regularity, namely stability in the rate of increase in the death rate. This stability, often called the Gompertz function, appears now around age 45 and persists for twenty years or more thereafter. It is ordinarily explained as evidence that intrinsic factors have intervened in a more compelling manner, casting the mortality risk into two terms: aging and vulnerability. The implication is that the aging term increases at a stable rate, hence that the vulnerability term decreases at a stable rate. What remains unobserved is the point or the level at which the aging term intervenes. Closer scrutiny of the Gompertz function across populations, and of biological theory concerning the function, suggests that the aging term may increase in a trend stable manner rather than at a stable rate. That is, there may be interactions between aging and vulnerability, or trade-offs within the heterogeneity of cohorts, that combine with aging to produce the Gompertz function. Populations age at different rates, which may be a function of differences in the degree of vulnerability accumulated before age 45 and of differences in the way that mortality shapes the composition of cohorts and therefore of populations over time.

In the third stage of the life course the evidence is sketchy. That stage deals with ages to which few individuals survived in most historical populations and with a part of the life course in which age exaggeration seems to distort most data sets. There, too, mortality curves display an important regularity, and an historical trend. The regularity consists of the substitution at advanced age of an arithmetic increase for the Gompertz or geometric increase in the mortality risk, so that the q_x function begins to resemble the exposure time function sketched in Figure 1.4 as curve T. That is, the number of survivors at advanced ages appears to diminish at something approaching a regular arithmetic rate from the age at which the Gompertz function ceases to apply until the end of the human life span. This arithmetic regularity does not always appear in pre-twentieth-century mortality curves, presumably because the age evidence is faulty rather than because survivorship has been closed in the sudden and catastrophic depletion of the population suggested by the pre-twentieth-century curves in Figure 1.4. The historical trend consists of a peregrination in the point at which the Gompertz function gives way to the arithmetic function. Over time the age at transition has risen, as appears from Figure 2.1. The rise has been interpreted here as an historical movement toward the later preservation of heterogeneity. As mortality declined and life expectancy increased, the relationship between mortality and morbidity shifted, and the leading effect of the shift was to ensure that people with a higher risk to morbidity lived longer.

Jones misinterpreted the content and implications of the mortality decline by adopting an intuitive assumption that the mortality risk is a direct and parallel representation of the morbidity risk. The transition from a high to a low mortality regime and the lower risks of the low mortality regime created, or widened, the gap between chronologic and physiologic age. But physiologic age is not equivalent to vitality. It is a measure of the capacity to survive rather than of the capacity for health and, as a measurement, is influenced by the duality of physiologic age itself. A gain in physiologic age may, at the individual level, signal an increase or a decrease in the amount of sickness that will occur in the remaining term of life. At the aggregate level the leading effect of longer average life spans has been to increase the number of new survivors, to ensure that more of the population has survived to ages at which propensities to disease present at birth and the accumulation of insults through life will produce ill health.

Animal models and reasoning from analogy to human counter-parts suggest that humankind's adaptation to the environment remains something less than optimal. Animals brought from the wild into a zoo live longer and display gains in life expectancy similar to those exhibited by human populations passing from the mortality risks of paleolithic or neolithic civilization to those of civilizations more successful in curtailing mortality. Transferred to a laboratory, where morbidity and mortality risks may be more thoroughly monitored and controlled, insects and small animals display still further gains. These gains comprise increases in life expectancy and life span but also increases that make the distinction between intrinsic and ex-trinsic risks more difficult to draw. The distinction between gains in life expectancy and in life span becomes still more vague. Environ-mental control on the order of what can be achieved in the laboratory with animal subjects implies the elimination of illness and injury hazards, including all elements of the vulnerability term, or at least all elements except the comparatively small hazard consisting of genetic malformations that are not now susceptible and present no likely prospect of becoming susceptible to treatment. The animal model therefore suggests the plausibility of finding the means to push life expectancy at birth not just to the modal age of death, which is perhaps 85 years, but to the human life span, which is 110 years or somewhat more. Indeed the animal model, interpreted in the light of insult accumulation, implies that still higher life expectancies might be achieved by creating human prospects in which, for the first time, it could accurately be said that the individual or the cohort has never been sick a day in its life.

Conquest of the space of life brought humanity into confrontation with a fresh problem. To the degree that we have begun to see the nature of the problem – and that is as yet a limited degree – the conquest assured a longer period in which intrinsic and endogenized sources of ill health would begin to hold sway. In the high mortality regimes of the past most people died from the effects of virulent infections. They died before experiencing the effects of propensities to disease present at birth and additional propensities acquired during lives exposed to illness and injury. The mortality decline pushed the risk of death into ever-diminishing portions of the survival rectangle. The cost of that conquest of space was to add years of life in which the effects of disease propensities and insult accumulation would be felt. To see the implications of this process more clearly, it is necessary to consider the risk of sickness as something distinct and distinguishable from the risk of death.

3 Sickness Risk

> Most Men know when they are ill, but
> very few when they are well.[1]

Imagine a continuum beginning at wellness—the hypothetical state in which an individual exhibits no pathological or behavioral signs of disorder. Toward what state does it extend? The obvious answer would be death caused by pathological or behavioral stress. Although the mortality-oriented definition of this counterpart of wellness has undeniable value, and leads to an assessment of the risk of death presented by any new insult, most sicknesses do not now and have not, except perhaps in unusually virulent epidemics, been resolved in death. Most sicknesses are resolved in something called recovery, in which the individual resumes activities engaged in before the insult, perhaps with reoccurrences. Other sicknesses do not end. They become submerged by convalescence, by coincidental illnesses, or by aging itself. Sickness is an aspect in most deaths, but the contrary is not true. What is more, many public health and medical measures that influence the risk of death may have little influence on the risk of falling sick or remaining sick. Sickness requires its own evaluation.[2]

But what is sickness? Again imagine a continuum, this one extending from the state at which an individual exhibits some signs of pathological or behavioral stress, even if those signs can be detected only through intensive scrutiny, toward a state of incapacity to perform basic functions, such as feeding or dressing oneself. To admit the existence of this continuum is to recognize the difficulty of deciding how sickness is to be identified and measured. All of us appear to fall at one or another point along this continuum. We are all either already sick, or potentially sick from existing propensities and signs of stress. But we are all sick only according to an extreme definition. In fact, most of the time we adequately perform not only the basic functions of caring for ourselves but also a wide range of other functions. This is true today, and it was true in historical societies, too. The problem therefore is to identify thresholds at which individuals pass from a state of capacity to function to a state of incapacity.

A further complication exists in the fact that individuals react in different ways to what appear to be identical levels of pathologic and behavioral stress. This book is a study of aggregate experience. To proceed, it is necessary to adopt an assumption: sensitivity to stress is normally distributed within any large population at any given time. Over time societies may change their sense of whether a given stress leads to incapacity to function. But at any one time the collection of individual judgments about all existing levels of stress will rise to a peak at a certain collective definition and decline thereafter. This is not a contentious assumption. Normal distributions are regularly observed in large populations. Of course, individual responses to the stimuli of pathological and behavioral stress vary from aggregate averages.

Confronted with a phenomenon – sickness – that exists as a continuum rather than a series of discrete components, we must find ways to distinguish stages within the continuum. Two useful approaches have been devised. One of these, as old as medicine, organizes pathological states according to leading characteristics – signs and symptoms – which are called diseases. Today, the classification of a population's ill health proceeds by clinical analysis, which seeks to identify disease states in order to diagnose them. In some countries diseases considered important for epidemiological reasons – notifiable diseases – are reported by public health officers to central statistical offices, which in this way collect data about the incidence of these diseases. For much of the history of medicine, diagnosis has proceeded from the assumption that most diseases have physical origins and that the leading manifestations of disease are also physical. Since the late nineteenth century, this assumption has been questioned, and the view has emerged that many disorders have behavioral origins and effects. These disorders, too, are classified as disease entities. To follow this diagnostic line, which assesses ill health within a cross-section, is to be led toward an inventory of all disease states manifested, an acknowledgment of multiple conditions in many individuals, and an ordering of these diseases. The diagnostic approach organizes information in a way that is intended to assist therapeutic and epidemiologic ends and perhaps to assess the risk to life posed by disease.[3] A second approach eschews diagnosis and uses as a definition of sickness the concept of capacity to function. The form functioning takes may be readily visible, such as the capacity to feed or dress oneself or to perform the tasks required in an individual's work, or it may be internal, and therefore measurable only by biochemical, physiological, or behavioral assessment. Ill health is graded according to whether ordinary functions are compromised.

Functional assessments are not new, but the twentieth century has seen considerable development in the effort to collect data about them. Some assessments seek to determine the degree to which a physiologic function, such as blood pressure or basal metabolism, departs from the parameters of ordinary performance according to existing information about the distribution of the function among individuals in adequate health. In this way, functional assessment offers a way to grade malfunction and to estimate the likelihood of future disease episodes in cases in which a certain compromise of function has previously been identified statistically and probabilistically with disease. Another category of the assessment of function is organized around the social costs of disorder. Measurements of hospital bed use, consultation of physicians, restriction in ordinary activity, and time lost from work or school produce data useful for predicting the demand for medical services, assessing the social and economic costs of ill health, and forecasting trends in these costs.

Neither the disease list nor the functional disorder list are entirely discrete, but collection in these categories makes possible the organization and interpretation of otherwise chaotic data. For enquiry to proceed in this way, it would be useful to preserve fixed definitions of each disease or functional disorder. In reality, fixed definitions do not exist for two major reasons: research continuously produces new information about disease and functional entities and about ways in which these entities should be perceived, and medical opinions change. The list of diseases discussed in pathology texts changes over time, often through the subdivision of existing entities. A sign of this, one of particular concern to historians and epidemiologists, is the lengthening and refinement of the list of notifiable diseases and of diseases given as cause of death. The lists grow not so much because new diseases are discovered as because the complexity of existing diseases has been further penetrated. For example, the designation 'old age', which satisfied the nineteenth-century Registrar General of Births, Deaths and Marriages in England and Wales as a way to account for many deaths among the aged, has given way to increasingly refined categories. A similar process exists in the functional approach. Physiologic and biochemical research identify functions that should be measured, and research in sampling procedure shows how to extract superior information from respondents.[4] In short, the phenomena being measured may not change, but the way in which they are perceived does change.

Some functional disorders are more susceptible to redefinition than others. For example, hospital bed use, on which some data might be collected for the past four or five centuries, is affected by the role assigned to the hospital, the designation of pathological and behavioral disorders that warrant hospitalization, and the demand for beds (which is partly a function of population size, age distribution, and the standard of living). Each of these variables has changed radically over time, and continues to change, to such a degree that it is difficult to see how hospitalization data could be standardized. Many early modern hospitals refused to accept individuals with diseases believed to be contagious, whereas many present-day hospitals focus on treatment and isolation of individuals with infectious and communicable disorders. Measurements of physiological and biochemical function also provide evidence of limited value to the historian, chiefly because the procedure of measurement is for the most part a recent technique, but also because the significance of the quantity measured continues to change as more is learned about the meaning of these signs. If measurements of functional disorder adhered over time to fixed definitions, it would be comparatively simple to arrange these measurements into a hierarchy and to assess changes over time in the level of ill health associated with a given functional limitation. Since fixed definitions do not prevail, it is necessary to proceed in another way. A category of function is needed about which data have been gathered for a long time and in a way open to adjustment to a common standard. The category that most nearly satisfies these needs is time lost from work because of ill health.

Ill health is an event that does not lend itself to direct observation. All the ways by which it is identified for study only represent manifestations of an underlying phenomenon. Thus a pathologic or a behavioral diagnosis gives an identity to a state of disorder, an identity that is manifestly useful. But the underlying disorder is more complex than its diagnostic identity suggests. Moreover, all identifications involve a certain risk of error. Diagnoses made represent only a part of the complete number of disorders within a population, and diagnoses of notifiable diseases reported represent only a part of the diagnoses made. Work time lost because of sickness is not ill health itself but a manifestation of ill health. In the most common case encountered in historical sources, this manifestation represents a judgment by a third party that an individual was unable because of pathologic or behavioral stress to perform the work required in the occupation he or she had been following. To acknowledge a state of functional incapacity is, in its own way, a diagnosis, one in which the objective is not disease identification and treatment but something closer to a distinction between clinical and subclinical disorder. At any rate a decision has been made, and not all third parties – physicians or workmates – would arrive at the same decision. Nor would the same decision necessarily be reached at different times or in different cultures. These real and potential sources of confusion about threshold, definition and identification require constant attentiveness to the characteristics of the proxy for ill health, be that proxy a diagnosis or an insurance claim. The great advantage of using sources about work time lost is that they reveal the scale and leading characteristics of the population at risk to sickness. Other sources often report cases of ill health but seldom reveal the size or other characteristics of the population among which these cases have occurred.

Work time lost means a sacrifice of income, and it is this feature that has produced historical records. These consist of financial accounts recording payments into and out of a fund used to compensate members for lost work time, together with ancillary information – rules – explaining how episodes warranting compensation were to be identified. Individuals came under observation when they purchased insurance, and they entered the pool of people in ill health when they were incapacitated for work and thereby earned benefits.

Wage insurance funds of this sort have been traced to classical antiquity, but the earliest known financial accounts date from the seventeenth century. During the nineteenth and twentieth centuries, the state involved itself in these activities, first regulating the management of existing funds and then taking over some of their compensatory functions. Since the late nineteenth century, the data provided by financial accounts have been supplemented by intensive surveys of the health experience of selected communities and, more recently, by random population surveys of the incidence of work time lost, sometimes measured in terms of diagnosed disorders and sometimes as events or prevalences. In every case, from fund to fund, from fund to survey, and from survey to survey, a different form of the phenomenon of work time lost is under observation.[5]

To be compared in a useful way, the different data sets must be adjusted to a common standard. As is the case with diagnosis, this is a particularly difficult task. The problem is not to reconstruct the disease profile of past populations, finding counterparts in the modern lexicon of the pathology textbook for historical diseases. It is instead to reconcile valuations of function and variations in the terms of the insurance contract or in the millieu of work. Whether ap proached via diagnosis or function, the history of ill health shares an abiding problem of perception: when individuals, physicians, or detached observers declare themselves or someone else ill, do they mean more or less the same thing over time? Or do judgments about the threshold separating health from illness change over time? This is not an easy question to answer. By the very nature of the matter, an objective standard is lacking, and the subjective influences that affect judgments – which are social, economic, cultural, and psychological – themselves change. Assuming that judgments about the threshold between health and ill health change from time to time in the case of diseases and functions, the key issue becomes how and in what way changes in the perception of threshold affect what statistical data suggest about the trend of ill health. For example, Ralph Josselin, living in the seventeenth century, treated colds as lightly as most modern sufferers do, refusing to curtail his activities. But he also insisted on preaching each Sunday while ill with a long and otherwise incapacitating swelling and ulceration in his left leg.[6] Present-day sufferers of something like Josselin's leg ulcers less often need feel compelled, as Josselin did, to work while so seriously ill. Since little is known about changes in perception, the 'true' sickness trend between Josselin's era and our own would not be apparent even if we possessed information about sicknesses that seemed to be similar. The very long run trend cannot be determined in so simple a way. But we can pursue an alternative strategy, which is to search for trends that seem to be undisturbed by perceptual changes and to examine their course over the very long run.

This chapter will consider a series of figures and tables that depict some aspects of sickness risk. In each instance, the data set(s) on which a figure or table is based has been selected because it provides an illustration that can be generalized. How broadly the forms to be encountered can be generalized is not yet apparent. Certainly, these forms will not apply to all other populations, especially not regarding specific morbidity levels. But the figures and tables will be broadly representative of the way in which sickness risks of the same type will occur in other populations.

SICKNESS AND AGE IN MALES

The incidence of ill health is influenced by many forces, but one of these – age – exerts more effect than any other.[7] (It is useful to distinguish between the contribution made by aging to the risk of death or ill health, and the association between age and ill health or mortality rates.) The image most authorities seem to have of the association with age is best represented by a vaguely defined figure with a U shape. The risk of ill health is high in infancy and early childhood. It declines to a low point in adolescence and rises gradually thereafter to a second peak in old age. But the idea of expressing morbidity risk as a curve, using something akin to the function of the life table that assesses mortality risk, is itself still uncommon. Whereas the idea of measuring expectation of life and using that measure to compare the quality of life between two societies is familiar, the health counterpart – a health expectation – is unfamiliar.

The reasons for vagueness about and unfamiliarity with the age distribution of health risks arise in part from the ambiguity of ill health. Like the mortality risk, the morbidity risk may change over time, so that comparing any two measurements of it gives the impression of failing to obtain a reliable estimate. In mortality, that variability is reconciled by comparing measurements over time, usually by comparing life expectancy at birth. Health in the United States (it is said) has improved since the nineteenth century, and the evidence for this is higher life expectancy.[8] Yet health in the US is not as good as it might be, because still higher life expectancies occur in some other countries. The morbidity risk adds another form of ambiguity, a form arising from the difficulty of selecting a single standard for distinguishing health from ill health. Different standards usually preserve resemblance to a U, but the sides of the U change their angles. Lacking a preferred standard, the morbidity risk has not been measured in a fashion analogous to the mortality risk even though the measurement of risk in this way is necessary in order to calculate the future stream of health risks in a population, which is the basic element in an expectation.

Once a standard has been selected, the morbidity risk curve acquires definition, and its movements across time can be plotted. These properties appear in modern health surveys, which sample several health indicators within stratified random samples of national populations. They appear with still better definition in actuarial investigations of time lost from work among the members of sick funds in the nineteenth century. The actuaries studied only the experience of insured people, so that their reports do not speak to the level of sickness in the overall population. This is an important limitation, but it is compensated for by other qualities of the actuarial reports. They deal with vast numbers of males, numbers large enough to follow experience age by age rather than in broad age groups, and they preserve consistent standards of measurement over time, standards elaborated in rules that distinguished claims warranting compensation from those not. The actuaries also investigated environmental and socioeconomic characteristics to see how factors other than age influenced sickness risk.

The practical objective of actuarial investigation was to measure work time lost to illness and injury, i.e., sickness. The theoretical goal was to discover a putative 'law of sickness' – an age-specific schedule that the actuaries expected would obtain in any large population properly surveyed. Discovery of the law would allow projection of claims in a given sick fund without requiring information about claims experience. Therefore the actuaries were chiefly interested in measuring the amount of time a given population would lose to sickness per member per year, which is to say, the duration of sickness episodes. It is useful to think about this form of sickness as the *risk of being sick*, or the *duration risk*. This risk measures sick time as a proportion of time at risk.

The Risk of Being Sick

Alfred W. Watson directed the largest actuarial investigation, which detailed the experience of the Independent Order of Odd Fellows Manchester Unity from 1893 to 1897. His report recounted claims in a friendly society with an average of more than 600 000 members in each year of the five-year survey period, one whose membership – males only – was concentrated in England and Wales and ranged across ages 13 to 100. This survey remains the largest single data set ever compiled in the United Kingdom. Figure 3.1 portrays the age-specific risk of being sick indicated by Watson's investigations (curve A) and compares it to some other sets of experience: the Odd Fellows from 1866 to 1870 (curve B), and three friendly societies operating throughout the Australian state of Victoria from 1903 to 1907 (curve C). Sickness is measured as weeks lost per year at each age in the aggregate membership. The graph provides sickness rates only for ages at which large numbers of men belonged to one or another society.

The curves in this graph suggest an age schedule with several interesting properties. First, the patterns confirm the degree to which age influences the sickness rate. Both in young adulthood, when the age-specific sickness rates are low, and in old age, when they are

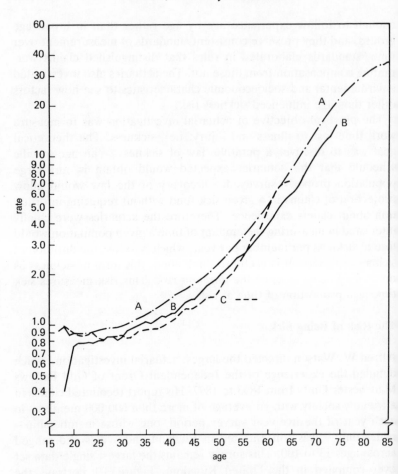

FIGURE 3.1 *The risk of being sick*

SOURCES [Henry Ratcliffe], *Independent Order of Odd-Fellows, Manchester Unity Friendly Society: Supplementary Report, July 1st, 1872* (n.p., n.d.), pp. 12-13 and 120; Alfred W. Watson, *An Account of an Investigation of the Sickness and Mortality Experience of the I.O.O.F. Manchester Unity . . . 1893–1897* (Manchester, 1903), pp. 138-9, 210, 212; A.M. Laughton, *Methods Employed in Investigation of Experience Rates of Sickness, Mortality and Secession and Monetary Tables Based on Experience* (Melbourne, 1912), p. 22.

high, the probability of being sick can be estimated more satisfactorily for any large number of individuals from information about their present age than from any other known statistical characteristic. However, even the experience of large populations, here ranging in size from 75 000 (curve C) to 600 000 males (curve A), does not produce curves that are entirely smooth. Each population is divided by the ages represented in it. When small numbers are at risk at each age, which occurs especially in curves B and C, irregularities are more numerous. These are an unavoidable result of subdivision. The actuaries dealt with irregularities by smoothing the crude data at their disposal, adopting one or another procedure for averaging age-specific data over several ages. Unsmoothed series are given here in order to show how much variation occurs even in large surveys and to underscore the kind of information that is lost in sampling procedures using small populations.

Second, the risk of being sick is influenced by other factors than age. The two Odd Fellows surveys, separated by twenty-seven years, show a similar distribution of age-specific risk, but indicate that sickness rates were higher during 1893–97 than during 1866–70. The difference can be attributed to as yet unidentified factors specific to the time at which the surveys were made (such as the disease profile, or the mixture of occupations, residential patterns, or income levels among insureds). Curve C begins and ends at rates similar to those of the Odd Fellows from 1893 to 1897, but for most of its course shows rates lower than those of either Odd Fellows survey. This comparison suggests that the risk of being sick may also be affected by differences in the rules applied to distinguish incapacity or in the characteristics of the populations under study. The nineteenth-century actuary's hope of discovering a law of sickness failed because of the influence of these additional factors. Sickness rates inferred from the experience of any two populations are unlikely to describe exactly the same curve.

Third, in the curves in Figure 3.1, both irregularities from age to age and disparities from curve to curve are most pronounced for early ages, from 17 to 35. On the basis of the data used to sketch these curves, it is not clear whether the risk of being sick rises gradually from a floor in adolescence or whether the distribution of this risk by age should be seen as a U curve. This issue is unclear in Odd Fellows and Australian friendly society experience because so few individuals joined before age 18 and because those who joined were usually ineligible for sickness benefits for six months after joining (the 'initiation', a period after which insurance rights were vested).

Fourth, Odd Fellows experience during 1893–97, which is the only data set dealing with large numbers of individuals at advanced ages, gives the impression that the rate of increase of the risk of being sick slowed between ages 70 and 80 and, thereafter, leveled off or declined. It is particularly difficult to assess risk at these ages in historical populations, because smaller proportions of each cohort survived to advanced ages, and because the friendly societies offered benefits for time lost from work. For the individuals represented in these three curves, employer-funded or state-funded retirement programs remained a hope for the future, and retirement from work had to be financed by the individual. The actuaries suspected that some elderly individuals used benefits as a pension. These individuals remained members of the sick fund and drew benefits under the assumption that they might recover and return to work. But, as age increased, so too did the proportion of members continuously sick. For advanced ages, it is difficult to distinguish episodes of sickness from age-related disability.

Fifth, these curves suggest that, between about ages 45 and 70, the risk of being sick, like the risk of dying, increased with age in a stable manner. In Chapter 2, it was noticed that different mortality rate series indicate that, for certain ages in adulthood, the death rate increases at a stable rate. The biologist Alex Comfort, who took the Gompertz function to be evidence of the existence of a distinct process of senescence operating with the mortality risk, hypothesized that morbidity data would reveal a similar function. The curves in Figure 3.1 seem to bear out Comfort's hypothesis. Curves A and B depict a stable rate of increase from about age 50 until about age 70. In those populations, the sickness risk doubled about every eight years, approximately the same doubling time observed in mortality series from late-nineteenth-century Britain. Curve C, which deals with Australian experience, also suggests a stable rate of increase for the smaller part of the age spectrum for which data are available but with a shorter doubling time: about seven years. Like the Gompertz function observed in mortality series, Figure 3.1 suggests that the morbidity form of this process will occur in different populations but will vary according to environmental factors. The strength of the aging term in morbidity remains unmeasured.

The Risk of Falling Sick

The sickness risk can also be considered according to the number of episodes or sickness events that occur within a population in a given period of time, a concept expressed here as the *risk of falling sick* or the *event risk*. If the age-specific average duration of sickness episodes were stable, then the risk of being sick would coincide with the risk of falling sick in the same population. Curves representing the two risks would appear at different points on the morbidity schedule because the risk of being sick would count days (or weeks) per year and the risk of falling sick the smaller number of events per year. If, however, the duration of sickness episodes itself changes from one age group to another because of factors unrelated to age, the two will diverge. To describe the risk of falling sick and begin to identify its form, it is useful to consult another actuarial report, one drafted by Francis G.P. Neison, Jr., who surveyed experience in the Ancient Order of Foresters Friendly Society for the five years beginning 1 January 1871. In that period, the Foresters had somewhat less than half as many members as the Odd Fellows during 1893–97.[9] For present purposes, the leading effect of this smaller membership is that fewer individuals are represented at all ages but especially at age 18 and at age 77 and above.

In Figure 3.2, curve D depicts the risk of being sick as inferred from Foresters experience during 1871–75, curve E the mortality rate at each age, and curve F the risk of falling sick. Curve D is expressed in the same manner as curve A in Figure 3.1; it sketches age-to-age changes in the average quantity of time lost from work because of sickness. Curve F assesses the risk of falling sick by sketching the proportion of all members who experienced an episode of sickness at each age.[10] Comparing it to curve E, we notice at once that the risk of falling sick was much higher at all ages measured than the risk of death. Since episodes of sickness are more numerous than deaths, reliable morbidity rates can be obtained from smaller populations than would be necessary to derive mortality rates.

In Figure 3.2, the risk of being sick reaches a floor at ages 23–24 and the remainder of this curve also follows the same form as the curves in Figure 3.1. In the Foresters series, the rate of increase stabilized at about age 50 and remained stable thereafter, although with some more irregularities that may be attributed to the smaller number of members at each age. In short, curve D repeats leading

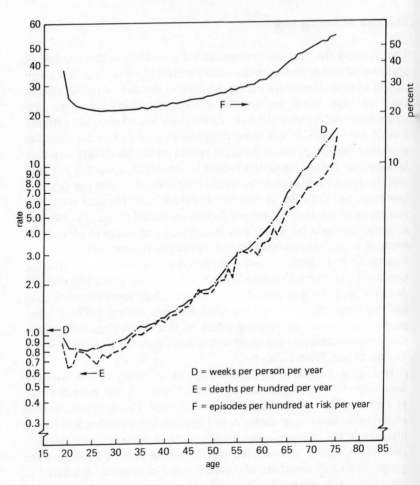

FIGURE 3.2   *The risk of falling sick compared to the risk of being sick*

SOURCE   Francis G.P. Neison, Jr., *The Rates of Mortality and Sickness According to the Experience of the Five Years, 1871-1875, of the Ancient Order of Foresters Friendly Society* . . . (London, 1882), pp. 35-6 and 55-6.

features of the risk of being sick already identified. The new information in Figure 3.2 consists of evidence about the age distribution of the risk of falling sick. In the Foresters experience, this risk reached a floor during the age band 25–34. Thereafter it rose much more gradually, resembling half of a shallow bowl more closely than the right side of a U.

Here is a leading explanation for the vagueness of the morbidity curve as usually conceived. Unless a distinction is made between the risk of being sick and the risk of falling sick, two basically dissimilar kinds of experience will merge. Once the distinction is made, it becomes clear that the average duration of sickness episodes changes with age and that these changes influence representations of the morbidity risk. For example, at age 29 when, in the Foresters series, the probability of falling sick was lowest (curve F), the average duration of this smallest proportion of episodes had already increased to the point at which the risk of being sick was noticeably higher than at its floor. The 20-year-old of the Foresters survey was more likely to fall sick but also to recover (or die) more rapidly than the 29-year-old. At age 65, the likelihood of falling sick was only 1.9 times greater than at age 29, but the likelihood of being sick was 7.7 times greater. The risk of being sick rises with age much more rapidly than the risk of falling sick because of the increasing average duration of all episodes. In the populations considered in Figures 3.1 and 3.2, the two risks declined together in very early adulthood, and rose together (although at different rates) from about age 35. Between some point within the age band 19–24 and age 35, the two risks moved in opposing directions.

Childhood and Early Adulthood

In the British friendly societies and in parallel groups in other countries, ill health acquired a definition from the capacity of the individual to perform functions associated with work. The sickness rate derived from the experience of those societies is a statement about aggregate incapacity in the part of the population with employment. That part included individuals with jobs, people temporarily or permanently incapacitated and receiving friendly society benefits, and people temporarily out of work but still eligible for benefits. Work – regular and full-time participation in the labor force – was characteristic of most men in Britain at ages 18 and above. But it was not characteristic of younger males. In general, the degree to which the capacity to work serves as a standard for distinguishing health from ill health diminishes as attention shifts from age 18 toward childhood and infancy. Smaller and smaller parts of the population come under scrutiny in consulting friendly society records for information about sickness rates at lower ages, and those parts become less and less representative of the overall population. Moreover, adolescents and children who worked regularly enough to warrant joining friendly societies held distinctive socioeconomic characteristics, which are likely to be reflected in health statistics, and these groups may also have been chosen for work because of other characteristics (e.g., height, orphaned status) with implications for health.

If work sometimes separates the population into groups with different characteristics likely to influence health status, it also serves as a bridge between health experience at age 18 and at each lower age. A comparison between the working 18-year-old and the working 17-, 16-, and 15-year-old would not manifest these different characteristics as clearly as would one between the working 18-year-old and the 10-year-old. But the association of some adolescents and children of each age with work lends an underlying unity to the standard against which health is measured. That is, the gradual shift of nineteenth-century adolescents into work between 12 and 18 helps redress the gap otherwise created by an abrupt movement into work. Even if the friendly society records cannot adequately capture the form sickness risks take from childhood into adulthood, the evidence they supply is useful because of this bridging function.

The sources consulted so far in this quest for information about basic forms of the sickness risk leave unanswered some questions about sickness risks in late adolescence and early adulthood as well. The leading problem is technical: how should the population at risk be counted in a stage of life during which young men joined and left the friendly societies, in turn expanding and shrinking the denominator of the fractions created to derive sickness risks. In the societies surveyed so far, most young men joined between ages 18 and 25. The issue of measuring numbers at risk is important because of the suggestion, from the mortality curves so far examined, that these risks take the form of a misshapen W with a lesser peak around age 20.

Especially toward the end of the nineteenth century, Odd Fellows and Foresters branches added juvenile counterparts. Throughout the century, separate friendly societies were organized for people not yet 18. In 1896, William Sutton, actuary to the Registrar of Friendly Societies, published a body of data about sickness experience at younger ages. He interpreted the information he had gathered in a way that diminished the effect of entrances and exits and that supplied some information about sickness risks for ages 9 and upward. [11] Figure 3.3 sketches curves for the risk of being and falling sick from Sutton's data, which relate to experience in some registered friendly

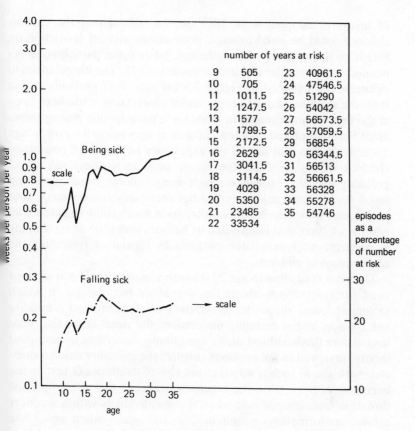

FIGURE 3.3 *Sickness risks at ages 9–35 (males only)*

SOURCE W[illiam] Sutton, *Special Report on Sickness and Mortality Experienced in Registered Friendly Societies*, House of Commons, Sessional Papers, 1896, LXXIX, 1134–9.

societies in England and Wales from 1876 to 1880. The sickness risks, like the mortality risk, reveal an interim peak, which occurred at age 19 in these two populations. From that age forward, the sickness risk declined, reaching another low point at ages 22–25 in the measurement of duration (the BS curve) and at ages 27–28 in the measurement of event risk (the FS curve).

From age 19 and younger, the number of individuals under observation diminishes rapidly and their association with work becomes increasingly problematic. Parliament restricted child labor in a series of measures adopted from 1802 on, but throughout the century children could be hired in some occupations without restriction on length of the workday. Nevertheless, labor force participation remained uncommon for children younger than 12. The irregularities in sickness risk indicated in Figure 3.3 for ages 9–17 probably derive from the small number of people under observation – numbers given in the figure – and changes in labor force participation among them. Since Sutton reported on a few children at ages below 9 – even at age 1 – it is obvious that not all the experience he consulted concerned children with jobs. Still, the minor peak in sickness risk at 12 probably identifies an age at which many children began work and faced work-related risks they had not previously encountered. That peak seems to be specific to populations in which children entered an adult work force and confronted its hazards with little or no training or preparation. It was later curtailed by legislation restricting the employment of children.

The peak at or close to age 20 is another matter, for it may signal a need for reservations about the degree or the manner in which biological forces shape the distribution of mortality and morbidity risk by age, and it certainly undermines the usual claim that adolescents are the healthiest of the age groups. According to biological theory, reviewed in the previous chapter, the mortality risk is associated with age in such a way that the risk of death peaks first at the beginning of life – when the organism's capacity to resist exogenous threats is undeveloped and when many individuals within a cohort exhibit malformations – and next in old age – when aging has undermined the capacity to resist exogenous and accumulated hazards or to repair damage. This distribution of risks implies a U-shaped curve, as mortality risk is usually described, or, more accurately, a curve shaped like a check mark or tick.

Figure 3.3 – and other data sets that confirm the existence of an interim peak in the morbidity risk around age 20 in nineteenth-century British populations – indicates that the morbidity risk, like the mortality risk, does not take the shape of a modified U or a tick but resembles a misshapen W. [12] When mortality and morbidity data are examined on an age-by-age basis, both rates are seen to increase more rapidly between age 11 or so and age 20 than they do at any point again until middle age. Compared to infancy and old age, adolescent risks remain low. But both their level and their rate of change indicate significant health problems.

The interior peak may be entirely a function of environmental hazards that are particularly intense in late adolescence, but the explanations offered for this phenomenon in cases where it has been observed in mortality series usually specify circumstances related to time and place. For example, the US population of 1979–81 displayed a marked shift in the survival curve around age 20 (Figure 1.4). Sometimes called the 'trauma bump', this phenomenon regularly appears around age 20 in twentieth-century US life tables. [13] Considering only white males, the group in which the undulation is most in evidence in recent US experience, the risk of death peaked at age 23, declined slightly until ages 28–32, and then resumed its increase. This feature of the US life table is usually explained not by an association with employment but as an effect caused by motor vehicle accidents and access to automobiles on the part of adolescents. [14] Since automobile accidents are still a leading cause of ill health as well as death in this group, the mortality peak would presumably find its counterpart in an age-by-age representation of morbidity among US white males. The issue, however, is whether automobile accidents are a cause or an effect of an unidentified behavioral or environmental risk.

In its manifestation in nineteenth-century British populations of working youths, the W's interior peak in the sickness risks might also be explained by factors peculiar to place and time. Most young men took up jobs in the adult world at those ages, often jobs that involved particular hazards for inexperienced hands. The new workers faced a sudden and temporary period of increased risk of occupational injury, a risk that diminished as they learned more about their jobs and the hazards associated with them. The increased risk around age 20 may also have derived from exposure to typhus and typhoid fever. Those diseases, which appeared together in the British cause of death registers until 1869, constituted two of the leading causes of death in the period covered by Sutton's surveys. [15] They are known as diseases with a marked age intensity in which mortality rates usually peak in early adulthood. But in Japan and Sweden early in the twentieth century, the same W-shaped curve was explained as an effect of tuberculosis.[16] The appearance of this peak in successive surveys of morbidity and mortality makes it unlikely that any one of these environmental factors – job initiation in hazardous occupations, typhus and typhoid fever, tuberculosis, access to automobiles – will provide a satisfactory explanation. Instead the rise of mortality and morbidity rates to a peak around age 20 may be a function of age-related factors, such as emotional instability and risk-seeking behavior. The biological model should be interpreted broadly to accommodate psychological factors. Recent research links higher adolescent mortality risk to depression, a condition believed to have biochemical and psychological origins but one associated more often with violence against the self (suicide) and property destruction than with the generalized morbidity and mortality suggested by the historical evidence.[17] Or the environmental interpretation might be recast as a change in exposure to disease rather than in specific diseases experienced.

In the nineteenth century and since, most authorities have assumed that the age distribution of the morbidity risk early in life could be inferred from mortality data. The risk would be highest immediately after birth and then diminish rapidly. That assumption requires merely that the case fatality rate preserve a more or less consistent decline in the passage from the diseases of infancy to those of late childhood. Cause-of-sickness data that refer to work as a standard obviously have little utility for this age group. Young children, even infants, were sometimes enrolled in friendly societies and claimed sickness benefits, but it is obvious that their claims were judged on another basis than capacity to work. What makes sickness so difficult to assess at these ages is the absence of any standard that might be used during a phase of life in which functional capacities and disease risks change rapidly and radically.

Useful data sets are rare. Further, each one has its own characteristics, so there is seldom a significant degree of consistency between surveys in the definitions or methods applied to gather observations. The numbers surveyed are often small and the populations atypical. What is more, not all authorities agree that the morbidity risk should be expected to parallel the mortality risk. Case studies often report an increase in morbidity between infancy and age 1.

In a study of nutrition and infection among Guatemalan villagers from 1959 to 1964, the mortality risk peaked in infancy but the morbidity risk at ages 1–2. The morbidity peak was associated with six to twenty-four months of age, when Mayan children of a highland region were weaned, and it appeared in measures of episodes and the duration of all illnesses observed in home visits made every other week. The research team associated this peak with nutritional deterioration linked to weaning rather than with stress on the immune system, another effect that might be cited to explain a sudden change in morbidity risk around age 2. However, they observed significantly lower morbidity rates through age thirty months in the control village, Santa María Cauqué, which was supplied with neither dietary supplements nor medical treatment, than in two treatment villages. A subsequent study in the control village from 1964 to 1969 reported a stupendous disease load among weanlings: illnesses and injuries, mostly diarrheal and respiratory diseases, occurred at a rate of 20 to 22 per person year, nearly five times the rate observed in the same village from 1959 to 1964.[18] Other researchers, too, have found the weanling months to be fraught with risks to life and health and have suggested that, in poorly nourished populations, morbidity risk peaks in harmony with growth retardation.[19] But it is not clear that they have found a common standard for measuring morbidity across the early months of life, or whether they have been misled by intervening factors, such as the willingness of mothers to expose infants and young children to visitors.

Other studies, dealing mostly with economically developed regions, suggest that morbidity risks parallel the mortality rate in infancy, and these studies point to distinctive passages – from breast-feeding into protracted weaning, entry into kindergarten and school – that mark transitions within a general pattern of declining risk.[20] The transitions are more sharply defined in small case studies in which many children are weaned or enter school at the same age in months than in aggregate studies in which the passages from one status to another are dispersed across months or years. The degree to which each passage influences the sickness risk varies according to many environmental circumstances in a way that suggests that cultural and social rather than biological factors have the greatest impact.

The net effect of this review is to leave the shape of the morbidity risk in infancy and early childhood in doubt. Environmental factors, such as cultural habits regarding weaning and socialization of children, demonstrably affect health, but their effects are not concentrated in a clearly marked age pattern. It seems apparent that the morbidity risk, like the mortality risk, declines to a low point at an age between 5 and 15. But the age at which the morbidity risk is lowest may not match the age of lowest mortality risk, which the data assembled for Figure 1.4 suggest to be 11. More uncertain still is whether the morbidity risk rises again – at least in societies where infants are breastfed – after the first six or twelve months of life or whether this risk at ages after six months may equal or exceed its level in the first month of life. The morbidity risk curve may be comparatively flat for the first year or eighteen months of life, or it may decline sharply from the immediate neonatal period.

SICKNESS RISK IN WOMEN VERSUS MEN

Female life expectancy has exceeded male life expectancy for most ages and in most European populations since the seventeenth century. In the twentieth century, the differential has increased and become more consistent. But it has never attained the degree of regularity that would suggest that biological factors dominate its terms, a suggestion that arises from the animal analogy – female longevity exceeds male in virtually all animal species – and from social history – specific instances of greater male longevity can be explained plausibly by sexual bias. Infanticide has sometimes been practiced selectively against females, and lower female than male life expectancy at ages 10–20 has been explained as an effect of the nutritional deprivation of girls. Variability in the sex differential indicates that behavioral and risk factors play an important role. Their effect shifts over time, and it may also be true that the interplay between biological and environmental forces changes as environmental forces shift.[21]

In some nineteenth-century societies, women faced higher mortality risks before and during childbearing years. Because the risk at those ages is low for both sexes, this differential rarely showed up in lower female life expectancy at birth. For example, in England and Wales in 1861, female *mortality* exceeded male only at ages 5–19 and 25–34, but female *life expectancy* exceeded male at all ages. This pattern appears in Figure 3.4 in a comparison of mortality rates of men and women who belonged to certain friendly societies in England and Wales during the period 1856–75. In the quinary age groups from 10–14 to 35–40, females died at higher rates than males (but the differential closed with the onset of childbearing years). After 35–40, male death rates remained higher than female until ages 70–74. The male disadvantage at higher ages sufficed to make male life expectancy at birth lower than female.[22]

Nineteenth-century observers usually attributed higher female life expectancy at birth to the higher risks of occupational mortality that men faced. But it is not apparent that this is a sufficient explanation or that the differential observed in the nineteenth century more

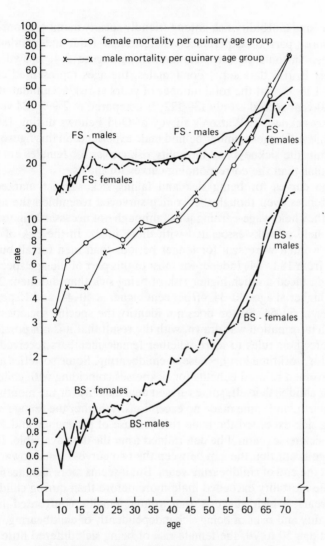

FIGURE 3.4 *Sickness and mortality risks by sex*

SOURCE Sutton, *Special Report*, 4–15tt.

closely approximated the natural or biological effect, as is sometimes implied.[23] Women often worked at wage-earning jobs in nineteenth-century Britain, and women with jobs often joined friendly societies, but few affiliated societies accepted women in large numbers. Tables addressing morbidity risk among friendly society members consist for the most part of experience amalgamated from independent societies. Sutton's report, summarized in Figure 3.4, provides the largest British data set.[24] For females, the ages represented extend from 1 to 93, but the total number of years at risk accumulated over the 20-year record is only 139 122, as compared to 2 995 724 years at risk to sickness in Watson's survey of Odd Fellows during 1893–97 and the still larger number behind male experience in this figure.[25] As a result, the sickness and mortality risk curves for females are more irregular than the corresponding curves for males.

The curves for being sick and falling sick suggest marked sex differences even though the women surveyed resembled the men in that they held wage-earning jobs (although not necessarily in the jobs they held or risks associated with those jobs). In the risk of being sick, women were sick for longer periods than men for all but two ages from 18 to 54. Indeed, for most of this part of the age spectrum, women faced a much higher risk of being sick than did men: 27 per cent higher at ages 30–34, 46 per cent higher at 40–44, and 15 per cent higher at 50–54. Sutton does not identify the specific societies from which information was drawn, with the result that it is not possible to explore their rules to learn whether female members received benefits for worktime lost because of childbearing. Some societies admitting women refused benefits for sicknesses coinciding with childbirth or for childbirth itself, some refused benefits only for the month after childbirth, and some made no exceptions. Whether the female risk of being sick exceeded the male risk because of pregnancy and associated sicknesses cannot be determined from the data available. It may be significant that the gap between the two curves closed toward age 50, at the end of childbearing years. But it seems more significant that female mortality exceeded male more before than during childbearing years, which suggests that young females confronted higher mortality and risks of being sick independently of childbearing. From about age 50 to 70, the female risk of being sick differed little from the male risk.

In the risk of falling sick, the sex differential was reversed. Women fell sick less often than men. With the exception of a few ages between 33 and 42, women experienced fewer episodes of sickness than men, but each episode was longer enough on average to produce a higher risk of being sick. In terms of the proportion of men and women who were sick, male rates exceeded female rates by 2 per cent at ages 30–34 and 40–44 and by sharply higher margins at earlier and later ages between 18 and 54. At ages 50–54, for example, the male rate was 18 per cent higher.

The same pattern appears in data accumulated by Austrian authorities for the period 1891–95 regarding 6.3 million years at risk among males and nearly 2 million among females. Measured by duration, female sickness rates exceeded male rates for all ages from 16 to 84. Measured by episode, males fell sick more frequently than females at all ages when pregnancies are excluded, but less frequently to age 43 when pregnancies are not excluded. The Austrian data suggest that work-incapacitating sickness occurs less frequently among women but that childbirths may conceal the form of this underlying sickness risk.[26]

This variance between the risk of falling and being sick may provide an important clue about how to interpret the relationship between morbidity and mortality. In insult accumulation theory, prior sickness is expected to influence later experience and the timing of death. Women would not be expected to experience more sickness than men yet live longer unless the additional sickness influenced insult accumulation to a lesser degree or was unrelated to it. The data in Figure 3.4 suggest that females enjoyed longer life spans than males because they accumulated fewer insults at most ages. The high female risk of being sick can also be interpreted as evidence that women convalesced more deliberately from the sicknesses they did suffer. It is also plausible to suggest that these women returned to work after longer periods of recuperation because their economic burdens were lighter (that is, fewer families depended on female breadwinners). If convalescence time is related closely to the quality of repair, female life expectancy may have been greater because of superior health care.

Plausible explanations for the sex differentials in mortality and morbidity are not difficult to suggest, but they are difficult to demonstrate. That difficulty increases when experience in these friendly societies is compared to morbidity and mortality among US females in the period 1958–81. The US health surveys, which measure the incidence and point prevalence of functional impairment and some specific diseases, regularly indicate higher female than male morbidity rates. The leading authority on US experience, Lois Verbrugge, finds that women report 20 to 30 per cent more ill health from acute conditions and non-fatal chronic diseases than do men of the same age, and more short-term disability. Men report more life-threatening diseases and more permanent disability. That is, women are sicker in the short run and men in the longer run; women experience more sickness but men have more serious health problems. Verbrugge explains the differential chiefly by exposure and lifestyle, and to a lesser degree by psycho–social factors (that is, sex differences in perception of or response to symptoms) or the idea that the differential should be attributed to a greater propensity of women to adopt what sociologists call the 'sick role'.[27]

The two patterns, one relating late-nineteenth-century British experience among women with jobs reporting work incapacitation, the other twentieth-century US experience in a cross-section of the female population, appear to be at odds. But Verbrugge's explanation of recent US experience also suggests a resolution. She argues that morbidity reported in the US surveys constitutes only a portion of all ill-health episodes. In the unobserved portion–episodes affecting work for less than a day and illnesses unreported altogether – Verbrugge believes that female ill health probably exceeds male to a still greater degree. The friendly societies applied a more stringent standard to distinguish sickness from health (incapacitation for work lasting at least three days) than the standard used in the US health survey (restriction of ordinary activity lasting a half day or longer) or than Verbrugge applied to hypothesize the distribution of shorter and unreported episodes. Taking those differences into account, women appear to experience more sickness, but their episodes are less serious in that they are less often life-threatening. Under the conditions obtaining in these populations, women lived longer because they accumulated insults more slowly.

Verbrugge's interpretation suggests a further modification in insult accumulation theory, one that demands diagnostic information in order to gauge the seriousness of sicknesses. This is an illustration of the need to combine diagnostic and functional approaches. Even so, it does not settle how diseases should be graded for severity. The threat different maladies pose to life changes with therapies, coincidental disease risks, and exposure. Nor is it apparent that threat to life is the appropriate way to gauge degree in insult accumulation.

Concerning other issues raised earlier in this chapter, Figure 3.4 shows that, for the women observed in the friendly society surveys, too, the sickness risk takes the form of a misshapen W. Between ages 9 and 35, the risk of falling sick peaked at age 19, reached a second floor at ages 26–27, and thereafter increased more slowly than among the male friendly society members to whom this experience is compared. The female risk of being sick also peaked at age 19 but reached a second floor immediately thereafter (ages 20–23) and then increased so rapidly that the risk at all ages from 27 up was higher than that at 19. In this instance, too, the decline in the risk of falling sick exceeded the decline in the risk of being sick. Among men and women, there is evidence of an undulation in the rate of insult accumulation in the ages associated with late development and early adulthood.

SICK TIME, HEALTH TIME

Age is the dominant but not the exclusive factor in the distribution of sickness risk and, as a force in distribution, age exerts its effects in ways that change over the life course, over time, and according to the way sickness is distinguished or perceived. This section will consider three aspects of perception: the distribution of sickness durations, the division of sicknesses between those resolved in recovery and those resolved in death, and lifelong experience with sickness and health. These issues, too, can be approached via the experience of male members of friendly societies in the United Kingdom in the second half of the nineteenth century, because those surveys present data in the forms necessary to make these distinctions.

Duration

Sickness episodes may be acute, which is to say that they may be of sharp and short course, hence resolved in recovery or death quickly, or they may be chronic, which is to say long lasting, even permanent. Common sense points to the need for such a distinction, but there is no settled opinion about when, in the duration of an episode, acute becomes chronic. Some authorities divide acute from chronic by distinguishing episodes lasting less than six months from those lasting six months or longer. Others prefer three months (that is, 13 weeks). Still others divide elsewhere. The division itself is an historical artifact, for it is influenced by the profile of diseases to which people are at risk as well as by therapy. For the high mortality regime of early modern European experience, there is considerable sense in adopting a division close to the one made by the physician George Cheyne: 40 days (six weeks).[28] Most acute disorders are resolved more quickly than six or three months, and a division at six to eight weeks would cover most of the leading causes of death into the eighteenth century, including typhoid fever and plague which, without treatment, may linger about eight weeks.[29]

Still, many infectious diseases common in the eighteenth century and earlier manifested themselves in ways that made the distinction between acute and chronic inappropriate. To call an illness 'a fever', a common diagnosis, was to avoid the issue of whether the ailment would have a brief or a prolonged clinical course. Many diseases appeared not as discrete episodes but in association with other ailments, acute or chronic, that the physician was poorly prepared to differentiate.[30] Furthermore, chronic diseases often include periods of remission in which, although the disorder continues and may be recognizable to a clinician or to the sufferer, the individual resumes ordinary activity. Chronic episodes also hide behind acute episodes of sickness in any reconstruction based on diagnosis, and acute diseases hide behind chronic. A division at eight, 13, or 26 weeks is meaningful when the issues that prompt it refer to function rather than diagnosis. For other purposes, however, it is more helpful to categorize diagnoses, and that is the approach usually taken in twentieth-century health surveys.

Both the onset and the resolution of sickness are often ambiguous events. Everyone is familiar with the often inchoate origins of many ill-health episodes and with the subjective elements involved in deciding when to resume ordinary activities after sickness. These ambiguities trouble all measurements of sickness time. In the friendly societies they were handled in a certain way. Sickness began at the conclusion of a waiting period during or after which the individual consulted a physician or was visited by an officer of the society (or both). From the society's perspective, the purpose of consultation and visitation was to determine whether the episode warranted compensation. Sickness ended when, during a process of regular consultations or visitations, the member was judged to be able to resume work or, in most cases, when the individual resumed work of his own accord and notified the society. From this procedure it is apparent that friendly society records would not include episodes or periods of sickness lasting less than the waiting period, which was usually three days to one week long, and that they also would not include episodes lasting after the resumption of ordinary activities except in those cases in which the individual once again entered a claim. The missing information is important, for brief episodes are the most common. The important point, however, is the consistent exclusion of those episodes in the insurance records, and their inclusion in most twentieth-century health surveys. The risk of acute sickness declines as age rises, and the risk of chronic sickness rises with age. [31] As a force influencing the risk of being sick, aging slows down the pace at which sickness episodes are resolved and exposes the individual to a changing group of disorders. In young adulthood, sicknesses are resolved more quickly: they tend to be acute disorders, and young adults have stronger powers of recuperation. At advanced ages, sicknesses are resolved more slowly: they tend to be chronic disorders, and older people have more limited powers of recuperation.

These characteristics appear in a clear way in the experience of the Odd Fellows during 1893–97. [32] Figure 3.5 divides sick time into five durations – weeks 1–13, 14–26, 27–52, 53–104, and 105–260 – for alternate quinary age groups from ages 20–24 to 80–84. [33] Considering the extremes, at ages 20–24, 80 per cent of all sick time occurred within weeks 1–13 and only 2 per cent within weeks 105–260, [34] but at ages 80–84, the proportions were reversed: 5 per cent of sick time fell within weeks 1–13 and 76 per cent within weeks 105–260. From these distributions, we can infer that at young adult ages the leading risk consisted of the risk of being sick for a short time, that at advanced ages the leading risk consisted of protracted sicknesses, and that the two types of risk were approximately equal at ages 55–59. For younger age groups, sick time was concentrated in the shortest term because recoveries were concentrated in that term, while for higher age groups sick time was concentrated in the longest term because recovery was slower and less frequent. That is, recovery was also a function of age in this late-nineteenth-century population.

The risk of being sick for intermediate terms was much smaller for all ages than the risk identified with the leading term at each age, and it shifted from one quinary age group to the next within narrow boundaries. Although these intermediate terms together account for 35 per cent of the time covered in a five-year survey, they did not at any age account for 35 per cent of claims. The two leading terms, weeks 1–13 and 105–260, together account for 65 per cent of the time covered, and more than 65 per cent of sick time at all ages.

Sutton's report on 1876–80 subdivides claims lasting thirteen weeks or less into three categories, weeks 1–4, 5–8, and 9–13. [35] Table 3.1 shows the proportional distribution of claims in these terms and in term 105–260. [36] In this population, too, sicknesses were concentrated in extreme terms, and within the shortest term, 1–13 weeks, they were concentrated in weeks 1–4 for all ages. To appearances, sicknesses tend to be brief or protracted.

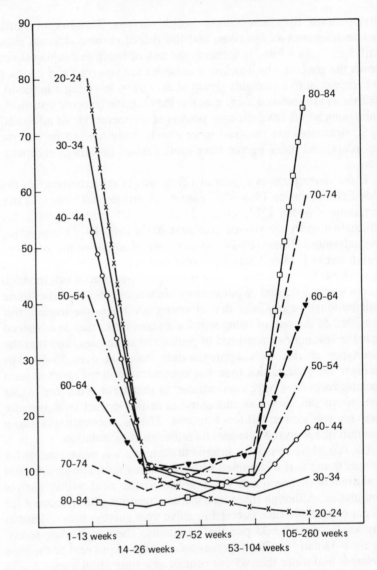

FIGURE 3.5 *Durations of sick time*

SOURCE Watson, *Manchester Unity*, pp. 19 and 138–41.

TABLE 3.1 *Proportions of sick time in extreme terms*

Age	Weeks 1–4	5–8	9–13	105–260
20–24	56.7	14.3	7.9	3.8
25–29	53.7	14.2	8.1	5.3
30–34	48.8	13.8	8.1	9.2
35–39	43.8	13.6	8.2	12.6
40–44	40.4	13.5	8.3	15.2
45–49	35.9	12.7	8.0	19.1
50–54	31.3	12.1	8.0	21.4
55–59	24.9	10.9	7.7	27.7
60–64	19.0	9.2	7.0	33.9
65–69	12.9	6.9	5.7	42.2
70–74	8.5	5.1	4.4	52.4
75–79	5.4	3.5	3.3	63.1
80–84	3.2	2.2	2.1	71.6

SOURCE   Sutton, *Special Report*, 1134–51.

Another way to show that episodes of sickness become more protracted as age rises is to examine the age-specific duration of sickness claims among only those members who entered claims. Table 3.1 was constructed by dividing the total number of weeks of sickness by the number of years at risk at each age, thereby giving values for the risk of being sick within the total population at each age. For this purpose, attention shifts to measures calculated by dividing the number of weeks of sickness by the number of individuals entering claims. Table 3.2 shows average durations for two populations, Foresters in 1871–75 and individuals included in Sutton's 1876–80 survey. Each pair of figures is similar, and these average durations increase with age in the expected way. It is also noteworthy that the pace of increase in the average duration of sickness episodes quickened appreciably after ages 60–64.

Recovery or Death

Sickness episodes have two possible outcomes, recovery or death. The two possibilities are common to all historical periods, but the distribution between the two has changed over time. In historical populations with a high mortality rate that are also especially prone to suffer acute diseases with high case fatality rates, such as seventeenth-century Europe, the outcome of many ill-health episodes will be quick and the number of deaths will take a prominent

TABLE 3.2   *Duration of sickness by age (in weeks per claimant)*

Age	Foresters 1871–75	Some registered societies 1876–80
20–24	3.6	3.8
25–29	4.0	4.1
30–34	4.5	4.6
35–39	5.2	5.3
40–44	5.9	6.0
45–49	6.8	6.9
50–54	8.4	8.2
55–59	10.9	10.5
60–64	13.5	13.6
65–69	18.4	18.6
70–74	22.9	24.6
75–79	29.4	30.3

SOURCES   Neison, *Foresters*, p. 40; and Sutton, *Special Report*, 1134–51.

place beside the number of recoveries. For most age groups, the risk of being sick will be comparatively low because of the shorter average duration of these episodes. In contrast, a population with a low death rate and more chronic than acute diseases, such as late nineteenth-century Britain, will face a higher risk of being sick. Even though the case fatality rate of its chronic diseases may be as high or higher than the case fatality rate of acute diseases suffered in the other population, its diseases will be resolved much more slowly. Some individuals who entered a survey period with protracted sickness, or who became sick during the survey, will not have died until after the survey concluded. At the same time, the survey would include the deaths of individuals who fell sick earlier.

Among members of British friendly societies, episodes resolved in death lasted significantly longer at all ages than those resolved in recovery or those lasting through the survey period. This character-istic, which is shown in Table 3.3, is partly an effect of the way in which age influences sickness durations and partly an effect related to the mixture of disorders suffered by these particular populations. In Table 3.3, Foresters from 1871 to 1875 are divided into two groups, those whose sicknesses ended in recovery or lasted throughout the survey period, and those whose sicknesses ended in death. Average durations are given for each age group, and the two columns may be

TABLE 3.3   *Sickness durations divided by outcome (in weeks per claimant)*

Age	Sicknesses resolved in recovery (1)	Sicknesses resolved in death (2)
20–24	3.3	10.0
25–29	3.6	11.0
30–34	4.0	11.3
35–39	4.6	11.5
40–44	5.2	12.1
45–49	6.1	12.6
50–54	7.5	14.3
55–59	10.0	15.0
60–64	12.1	18.8
65–69	17.5	20.7
70–74	22.1	24.8
75–79	31.1	26.9

SOURCE   Neison, *Foresters*, pp. 82–5.

compared to the Foresters column in Table 3.2, which gives the average duration of sickness in both groups together at each age.

Even though the group of Foresters who died within the survey period includes some individuals who died suddenly, or who died from illnesses and injuries not lasting longer than the waiting period,[37] it is at once apparent from Table 3.3 that death in this population was usually associated with extended sickness. Although the average duration of episodes rose in both groups with age, the pace of increase was markedly higher among those who recovered or remained sick. In that group, the average duration of sickness episodes was more than nine times greater at ages 75–79 than at ages 20–24, but among those dying this ratio was only 2.7:1. Among members who recovered or remained sick, episodes lasted one-third as long at ages 20–24 than among members who died, but the more rapid increase of these durations continued to the point at which, at ages 75–79, those who recovered experienced longer average sicknesses than those who died. That is, the risk of dying while sick was closely associated with the duration of sickness in lower age groups, but at higher ages each episode was, on average, as likely to result in death as in recovery or continued sickness. Even though column 1 in Table 3.3 includes a number of individuals with long-lasting or permanent disabilities, such as lost or broken limbs, blindness, lunacy, paralysis, and rheumatism,[38] these durations are much shorter than those in column 2. Another survey, by Francis G.P. Neison, Sr, which deals with members of Scottish friendly societies from 1831 to 1842, distinguished sicknesses immediately preceding death from other episodes among the segment of members dying.[39] It showed that sicknesses immediately preceding deaths were also longer at most ages than prior sicknesses.

Several inferences follow from these observations. Extended sickness – the failure to recover – sharply increased the risk of death in about the first half of adulthood. Longer sicknesses, taking all illnesses and injuries together, undermined the individual's capacity to survive, and deaths were associated with both the duration of an episode and with age. That is, among young adult males in nineteenth-century Britain belonging to friendly societies, death was dominated not by acute disorders with high case fatality rates, but by chronic disorders. Those who were sick fell into two distinct groups. This division is likely to be a function of the disorders suffered, a matter we are unable to explore because the friendly society surveys include so little diagnostic information. It is also likely to be a function of the health status that members who died carried into their terminal sicknesses.

Lifelong Experience

Every life is a story of states of health, good and ill, ending sooner or later in death. The sickness rate characterizing a certain population is an expression of time spent in each state, and can therefore be used to infer experience over a hypothetical adulthood lived entirely within a survey period. This is an artificial construction because friendly society members in each survey belonged to a number of different birth cohorts, each with a distinctive mortality and morbidity experience. Considering sickness in this way is akin to investigating mortality in a period rather than a cohort life table. This is the same approach used earlier in this chapter; the difference is that here quantities will be presented for each quinary age group and they will also be considered collectively.

Table 3.4 draws on Neison's survey of Foresters experience during 1871–75 to derive proportions of sick time and health time.[40] It shows the degree to which health time exceeded sick time at all ages, and most especially at ages 20–24 to 60–64. Even at 80–84, at which point

TABLE 3.4   *Sick time and health time among Foresters*

Age	Sick time	Health time	Age	Sick time	Health time
20–24	1.6%	98.4%	55–59	6.2	93.8
25–29	1.6	98.4	60–64	8.8	91.2
30–34	1.9	98.1	65–69	15.3	84.7
35–39	2.2	97.8	70–74	23.0	77.0
40–44	2.6	97.4	75–79	33.8	66.2
45–49	3.3	96.7	80–84	40.1	59.9
50–54	4.3	95.7			

SOURCE   Calculated from Neison, *Foresters*, p. 43.

Foresters included some individuals still working regularly, some working occasionally, and some incapacitated for work and drawing continuous benefits, nearly 60 per cent of the members' time was available for work.[41] Over this hypothetical adult life, sick time accumulated to a total of 377.5 weeks, or 7.2 years within 65 years at risk. That is, about 89 per cent of this portion of the hypothetical average member's adult life was spent in a state of capacity for work and about 11 per cent in a state of incapacity. This table also shows that the percentage of health time dropped gradually from one quinary age group to the next between 20–24 and 60–64, and then dropped sharply. Through ages 60–64 this hypothetical life accumulated 84.7 weeks (1.6 years) of sick time, an amount equal to 3.6 per cent of time at risk. But from 65–69 to 80–84 ill-health time jumped to 28 per cent of time at risk. Sick time between 60 and 69 surpassed the total accumulated from 20 to 59, and sick time between 70 and 79 surpassed the total from 20 to 69.

The figures in this table, which are similar to experience in other friendly societies,[42] help explain both the subsequent rise of a practice of involuntary retirement, in which the retirement age was fixed at some point between age 60 and 70, and a suggestion from the actuaries that sickness benefits might be transformed into a pension at some point between these ages. The actuaries recognized that the risk of being sick increased so rapidly after ages 60–64 that reduced benefits might be distributed to the entire membership living beyond age 64. Although this suggestion appears repeatedly in the actuarial literature, it was not adopted in most British friendly societies until the end of the nineteenth century. Friendly society members resisted, apparently because they believed they remained able to work. They

understood that a pension given all members after a certain age
would either have to be inadequate to meet living costs without
additional income or, if paid at a higher level, would have to be
funded by increased premiums at lower ages.

Table 3.4 can also be seen as a basis for re-examining the issue of
changes over time in the span of the working life and the aggregate
quantity of time available for work. In present-day populations,
incapacity for work is associated with the age of involuntary retirement, often 65, and the portion of the population consisting of
dependents is measured by comparing the number of individuals too
young to work and those past retirement age to those of working
ages. The idea of involuntary retirement is chiefly a twentieth
century concept, at least in its application, as is also the notion that
working life may be held to begin toward the end of physical development, at about age 20. From an historical perspective, dependency is
a more complex phenomenon, in that ages of entry into and exit from
work, the proportion of the population living at all ages, and perhaps
also the proportion of those at working ages who were able to work
have changed over time. These changes influence the dependency
ratio and judgments about optimal ages for entry into and retirement
from the workforce, and they influence the way in which dependency
is measured. Just as the passage from a high to a low mortality regime
extends the average length of working lives, the passage from a high
to a low morbidity regime may significantly affect the quantity of time
available for work.

Heterogeneity

The curve of health time sketched in Table 3.4 averages experience
with being sick, a phenomenon subject to substantial variation in
individual cases. This variation is also apparent when we consider
data presented earlier about the risk of falling sick. From Figure 3.2
we see that one-quarter or fewer Foresters fell sick at each age from
19 to 47. Some of those episodes represented more than one claim
entered within the survey period by the same individual. The data do
not show whether the individuals entering claims in one period
represent a random distribution of all members or a distribution
influenced by prior sicknesses. The actuarial reports deal only in
aggregates, but it is possible to learn something about the scale of
variation by considering the records of a small independent friendly
society, the Guild of St George, located in Carrington (Cheshire)

TABLE 3.5 *Sickness as a proportion of time at risk (by age)*

Case	–19	20–29	30–39	40–49	50–59	60–69	70–79	Aggregate
M.A.M.B.	1.3	9.3	8.3	13.8	11.2	6.9	60.9	16.5
(female, joined 1883 at age 16, died 1945 at age 78)								
J.E.A.	0	2.4	4.9	5.1	3.8	20.2		6.6
(male, joined 1883 at age 15, died 1937 at age 69)								
A.H.	0	1.2	1.4	0.3	0.4	0	0.6	0.6
(female, joined 1881 at age 18, died 1943 at age 79)								
J.T.	1.3	1.0	1.9	0.7	1.2	1.5	0	1.2
(male, joined 1891 at age 16, died 1945 at age 70)								

SOURCE Cheshire Record Office, Chester, DDX 186.

England), near Chester. Members of the Guild of St George come under observation in 1873, when the roll contained 53 men and 102 women, and the records extend to 1946 (lacking information for 1885 only).[43] The cases selected for Table 3.5 deal with individuals who joined in 1873 or soon thereafter, at ages ranging from 14 to 20, and who remained members until their deaths. No member survived beyond age 79, and these cases represent the longest-lived members.

Even with this small body of experience, it is immediately apparent that aggregate averages of sick time and health time conceal noteworthy variations in individual experience. Consider the four individuals whose histories are summarized in Table 3.5. Each is an exception chosen for his or her representation of extreme experience, one male and one female member who lived long lives but with comparatively high proportions of those lives spent in sickness versus two other members who also lived long lives but with negligible amounts of sick time. The extreme cases serve as an antidote to all the other characterizations given in this chapter, which are based on aggregate averages. They suggest why many friendly society members aged 60–64 or more expected to continue to work. Sickness benefits constituted only a fraction of wages ordinarily earned, and, for protracted claims, all major friendlies reduced the benefit level to half or less. Even from 80 to 84, and certainly at lower ages, the time available for work provided the possibility of higher income, although to work at age 80 may have meant changing jobs or tasks.

Considering Table 3.4 in terms of the risks of being and falling sick, given in Figure 3.2 for Foresters, it is apparent that the increase of sick time from 20–24 to 80–84 was due chiefly to a rising likelihood of being sick rather than to a rising likelihood of falling sick. From ages

20–24 to 80–84, the risk of falling sick increased 2.7 times, but the proportion of sick time increased 25 times. At ages 60–64, health remained a prevailing expectation that all members might share, an expectation that would prevail all the more strongly among members who had experienced little ill-health time to ages 60–64. The sick-time distributions of Table 3.4 combine the experience of members dying and members surviving the survey period, 1871–75. Part of sick time to ages 60–64 had been accumulated by members who died. Among survivors to age 60–64, therefore, the figures in that table overstate actual proportions of sick time. The proportions also include the experience of individuals in ill health throughout the survey period, which further overstate sick time experienced by most members. And the few individual cases selected from the Guild of St George alert us to the likelihood that many members at ages 60–64 will have had little or no experience with sickness in the way in which the friendly societies distinguished it from health. That is, Foresters aged 60–64 are likely to have consisted of two groups, one made up of (or distributed toward) individuals already in ill health or with a considerable claims record and therefore with a reasonable expectation of future sickness, the other of individuals with little or no prior claims experience and therefore with a reasonable expectation of future health. The specification of an age of involuntary retirement between 60 and 70, which in Britain began in the decade after the last friendly society survey, may have faithfully reflected age-related shifts in average sick and health time. But those averages may be derived by combining experience from two distinct modal groups one prone to sickness and the other not.[44] This possibility is but one illustration of the degree to which the forms and modes of sickness as considered in this chapter, reveal aggregate averages but conceal a substantial and significant amount of variation from those averages

CONCLUSION

To approach ill health as a matter of functional incapacity is to see ways in which a fresh body of historical sources can be brought to bear. Like modern health surveys, these records identify the size of a population at risk to ill health and the time at risk. In a way seldom possible with other historical sources, they provide measures of the incidence of sickness. To call upon these sources is also to reorien the measurement of health experience in two important ways. First sick fund records distinguish a realm of ill health from a realm of health by identifying a threshold consisting of the point at which people participating in the labor force lose the capacity to engage in one of the fundamental activities of human experience, work. This mode of discrimination seldom coincides with explanations of the cause of ill health, both because diagnostic data are usually wanting in the sick fund records and because diagnosed disorders will occur in both realms even though they congregate in the ill-health realm. Second, these sources evaluate the severity of ill health in another way than do more familiar sources, which report death by cause and which sometimes also provide totals of diagnosed diseases. In the diagnostic approach, the severity of an ill-health episode is usually graded according to the likelihood that it will result in death, although this assessment is often implicit. Diseases are deemed especially important when they are identified with high case fatality rates. In the functional approach, severity can be graded according to either the risk of being sick, which measures the amount of ill-health time as a proportion of the time at risk, or the risk of falling sick, which measures the probability that the threshold will be passed. Sicknesses are held to be important whenever they threaten a substantial portion of the population at risk or whenever time spent in sickness constitutes a significant portion of time at risk. In the realm of function, too, risk can be distinguished in a manner analogous to case fatality rates. Among the Odd Fellows and the Foresters, the sickness that was likelier to be resolved in death rather than recovery was, for most ages, the protracted episode. Long sicknesses compromised vitality more seriously.

Like mortality, the risk of sickness is influenced more by age than by any of the plentitude of other factors that play some role in determining the level and trend that will prevail in a given population. Unlike mortality, the morbidity risk is not unitary. It retains an underlying similarity to the mortality risk, but the degree of analogy between the two depends on the form of morbidity singled out for investigation. Here attention has been drawn to two versions of functional incapacity: the risk of being sick, which is a measure of the duration of sickness episodes or the amount of sickness time accumulated within a period of time, and the risk of falling sick, which is equivalent to the epidemiologist's concept of disease incidence.[45] These two sickness risks vary – they move up or down the schedule – between any two populations, but each preserves a basic form. At least in the populations so far considered, the age distribution of the risk of being sick closely resembles the age distribution of the risk of death. In nineteenth-century working populations the association between sickness and age expressed itself in much the same way in the duration of illnesses as in the risk of death. In contrast, the risk of falling sick described a much flatter curve, bending the sides of the misshapen W downward.

Although it is generally appropriate to say that morbidity and mortality risks are especially high early and late in life, intervening risks do not take the simple form of a U curve. Instead, they move sharply upward in late adolescence, forcing the U into a W, and suggesting age-associated changes in risk during adolescence and early adulthood. Observers have explained the interim peak in the mortality risk around age 20 by different means at different times, but the persistence of this peak across time and in radically different environmental circumstances suggests the operation of biological as well as environmental forces.

Another regularity in the series consulted consists of the tendency of females to suffer longer sicknesses than males but fewer sickness episodes. Because, in modern times, women have consistently en joyed longer life expectancies than men, the sex differential in sickness experience seems to provide one way to pursue the issue of how sickness experience influences the timing of death and the likelihood of future sickness. If women accumulate serious insults at a slower pace, a possibility suggested by the lower female than male rates of work incapacitation, then higher female life expectancy might be attributed to a lower index of cumulative health problems. The data presented here are also consistent with an interpretation in which women convalesce more deliberately, perhaps repairing the insults they do suffer more completely.

We examine the life course as a series of episodes of health and ill health with the help of schedules of the duration and episode sickness risks that include reliable age-by-age information for the part of the life course extending from 18 or somewhat younger until 85. So far the data present themselves only in the form of experience within a few populations in the period of individual surveys, rather than the experience of successive cohorts recorded from birth or adolescence until old age and death. But the possibilities are apparent. We can formulate an expectation of health analogous to the life expectation based on mortality risks faced at each age, or, rather, we can formulate two expectations, one built on the risk of being sick and the other on the risk of falling sick. To follow even a few lives from

the Guild of St George is also to see that individual health experience, and eventually the experience of important historical groups,
can be reconstructed. Within the reconstruction lie opportunities to
discover how sickness experience earlier in life influences later health
and the timing of death.

Sickness risk as reconstructed from friendly society experience
provides a foundation for the examination of functional incapacity
and ill health in general across time, and for the comparison of
functional and diagnostic measures of ill health. The levels of morbidity found among Odd Fellows, Foresters, or other societies should
not be expected to apply to any other population but the friendly
society records furnish a scheme for comparison, comparison of
definition, of differentiation, and of experience.

4 Health and Sickness in Europe, 1600–1870

La mort ne pourra être appréhendée de
manière satisfaisante que par l'étude
globale de la morbidité.[1]
[Death can only be satisfactorily
understood by the comprehensive
study of morbidity.]

The history of mortality in Europe from 1600 to 1870 can be told as a
story of descent on an uneven slope. This era opened with crude
mortality rates ranging between about 25 and 40 per 1000 per year,
clustering at or above 30, in the regions so far studied. Between the
middle of the seventeenth and the middle of the eighteenth century it
is possible to detect signs of lower death rates, but the signs of decline
do not become especially strong until the 1740s. For some sixty to
eighty years thereafter, until about 1820, the descent was sharp and
the crude death rate fell to about 20 per 1000 per annum. The decline
ceased in the 1820s and did not begin again until the 1870s. Crude
mortality rates are only an approximate guide, but they identify three
broad mortality regimes: high, until about 1740; intermediate, circa
1740 to about 1870; and low, since about 1870.

Each stage of this passage is difficult to explain, but there is
considerable agreement on three points. The 1650–1750 retreat
should be attributed chiefly to a diminishing risk of death from
epidemic disease; the plateau of 1820–70 should be attributed to the
growth of cities and the breakdown of urban amenities (so that a
trend decline persisted but was matched by increases due to urban
filth and urban growth); and the early stages of the decline after 1870
should be explained chiefly by public health remedies applied in
cities. These are modest achievements toward understanding, and
even they constitute incomplete explanations. If the death rate declined between 1650 and 1820 chiefly because deaths in epidemics
occurred less frequently, why did such deaths occur less frequently?
In this chapter the purpose is not to answer such questions, but to
reformulate them in the way they must be posed if we are to see
death as an outcome of illness. This purpose draws our attention to
certain features of Europe's experience with death and the transitions

in this long history of declining death rates. The key features are two: the reign of infectious disease epidemics, and the way in which specific diseases cause lasting damage.

THE MORTALITY REGIME

Epidemics

Although vast, usually qualitative, and often difficult to interpret, the evidence about epidemics nevertheless shows that their frequency and intensity declined in Europe after the fourteenth century, the century of plague. This evidence unfortunately appears in forms that make it difficult to measure the pace of change. Studying sample locales in Italy, Del Panta and Livi Bacci report that, in the fifteenth and first half of the sixteenth century, mortality crises occurred at about one-half the intensity of the fourteenth century, in which the plague had reappeared. The decline continued after 1550. Counting as crises those years in which the number of deaths exceeded the average of surrounding years by 50 per cent, Livi Bacci provides the scale that follows.[2]

1580–1699	49 crises per 1000 years at risk
1700–1799	27
1800–1859	52

Until the nineteenth century, mortality crises – all of which were related to epidemic disease even though their causes sometimes included warfare and crop failure[3] – declined in part because they were to an increasing degree contained in the region affected, in part because later epidemics were milder, and in part because epidemics occurred less frequently. The increased frequency and intensity of epidemics from 1800 to 1860 gave way to a still lower incidence of crises from 1870 to 1909, the last period studied.

A similar pattern obtained in England. Counting crisis months rather than years and using a different technique to distinguish crisis from normal periods, Wrigley and Schofield report the scheme that follows.[4]

1550–74	14.6 crisis months per 1000
1575–99	13.4

1600–24	12.6
1625–49	12.9
1650–74	10.8
1675–99	10.0
1700–24	10.4
1725–49	16.2
1750–74	9.8
1775–99	9.2
1800–24	6.0

In the decennial version of these data, Wrigley and Schofield also report an increase from 1810–19 to 1830–8, at which point the series ends.

Although the regions studied for these chronologies – urban Italy and a sample of English parishes – may have been atypical of Europe, the scheme of decline captures what would be inferred about Western and Central Europe from other sources. With this scheme before us, it is easy to see that population growth should have been concentrated in the eighteenth century and after 1870, and that epidemics played a leading role in restraining growth before 1700 (especially before 1650 or 1660), during 1800–59 in Italy, and for some decades after 1830 in England. Considering only the mortality side, Europe's population grew in the long run especially because the hazards associated with epidemic disease diminished. The growth shows up in larger population figures and higher life expectancies.

In Geneva, too, mortality crises declined in frequency from the late sixteenth century into the nineteenth. This particular trend can be examined as it was experienced in three age groups – people dying at ages 0–14, 15–59, and 60 and above – in Figure 4.1.[5] This figure, which gives measures of variance rather than death rates, shows that decline in the frequency of crises should be considered in terms of age. Among Genevans aged 60 and above the variance declined slightly from early in the seventeenth century and the coefficients of variation fluctuated little. Decade after decade Genevans of those ages died at rates falling close to the mean. In the age groups 0–14 and 15–59, in contrast, the coefficients fluctuated further into the seventeenth century. Among Genevans dying at ages 15–59, the last major fluctuation occurred in the 1630s, but among people dying at ages 0–14, it came only in the 1680s. Different age groups became less susceptible to the sharply demarcated mortality crises of the sixteenth and early seventeenth centuries at different times. In this way, the

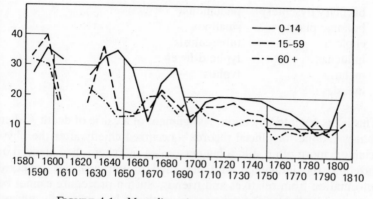

FIGURE 4.1   *Mortality crises in Geneva, 1585–1805*

SOURCE   Alfred Perrenoud, *La population de Genève du seizième au début du dix-neuvième siècle: Etude démographique* (Geneva, 1979), p. 424.

age pattern of deaths in Geneva is suggestive about changes in the profile of leading diseases and, specifically, about the disappearance of plague after 1640. As the profile of disease risks shifted, so too did the age distribution of infection and death.

The Reign of Infectious Disease

Infectious agents remained the characteristic causes of death and probably also of illness in Europe between 1600 and 1870. Thousands of agents are infectious for humans, for the term applies to all environmental organisms that can multiply in or on a host and produce a response. To these must be added an unknown number of diseases associated with congenital, toxic, degenerative, metabolic, neoplastic, and other causes. Twentieth-century lists of diseases are longer than their eighteenth-century counterparts, such as the more than 6000 given by the physician Jean Razoux in 1767.[6] Some diseases have probably emerged since then, and others have disappeared. But the wisest assumption seems to be that the two profiles largely overlap. The profile of diseases actually experienced has changed far more than the profile of diseases that might be contracted without public health, immunological, and chemical prophylaxes.

The leading causes of death, a comparatively short list, remain the best-known diseases of the high and intermediate mortality regimes.[7] They were:

bacillary dysentery	pneumonia
bubonic plague	smallpox
cholera	tuberculosis
influenza	typhoid fever
malaria	typhus
measles	

This list is open to objection. Assignment of a cause of death – when that was done for official records – occurred chiefly after the physician or, more often still, a lay person – a searcher – had glanced or gazed at the individual who had died or perhaps also collected information from relatives and friends. Such a procedure cannot be considered reliable. The cause(s) of death can be profoundly difficult to specify under the best of conditions. A 1977 survey in England and Wales showed that clinical opinion differed from autopsy findings half of the time.[8] In an age in which autopsies were uncommon, as they were until the nineteenth century, it would be absurd to suggest that the searchers identified the cause of death correctly by noticing some external signs after death, or even by the most diligent inquiries among people who had witnessed the sickness and the death.

Nevertheless, it is often claimed that these diseases are now and must then have been so obvious in external signs that, even if we have to admit the likelihood of confusion among them, we should expect them to have been readily distinguished from other possible causes. This, too, is an untenable position. The searchers, and the friends and relatives of the dead from whom they drew most information, noticed chiefly external signs of disease now understood as part of the acute phase response. Only four diseases on this list (cholera, dysentery, influenza, and pneumonia) are not associated with cutaneous lesions, usually macules (which are small, discolored spots), papules (which are raised macules), or maculopapules. Historians sometimes say that these lesions are specific to each disease and identifiable even to untrained observers, and they use that argument to justify a study of mortality from one listed cause over time. Even in well-marked diseases, however, diagnoses remain uncertain. Some victims do not display lesions, and others do not display them in the classic form. To take only one example, typhoid fever is described in a modern text as being difficult to distinguish (without isolation of *Salmonella typhi*) from other salmonella infections, pneumonia, tuberculosis, malaria, murine typhus fever, acute bacterial bronchitis, and several other diseases.[9] Should we suppose that identification was easier in the eighteenth century, when typhoid was neither generally distinguished from typhus in medical tracts nor conceivably to be isolated by its microorganism?

What is more, even the presence on a person's body of lesions in a classic and distinctive form, one that cannot be attributed to insect bites or other causes, is not sufficient to show that the disease causing those lesions was the cause of death. Given the frequency with which death was ascribed to diseases usually associated with lesions, we must suspect that there were many instances in which people suffered multiple illnesses but were recorded under only the one of them associated with skin lesions. More troublesome still is the concentration of causes in a relatively short list of diseases mostly causing skin lesions and having high case fatality rates, and the comparatively infrequent mention of other infectious diseases, even some we know are associated with high case fatality rates when untreated or treated by ineffectual means and suspected of having been prevalent in early modern Europe. That is, the list given above identifies some of the leading causes of death but it is certainly incomplete, and it is incomplete especially in two areas: diseases (infectious and non-infectious) not associated with skin lesions but capable of causing death in a significant number of cases, and diseases not associated with death or associated with death only through complications.

To test the diagnoses of the searchers or even those of medical experts is at the moment impossible. Early modern diagnoses cannot simply be translated or transcribed into modern terms, not only because diseases were described in the seventeenth and eighteenth centuries in imprecise ways. Even when reputedly excellent clinical records survive about individual cases or epidemics, modern medical authorities and historians often find themselves unable to agree on a diagnosis.[10] Nor have there yet been extensive studies of the physical remains of people who died then. Analyses of skeletal remains of paleolithic people suggest the presence of certain diseases – tuberculosis and syphilis are good examples. But that is not an important issue regarding cause of death in the seventeenth and eighteenth centuries. Tuberculosis, syphilis, and some other diseases that also leave skeletal damage are already known to have occurred then. The issues are the entire profile of disease and the relative intensity of diseases as causes of illness and death. Diagnosis at these levels requires access to tissue and fluids.

The apparently insurmountable difficulty of arriving at reliable diagnoses of even the leading illnesses causing death during the period 1600–1870 has prompted a number of other approaches in historical epidemiology. Ann Carmichael suggests that multiple conditions and secondary infections played a large role in deaths, a circumstance recognized in a de facto way by physicians who wrote about disease continuums as well as about discrete infections. From this perspective, the decline in the death rate at certain times implies a declining incidence of concurrent infections and perhaps also of complications. Some excess mortality – that is, some increase in deaths from other causes – continues to be observed in influenza epidemics, but Carmichael's idea is that this component of mortality declined because large-scale epidemics became less frequent and perhaps also because those that did occur involved fewer secondary infections.[11] Such a pattern might be observed in communities that began to isolate sick individuals or to quarantine sickly regions, and perhaps also where public health reforms such as drainage and lavation curtailed the population of insect vectors transmitting common diseases.

Clinical and biostatistical enquiries point up such antagonisms between diseases as Raymond Pearl's classic demonstration that cancers are less common in individuals with active tuberculosis. Mirko Grmek maintains that a history of sickness can be fashioned by observing the *pathocénose*, the profile of pathogenic states, which is shaped by antagonisms and affinities among diseases as well as by other forces. René Dubos argued that the mortality decline could be attributed to adaptation between pathogens and their hosts, a process that produces lower case fatality rates as unfamiliar diseases (e.g., the plague in 1348–50) become familiar, and that adaptation may also alter the age prevalence of some diseases (as it did of cholera). At the individual level, the relationship between host and pathogen is often antagonistic and results in a clinical manifestation of disease. But at the population level, the relationship must be symbiotic in order that both species survive. The host and the pathogen adapt to one another, though at the vastly different paces allowed by reproduction among microorganisms versus that among humans. They may also manifest changes that temporarily exacerbate the antagonism between them. For example, some microorganisms are unstable and are known to undergo changes that make them suddenly more virulent or less virulent. Such mutations have been proposed as a better way to account for specific episodes in the comparatively short time span of European mortality experience than the far more deliberate pace of

human mutation and adaptation. In theory, at least, microbial mutations might explain instances in which death rates rose or fell sharply
but for which no other reasons are known or seem plausible. And
they might also explain the long-run trend decline, in which case it
must be concluded that the mutations were skewed only toward those
mutations diminishing microbial virulence. Another possibility of
adaptation lies in some change in average levels of human resistance
to disease, such as might occur if a badly nourished population began
to eat more food or a sporadically malnourished population began to
eat regularly. Each of these interpretations offers a way to account
for the mortality decline of the eighteenth century, but the available
evidence is inadequate to permit a definitive choice among them.[12]

A WORLD OF TEN DISEASES

I wish to pursue another line of discussion that identifies a profile of
some leading causes of death and illness in order to examine ways in
which diseases in that profile shaped the experience of sickness. In
this approach, attention may be diverted from the effort to verify or
correct diagnoses given at the time or to fill out the list to include
especially causes not associated with cutaneous lesions. It can focus
instead on what might be called the vital statistics of illness: case
fatality rate, age prevalence, fatality curve, and clinical course.

Imagine a world in which only ten diseases occur. These ten would
include seven from the list of leading causes of death from 1600 to
1850 given above – bacillary dysentery, cholera, influenza, plague,
smallpox, typhoid fever, and tuberculosis – and three that might be
added to the list if, on the one hand, we knew more about illnesses
not resolved in death, and, on the other hand, we knew more about
deaths misdiagnosed because of the rarity of autopsy: the skin fungus
sporotrichosis, the round worm infection ascariasis, and atherosclerosis.[13] The first seven have already been identified as common diseases in Europe in at least some part of the period 1600–1850. The
latter three were more rarely and less conclusively identified in that
period but are diseases especially likely to have caused considerable
illness. The ten diseases are not intended to be representative or to
constitute the disease profile of any period. They have been chosen
because they will help illustrate certain points and because they are
not unrepresentative of diseases from that era.[14]

Nine of these diseases are infectious. The tenth, atherosclerosis, is a cardiovascular disease first linked persuasively to myocardial damage in nineteenth-century autopsies but described in earlier sources (such as Giovanni Lancisi). It increased dramatically as a cause of death late in the nineteenth and early in the twentieth century because it was more often recognized, a larger proportion of the population began to die at ages at which atherosclerosis is well developed, additional risk factors had developed, and perhaps also because the portion of the population whose diet and behavior made them significantly more susceptible had grown. Atherosclerotic plaque builds up beginning early in life, reduces blood flow, and may break off into clots, causing sudden death. Each of the ten diseases is distinctive in its vital statistics, as Figure 4.2 indicates by reporting case fatality rate, age prevalence, fatality curve, and clinical course.

If we put this information together with what is known or can plausibly be assumed about the chronology of these diseases, we begin to see more characteristics of the age of infectious disease. The major points of that chronology are two. First, in Europe plague was limited to the period up to about 1670 (occasional epidemics thereafter notwithstanding) and cholera to the period from 1830. Second, in the threat posed to health and life, some of these diseases waxed and waned in long cycles (smallpox, typhoid fever), influenza was probably recurrent in a two to three-year cycle, and the others probably remained persistent threats.

The data base remains incomplete. It does not, for example mention prevalence according to sex, income, way of life, nutrition geography, or climate – all important factors. But it is already complex enough to show that the single constant of this part of the era of infectious disease was the inconstancy of the disease threat. The face of disease varied from generation to generation, so that each cohort confronted a unique combination of assaults. Deaths among the members of one cohort were caused by many of the same diseases that killed people in surrounding cohorts. But the relative importance of diseases shifted perpetually and, more important, the disease episodes accumulated by survivors shifted continually.

What will bring this home but is so far missing is a sense of the prevalence of these diseases within this hypothetical population facing only the ten diseases. Disease prevalence is notoriously difficult to estimate because, even in societies with many physicians and populations attuned to health issues, many cases of disease escape

Disease	Case fatality rate[a]	Age prevalence	Fatality curve[b]	Clinical course[a]
ascariasis	low[c]	1–13	not applicable	chronic
atherosclerosis	variable	35 and over, esp. 65 and over	variable	prolonged, with sudden resolution
bacillary dysentery	1–25%	1–4, adults	2–4 days	1 week
cholera	up to 50%	none[d]	a few hours to a few days	1 week
influenza (Type A)	0.5–7%[e]	5–14 and all ages	1 to several days	1 to 3 weeks
plague	up to 60%	10–29	1st and 3rd weeks	4 weeks or longer
smallpox (variola major)	10–50%	1–4	2nd week	3–4 weeks
sporotrichosis (a fungus disease)	very low	adults	not applicable	prolonged
tuberculosis (pulmonary)	difficult to estimate[g]	infants young adults	variable	prolonged
typhoid fever	c. 10% average[f]	under 30 esp. 15–25	a few days to 2 weeks	1–8 weeks

NOTES a. In untreated cases; b. i.e., peak period of deaths after onset of symptoms in untreated cases; c. except with complications; d. in populations previously uninvolved with cholera; e. based on 1918–19 epidemic only; f. as of the early twentieth century; probably higher previously; g. many cases go undiagnosed or death occurs because of secondary infection

FIGURE 4.2   *A world of ten diseases*

SOURCES   See n. 14

notice. Some of the cases are subclinical and pass without disturbing the individual who experiences them. Subclinical episodes may nevertheless have deferred effects that are helpful (for instance, they confer immunity) or not (e.g., they cause tissue or immune system damage). Other cases are clinically manifest but are not called to the attention of medical authorities. In Europe between 1600 and 1800, the bulk of the population seldom obtained access to trained medical practitioners. The illnesses (and injuries) of those people escape our notice because the people themselves seldom saw physicians or entered hospitals, the major recorders. In some instances, prevalence can now be reconstructed by using the case fatality rate associated with a disease: if the smallpox case fatality rate among Genevans aged less than five years ranged between 10 and 17 per cent, 'then we can deduce that between 60 and 100 per cent of children were infected whenever there was a serious epidemic'.[15] But this technique can be applied only in a few instances.

Smallpox provides an example of prevalence at one extreme: its victims who survived acquired lifelong immunity, and most children acquired immunity. That is, smallpox was prevalent at ages 1–4 especially because that was an uninfected population without any acquired immunity and one no longer protected by antibodies provided by the mother, who had suffered smallpox in her own childhood and protected the infant until it began the weaning process around age one. Other diseases in the list of ten convey temporary immunity to certain strains or to the complex of related strains known under the name of the disease, some convey limited immunity, and some have no immune effect. In these diseases, the individual may fall ill when again exposed and may fall ill repeatedly over a lifetime. For example, the bacteria that cause bacillary dysentery and other shigelloses occur in several strains. Immunity following shigellosis seems to be specific to the strain and ineffective in poorly nourished people a year or more after the first episode.[16]

One way to compensate for the diverse nature of each disease is to apply what is known about prevalence in populations similar to those of Europe between 1600 and 1870. Such an application results in the information provided by Figure 4.3. The cumulative effect of this figure is a new awareness of how much of the population must have experienced and survived a long list of disease episodes. In this hypothetical world of ten diseases, an individual who was born toward the end of the seventeenth century and died 85 years later may have survived single episodes of five of these diseases (ascariasis, smallpox, sporotrichosis, typhoid fever, and tuberculosis), recurrent episodes of two (dysentery and influenza), and developed atherosclerosis secretly since childhood. The two diseases escaped – cholera and plague – do not appear because they were rare in the period specified.

To live in Europe between 1600 and 1870 was to face a series of vivid and recurrent disease risks. Although the feature most re-

ascariasis – general among young children, usually mild in effect except perhaps in untreated cases

atherosclerosis – prevalent in modern populations, developing progressively throughout life; perhaps also prevalent in earlier populations, although the pace of development in adulthood may have been slower

bacillary dysentery – general and recurrent among children and adults, with recurrence limited by temporary immunity to specific strains

cholera – general in affected areas but, despite the alarm caused by nineteenth-century epidemics, never prevalent throughout Europe

influenza – individual epidemics affect up to 40 per cent of a community and, since individuals may contract several strains and risk persists at all ages, individuals are likely to have several episodes over a long life

plague – the high case fatality rate suggests low prevalence except in sharply delimited places and periods, in which numerous deaths occurred

smallpox – so highly restricted in age incidence and so frequent in epidemic form before 1750 or so that it appears likely that most children living in towns, and cities experienced smallpox

sporotrichosis – prevalent among agricultural workers, among whom the fungus harbored in soil and vegetation entered through small wounds

tuberculosis – general in the adult population, though often in the form of inactive infection

typhoid fever – probably general among young adults

FIGURE 4.3   *Diseases and their prevalence*

SOURCES   See n. 14.

marked upon of this panorama of risks has been its intensity – the probability of dying in an epidemic – the most remarkable feature of it appears, in the formulation offered here, to be the probability of being ill repeatedly. Many people died in major epidemics, but even the diseases posing the gravest risks rarely carried off more than 10 per cent of individuals infected. If we examine those epidemics in terms of the time at risk – if, that is, we multiply the number of people in a community by the number of months in the years under observation, and divide the number of months in which epidemics of any kind prevailed by that product, and if we perform the same operations to derive an illness rate – a simple fact will at once be clear: epidemic mortality was much less frequent than illness, epidemic or not. Even in the age of infectious disease, illness was usually survived. This appears from our small world of ten diseases, which is skewed heavily toward diseases with high case fatality rates. It is all the more noticeable if we cast our mind's eye over the full range of diseases identifiable with the period from 1600 to 1870: rheumatism, arthritis, bronchitis, dental caries, ear infections, hepatitis, the common cold, bacterial meningitis, infected wounds, scabies, diabetes, pneumonia, cancer, scarlet fever, diphtheria . . .[17]

From this perspective – which is only the first perspective we shall take – the ordinary individual appears to have experienced both a continuing series of infectious diseases and the risk of concurrent infections. Up to half the individuals born failed to survive childhood, although this proportion began to decline during the seventeenth century and declined significantly during the eighteenth century. Epidemics caused fewer deaths, but it is not entirely clear whether this should be attributed especially to fewer epidemics or to milder epidemics. Did both the morbidity and the mortality rates shift as the rate of epidemics declined?

After childhood, the likelihood of death diminished rapidly, but the typical individual seems to have continued to suffer recurrent infections and other diseases. The rate of exposure – a factor linked especially to filth but also to other features of life – and the limited capacities of acquired immunity argue that disease was an ever-present threat, even if many episodes lasted for short periods. It is difficult to imagine this world in any other terms than the plentitude of its illnesses. And it is difficult to imagine it without drawing a parallel between health in economically underdeveloped regions in the present and health in underdeveloped Europe in the past. In the Third World, usually in locales with climates and population densities quite different from early modern Europe, health surveys report continuous exposure, high morbidity rates, and concurrent infections.[18]

Finally, Figure 4.2 shows that, in using sources that record sicknesses only if they last at least three to six days, as the sick fund records do, we will fail to detect many episodes of illness and injury and some episodes of disease ending quickly in death. Mild illnesses like ascariasis and sporotrichosis, many cases of tuberculosis and atherosclerosis, and subclinical infections in general escape notice because the people with those diseases did not always believe themselves sick enough to take time off from work. Other diseases in this list, especially bacillary dysentery but also some quickly resolved cases of influenza and typhoid fever, may have ended in recovery before the individual became eligible for benefits. And others, especially some cases of plague and cholera, will have resulted in death within the waiting period. They will appear in the sick fund records only as deaths, and they will appear as deaths that may, on the basis of vital statistics and in the absence of diagnoses, be attributed to injury or disease. In short, sickness will always have been more prevalent than any of the records at our disposal can be made to show.

THE LASTING EFFECTS OF DISEASE

Liselotte von der Pfalz – known as Madame – lived at the court of Louis XIV as the second wife and then widow of the king's brother, Philippe I d'Orléans, called Monsieur. An outsider – German – and, moreover, someone with a taste for satire and exaggeration, Madame wrote long letters and included in them physical descriptions of people at court. She expressed her taste for satire in a conventional manner, calling attention to physical deformities and damage. To Madame, Paul Pelisson-Fontanier, the Abbot of Gimont, seemed

an awful looking person, his face was all square from smallpox scars, white against a yellow background. His eyes were all rimmed with red, and there was something like wax in the corners and between the lids, on which he had no hair but only the raw flesh. His nose was broad, and the nostrils were wide open, also full of smallpox scars. His eyes were dripping continually, his mouth went from one ear to the other; [he had] rather heavy, altogether white lips, black teeth with many of them missing . . . He was quite monstrous, but most intelligent and very learned.

Madame herself survived smallpox in 1675, at the age of 23, and was also marked for life. She died in 1722 of a surgical wound from being bled and perhaps from other causes, too.[19]

As the historian Alfred Perrenoud noticed about Geneva, smallpox was at many times and in many places a disease that nearly every child suffered, although not always at a clinical level. The lasting signs of its presence were often seen and reported. So commonplace were facial scars that smallpox has become a metaphor for a population that bore, in many ways outwardly manifest, the lasting evidence of its diseases and injuries. Beggars, who congregated at churches and public squares and who opened the purses of passersby by the pity they evoked, often turned to deception to supplement whatever signs of disability they might honestly present. From such evidence, we obtain the impression of a people whose past experience with sickness and whose malformations were obvious.

This metaphor is not, however, especially apt to the idea that illnesses and injuries have lasting effects on later health. Smallpox scars bring to mind physical damage evident at a glance and, indeed, the damage smallpox may cause is chiefly external. It takes the form of healed lesions distributed on the face and from the mouth to the esophagus; lesions do not appear on internal organs unless smallpox is accompanied by a secondary infection. The external scars do not seem to be associated with lasting physical effects that make smallpox sufferers more prone to later illness or injury. The Abbot of Gimont may have suffered from the signs of his episode of smallpox for, even in an age in which such scars were common, he could still be described as 'monstrous'. But his suffering would have been emotional and will therefore be more difficult to verify retrospectively or to link to later ill health.

Evidence is needed about whether other illnesses and injuries of that era had lasting effects for physical health. Such evidence is extraordinarily difficult to obtain in a direct way from sources of the seventeenth and eighteenth centuries. In that age, the body was seldom probed for signs of disease, either while the illness was clinically active or after its course. Comparatively few people consulted trained physicians, who might have reported signs or symptoms suggestive about internal effects. When consulted, most physicians believed they could diagnose and identify useful remedies by visual inspection of a patient or even by letter on the basis of brief written descriptions. Few autopsies were performed and, in those performed, attention was rarely focused on the signs of damage that we have since learned to be most revealing about a subject's disease history. To explore the putative effects of diseases common before 1870, it is necessary to rely chiefly on evidence accumulated after 1870.

The Immune Response

One of the ways in which disease leaves lasting effect is immunological. Upon invasion by infectious agents, the individual with a healthy immune system produces disease-specific antibodies. In this way, the disease itself gives rise to an adaptation that diminishes the likelihood of injury or death and often also reduces the chances of a further episode of that disease. Some diseases provoke an immunity that is virtually complete and lifelong. Others produce partial or briefer immunity, protecting the individual from further assaults from the specific strain of the infectious agent encountered but not against all strains of the same disease. And still others provoke little or no immune response. Although the immune system may be disordered and even a source of illness, the immune response is usually ben-

ficial. It has loomed large as an historical force, protecting genera-
ion after generation from repeated episodes of some of the most
ife-threatening of infectious diseases, including smallpox and diph-
heria. To imagine the absence of an immune response while holding
everything else the same is to speculate that humankind could never
have aggregated into communities large enough to sustain infectious
agents.

Insult Accumulation

f the immunological effect of infectious disease is chiefly beneficial,
other effects are not. Many diseases cause structural or functional
alterations in tissue or cells. Some of these alterations are obvious
and are repaired, at least at a superficial glance, as illness gives way to
recovery. This is true with the maculopapular rash of rubella. Others
– such as smallpox – cause lasting damage but have no well-identified
effects for later health. Still others cause internal damage to structure
or function, damage that in most diseases came to be identified only
n the nineteenth or twentieth centuries, when autopsies were per-
ormed in large numbers and in a deliberate search for post-mortem
signs of disease, and when animal models began to be employed to
provide evidence about the physical effects of disease.

   One of the models for examining insult accumulation is derived
rom experiments with the effects of radiation on laboratory animals,
which is to say animals selected to diminish the degree to which
individual variations would distort species-level findings. Animals
that survived radiation exposure were found to carry lasting damage
that influenced their subsequent survival and capacity to resist later
insults, including those of other types. Each later exposure added to
he sum of damage from an insult that the immune system was
powerless to ward off. This particular model is limited in applica-
bility. A series of radiation doses may add cumulative damage, and
radiation exposure is often capable of adding increments of damage
that become manifest only many years later. But, speculation about
he direct and indirect effects of sunspot activity notwithstanding,
here is little reason to associate historical patterns of mortality in
Europe or elsewhere with changing radiation exposure. Moreover, in
he European environment, only frostbite displays a similar pattern
of damages that accumulate in the specific way that each episode
increases the likelihood of a future episode. Frostbite, which also
occurs at temperatures above freezing when wind speed is high, is

more likely if the individual has had a previous cold injury. But it is
identified with lasting tissue damage only in severe cases, which may
now be treated successfully but seem likely to have resulted in death
in most instances before the twentieth century.[20] Thus frostbite, even
if it was a more general disease in the past than it has since become,
would poorly serve as an example.

Much more apt examples are some of the common infectious
diseases within European experience, not smallpox but rheumatic
fever, typhoid fever, diphtheria, influenza, syphilis, tuberculosis, and
others. Each of these diseases is associated with lasting tissue damage
at different sites within the body and with different effects in a way
that can be shown by considering a well-developed model, rheumatic
heart disease.[21] Rheumatic fever is one of the complications most
common in group A streptococcal infections.[22] Some rheumatic
fevers, both clinical and subclinical, in turn cause rheumatic heart
disease, which consists of permanent damage usually to the mitral
valve on the left side of the heart. The damage occurs in the early
stage of infection. Its effects may be felt soon thereafter and cause
death, or many years later when damage suffered in childhood
(usually at ages 6–15) sharply increases the risk of death from heart
failure in middle age.

The incidence of rheumatic heart disease declined sharply after the
introduction in 1936 of effective chemotherapy in the form of sulfona-
mides and, later, penicillin. Three surveys of urban US school populations between 1920 and 1934 reported rheumatic heart disease at
rates from 4.3 to 5.0 per 1000, and this condition – determined by
auscultation, which cannot detect all cases of damage – was the chief
cardiovascular cause for rejection for service in the US military from
1941 to 1943, with a rate of 24 rejections per 1000 men. The difference between these rates, 4.3 to 5 per 1000 and 24 per 1000, can be
attributed to the fact that one population (recruits) had passed
through most of the ages at particular risk to rheumatic fever, and
probably also to the greater representativeness of recruits than
schoolchildren in these samples. The actual incidence of rheumatic
heart disease in the US around 1940 was probably closer to 24 per
1000. That is, one basis for backward projection is an approximate 2
per cent incidence of lasting damage.

The historical incidence of rheumatic heart disease must be estimated, and any estimation demands some assumptions. These could
build on twentieth-century studies, which explain that the virulence
of rheumatic fever changes over time; that lasting cardiac damage

ɔccurs in about one-third of rheumatic fever cases; that the pathogenesis of rheumatic fever remains unknown but is held to result from an interaction of factors associated with the agent, the host, and the environment; and that the strongest environmental associations consist of crowding and poverty (but not dietary deficiency). Several authorities have also suggested that scarlet fever – with tonsillitis, the streptococcal infection most closely associated with rheumatic fever – declined in virulence in England and the US toward the end of the nineteenth century, having been a common disease and a leading cause of death among children.[23] On these grounds, it seems reasonable to suppose that rheumatic heart disease was commonplace and a common cause of death in certain cohorts, and to speculate that in some historical cohorts the incidence of rheumatic heart damage may have been greater than 2 per cent of the adult population. If scarlet fever was especially intense between 1840 and 1880, as George Rosen suggests,[24] and if scarlet fever is to be more closely associated with rheumatic fever than other streptococcal and viral infections, then the cohorts that passed through the ages 6 to 15 during those 40 years seem especially likely to have suffered valve damage. That is, individuals born in England and the US between approximately 1825 and 1874 were prone to rheumatic heart disease, which would have been a leading cause of death some 50 to 60 years later (that is, 1875 to 1934). In earlier periods, streptococcal infections waxed and waned in incidence, which suggests long waves of rheumatic heart damage in preceding generations. But, by itself, rheumatic heart damage cannot account for a substantial part of mortality in England or the US or for trend movement toward lower death rates. Insult accumulation theory can be applied to interpret experience only if lasting damage can be identified with other illnesses and injuries.

Autopsy Findings

People who died between 1875 and 1934, in particular people whose lives had been characterized by crowding and poverty, were especially likely to be autopsied at death (even though the overall probability of autopsy remained low). They died in a period in which pathologists were keenly interested in understanding the signs of disease after death. In one well-reported sample, William Ophüls performed or participated in more than 3000 autopsies in San Francisco hospitals between 1900 and 1923. He examined tissue unrelated to the cause of death as well as related specimens, and he collected evidence about characteristics of his subjects: age at death, disease history, socioeconomic status, race, and sex. These data formed the basis for a statistical survey which showed that, within this unrepresentative population, the leading cause of death in infancy was congenital syphilis, 64 per cent of the population showed signs of tuberculosis, and few died from acute infectious diseases, but lesions from earlier infections were common.[25]

Ophüls reviewed earlier pathological investigations and used part of his population – 500 specimens – to investigate whether arterial disease in adulthood might be traced to infectious diseases experienced early in life. Previous investigations, often based on a combination of autopsy evidence and disease histories, suggested associations with certain diseases, and Ophüls sought to examine a larger number of individuals and collect information about health history more carefully. His method was to distinguish people who had suffered infectious diseases from those who had not, to compare arterial and aortal damage in the two groups, and to compare the age distribution of observed damage to the distribution that would be expected if arteriosclerosis were associated only with aging. Ophüls found that signs of arterial and aortal damage were marked in people with a history of infectious disease but absent in those without. Infectious diseases 'injure the arterial walls in such a way that they tend to earlier and more rapid decay', for example, by causing lesions where plaque builds up and promotes atherosclerosis. The process begins early in life and may continue for 20 to 60 years without overt signs or symptoms until a vessel's passageway is occluded or the lesion breaks off.[26]

Since the 1940s, most of the effort to reconstruct the population-level development of atherosclerotic signs has attempted to move backward from the life stage at which mature signs are plentiful, at ages 50 and above. Through prospective surveys such as the Framingham study, which follow a selected sample population through adulthood and comparative studies such as Ancel Key's seven-country comparison, which contrasted selected adult populations with distinctive characteristics, the research focus shifted from autopsy findings to the identification of risk factors. The leading risk factors for coronary heart disease are believed to be aging, excessive serum cholesterol, hypertension, smoking, inactivity, and emotional stress. These and other known risk factors account for about half of the risk of coronary heart disease. At the clinical level, they are combatted by surgical intervention and drugs, at the preclinical level by attempts to halt or reverse the process of insult accumulation, such as by dietary modification (that is, risk-factor therapy).[27]

The ways in which risk factors operate and accumulate suggest that developments at the cellular level and in childhood and youth constitute the most promising areas for the discovery of additional factors and means to interrupt the accumulation of damage, but Ophüls's particular line of attack has been given up. Individuals whose deaths are attributed to cardiovascular disease are now the least likely to be autopsied, and autopsies in general are now done less frequently and usually with narrower objectives.[28] In the sense meant by Ophüls, the need for evidence about artery and organ damage in childhood diminished sharply with the reduced incidence of infectious diseases in the twentieth-century population, including the portions of it reaching age 50.[29] Nevertheless, this line of enquiry has some important implications for retrospective analysis.

Ophüls's findings about the deferred or 'long' effects of infectious diseases, which elaborated and specified earlier findings, associated certain diseases with greater or lesser quantities of lasting damage to organs, arteries, and other tissue, especially to arteries and heart valves. Disease complications ceased to be seen as only or chiefly 'short' in effect – the manner in which, for example, an influenza epidemic increases the likelihood of fatalities from heart disease, or influenza activates tuberculosis or promotes schizophrenia, or a given disease, such as diphtheria, is associated with immediate complications. The leading diseases with long effects appeared to be streptococcal infections in general and rheumatic fever in particular, plus typhoid fever, diphtheria, influenza, and perhaps tuberculosis. That is, Ophüls and his predecessors detected the lasting effects of diseases that had been especially common in the general population of Europe and the US until late in the nineteenth or early in the twentieth century, and observed those effects especially in coronary disease. Each of several infections contributed its own damage – brief, persistent, or permanent – and the damage associated with each of them accumulated among survivors. Some damage, such as mitral valve scarring, could be linked directly to the later health and timing of death in autopsy subjects. But Ophüls did not attempt to deal only with damage associated directly with cause of death. He observed instead the accumulation of damage that may best be understood, in the language of the previous chapter, as increments to the vulnerability term. Parts of the body functioned less satisfactorily when damaged, but the system both adapted to and repaired damage. Insult accumulation theory suggests that the damage, and the allocation of resources to repair and adaptation, influences vitality.

Risk Factors and the History of Ill Health

Although the designation is distinctive, the notion of risk factors has been pervasive in historical discussions of general rather than disease-specific mortality. Until the eighteenth century, and once again between about 1820 and 1870, the city was recognized as a site of excessive mortality, requiring in-migration to maintain its population. Urban populations died at higher rates because the city was crowded and filthy, its streams and rivers polluted with industrial and human waste, its air thick with particles from wood and coal fires, and its streets strewn with waste. Medical topographers and geographers – forerunners of epidemiologists – sought to identify the full range of environmental factors associated with epidemic disease, and incriminated especially standing water, undisposed waste, foul air, and improperly buried human corpses. Physicians associated certain occupations with higher disease risks (for example, chimney sweeping with cancers) and warned that immoderate drinking and eating, or improper diets, damaged health. Much has since been learned about the way in which specific risk factors operate in particular diseases, arterial and otherwise, the effect of individual factors has been specified statistically, and the long process of damage accumulation has been observed. Luigi Cornaro, the pathologist Walford's example of an historical figure who discovered how to suppress aging by dietary means, ate about 920 calories per meal or per day, it is not clear which. But his restricted diet consisted of bread, meat, and broth with egg, in equal quantities, plus wine. Cornaro carefully avoided garden produce, vegetable soups, and fresh fruit.[30] The contrast between his diet and the diet likely to be recommended today by proponents of restriction suggests that Cornaro lived to about 100 despite what he ate. None of these changes in what is known or surmised provides reason to believe that risk factors did not operate also in exposure to and accumulation of damage in historical populations.

The key differences between the present-day population and its historical counterpart are two. First, the insult load has changed character. Except for cigarette smoking, each of the factors now associated strongly with a higher risk of coronary heart disease was present in the historical environment (although many risk factors associated with other diseases, for instance, industrial chemicals linked to cancer, may not have been). On balance, it is not apparent whether the risk factor load has intensified or diminished, but it is apparent that its elements have shifted and that exposure to toxins is different. To the eighteenth-century observer, toxicity was associated with naturally occurring substances, especially human and organic waste. To the twentieth-century counterpart, it is associated more closely with manufactured items, tobacco in cigarettes but not in all forms, industrial chemicals, and food additives. Second, and more important, the portion of the population arriving at age 50 has grown, and grown to the point at which the population now manifests damage on a vast scale.

In the aggregate, insult accumulation has become a more important effect on health as the likelihood of dying early in life from any given disease, injury, or environmental insult has diminished, and as the dying population has aged. Damage not likely to reveal itself in historical populations – in Sweden from 1751 to 1760, for example, less than half the population lived to be 40 – became apparent because life expectancy increased.[31] The physician observing the high mortality regime of before 1740 and the intermediate regime of *circa* 1740–1870 knew the deferred manifestations of insult accumulation well enough, though not the process itself. But the degenerative diseases most closely associated with insult accumulation occupied a comparatively modest place in inventories of the leading causes of death because so many people died of infectious diseases as they passed through the early stages of accumulation. Among older adults, the most common diagnosis for cause of death remained the indefinite 'old age'.

CONCLUSION

This chapter provides two conceptions of the sickness risk. One suggests that life consists of a series of confrontations with more or less discrete hazards from disease and injury. Diseases, which dominated the equation in the high mortality regime, seized people in batches large and small, killing certain numbers of them. Case fatality rates fluctuated, especially in a few unstable disease agents, but the largest part of the history of disease can be told as a history of exposure. It is, nevertheless, a complicated history. Exposure itself was inconstant, so that successive generations in the high mortality regime confronted something akin to a fixed exposure profile but an ever-shifting disease profile. Each cohort built its own history of disease experience, a history it carried forward as its size diminished in the manner shown by the life table's column of survivors (Chapter 1).

This is the conception that prompts curiosity about the leading causes of death in the high mortality regime.[32] To estimate the sickness burden for any cohort within this conception, it is necessary to identify the diseases causing death at a certain place and period, to find case fatality rates, and to associate the leading diseases with population characteristics – age, sex, residence, occupation. That information gathered, and interpreted sensitively in the light of what can reasonably be supposed about changes in the form and virulence of diseases known now in somewhat different form, leads to a profile of sicknesses that might have been fatal. It can also be interpreted, in combination with what medical texts, patient histories, personal memoirs, and other sources reveal about the identity and prevalence of non-fatal diseases, as the essential background for a reconstruction of sickness and as the gauge of the relative health of each historical community.

In this first conception, it is implied that the risk of death is a reliable but understated version of the risk of sickness. A parallel relationship between disease risk and death risk has often been observed in individual diseases and is implied by the idea of case fatality rates. The rates associated with any given diseases are usually found to be variable rather than fixed, but they are variable within a narrow range. Within the limits of that range, knowing the number of deaths from a given disease provides the information necessary to estimate the number of clinical cases.

The second conception in this chapter points to the prevalence of sickness episodes resolved in recovery. Even the most virulent diseases of the high mortality regime seldom caused the death of more than 10 per cent of the individuals who manifested clinical symptoms, and most diseases were associated with still lower case fatality rates. But it adds the evidence that recovery is often incomplete. Many diseases and injuries, and many contacts with the environment not perceived at the time to consist of ill health, have lasting effects, beneficial or harmful. Like the beneficial effects of immunity, the harmful effects may be temporary, lasting, or permanent and they may vary in degree. Adding deferred effects further complicates a full picture of experience at the level of a population and within its cohorts. If each cohort builds its own individual history of disease, it also builds its own still more individualized profile of insult loads, a profile conditioned by the insults its members have survived and by the intricate implications of each load for the insults yet to be faced through the remainder of its history.

The second conception also disturbs the relationship that can be supposed to exist between the mortality and morbidity risk. When insult accumulation is added in, parallelism gives way to an uncertain association. The importance of a cohort's prior disease experience is intensified and, with it, the importance of assessing how the composition of the cohort may have changed over time.

Consider the problem in terms of health endowment at birth and the health index accumulated by survivors. At birth, one historical cohort closely resembled another, its frailty – or susceptibility to ill health and death – was distributed across a spectrum influenced by inherited factors and fetal experience.[33] But, for the most part, the pattern of its sicknesses and deaths awaited determination. In infancy, each cohort lost up to a third of its members, and in infancy each cohort lost its virtual equality with other cohorts. Each began to acquire an insult load and an immunity profile peculiar to its experience, both features whose history is told more effectively by the diseases and injuries that the cohort survived than by those that caused heavy mortality. Everything else being equal, the higher the case fatality rate, the lower the degree to which exposure to any given disease conditioned the cohort's later health. As the cohort aged the role of its birth profile diminished and that of its exposure and insult profiles increased further. At every stage of life, the key factor in a cohort's future health experience consisted more and more of the illnesses and injuries its members had survived.

In the high mortality regime, however, the likelihood of survival was curtailed by the high scale and frequency of disease assaults. Every cohort was quickly winnowed so that about three-quarters of its members survived infancy, half to age 30 or so, and only a quarter to age 50. Insult accumulation, especially short effects, played a broad role in mortality at younger ages but a more restricted role in adulthood. No means exist to observe it directly, but the Gompertz function may offer an indirect view. In the earliest population for which this function has yet been reconstructed, a population in eighteenth-century England, a stable rate of increase in the death rate appeared around age 15 and persisted until about age 50. That is, the Gompertz function seems to have showed up and disappeared earlier than the pattern noticed in the previous chapter regarding nineteenth- and twentieth-century experience, when the function was identified with ages 45 and above. The implication of this peregrination through the life course is that the vulnerability term (as the insult index was designated earlier) was sufficiently greater in scale to bring the aging process into operation at an earlier age. Neither early modern nor nineteenth-century Europeans aged earlier than their modern counterparts in a chronologic sense, but their physiologic resources were depleted earlier.

Taken together, these two conceptions promote an interpretation about the trend of sickness risk and the relationship between morbidity and mortality between 1600 and 1870. A declining incidence of epidemic disease and a decreasing death rate after infancy suggest that the risk of falling sick diminished over time and, with it, the insult load accumulated by successive cohorts. In the long run, especially after about 1740, each age group from five until about 25 contained more new survivors, more individuals who would not have lived in the old mortality regime but who survived longer in the evolving regime. The rate of insult accumulation slowed, but its effects became more apparent. They were manifested in a sharper upward slope in adulthood of the risk of being sick as compared to the risk of falling sick. The pace of insult exposure and accumulation remained high enough that each cohort regained its equality to other cohorts around age 30. That is, the likelihood of survival increased at each age between five and 30 but not in infancy or old age. Life expectancy at birth increased because of the years added to life at intermediate ages. Within the years of life added to each cohort's experience, especially years at ages 25 or 30 to about 50, chronic and degenerative diseases became more common. That, at least, is the implication. Whereas in the high mortality regime the risk of falling sick had dominated the consideration of morbidity, in the intermediate regime it began to give way to the risk of being sick. Over time, the mortality rate and the risk of falling sick declined, but the risk of being sick increased.

Taken together, these two conceptions show also how quantitative and qualitative, demographic and medical, and diagnostic and functional approaches and information must be melded. Only in their merger can historians understand the life history of cohorts, the epidemiologic transition, and the persistent problem – a retrospective

nd prospective problem – of shifting disease profiles and population
haracteristics. And only in that merger can historians resume their
art of the dialogue with biologists in which the goal is to understand
uman population ecology.

5 The Experience of Sickness before 1870

> Health is generally measured by death-rates.[1]

Two types of sources inform us about the experience of sickness from the seventeenth century into the nineteenth. One consists of a complex assortment of beliefs and assumptions now held. These beliefs and assumptions are based on testimony about disease and death which is unambiguous in thrust and is usually held to be unambiguous in implication, too. Disease and death were rife, and mortality rates were high. The other source consists of case studies in which the by-now-familiar gauge, absence from work attributed to illness or injury, is used to measure the incidence and duration of sickness. Neither source will, by itself, give a satisfactory account. On the one hand, some of the beliefs and assumptions will be false but, in the absence of ways to examine the foundations of these beliefs and assumptions, it is extraordinarily difficult to decide which may be false. On the other hand, the case studies are few in number and represent small segments of the overall historical population at risk to sickness. Used together, the two sources can sharpen the questions asked and guide research.

BELIEFS AND ASSUMPTIONS

The things we believe to have been true of sickness experience in the past are sometimes difficult to track to their sources. They are also difficult to convert from the generalizations in which they now appear back into the experience that gave rise to those generalizations. This difficulty occurs because the beliefs and assumptions are based on general ideas about ill health while the surviving evidence consists chiefly of specific medical testimony about disease and death. The medical testimony focuses on diseases and the likelihood of dying, but it has limited value unless it can be linked to evidence about health and the likelihood of recovery from sickness. Although the metaphysical question – whence the beliefs and assumptions – has its

128

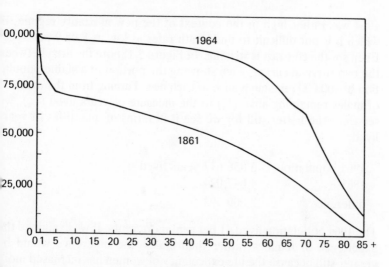

FIGURE 5.1   *Survival curves for males living in England and Wales, 1861 and 1964*

SOURCE   Samuel H. Preston, Nathan Keyfitz and Robert Schoen, *Causes of Death: Life Tables for National Populations* (New York, 1972), pp. 224, 268.

ascination, it need not trouble the way we proceed here. Rather than earching for explanations of the ways in which these particular eliefs and assumptions have arisen, let us instead summarize them.

The summary can begin with a contrast so sharp and compelling hat it conditions all views. The contrast is the familiar one between he old mortality regime and the new, but let us consider it in a new vay. The customary mode has been to compare crude or age-specific leath rates, showing how much higher those were in the old mortality egime.[2] In place of this, consider the contrast as it was made in Chapter 1, in terms of years of life lived in the new mortality regime ut not in the old. What did a high death rate mean in terms of years f life sacrificed to it? Figure 5.1 offers one version of the contrast, lrawing on the experience of males living in England and Wales in 861 and 1964. It gives a decidedly moderate version of the contrast, or the 1861 crude death rate was 23 per 1000 a year and the 1964 rate 2. That is, the death rate in 1861 – a year representing the intermedi- te rather than the high mortality regime – was already quite low in he context of the old mortality regime, in which crude death rates ad often reached or exceeded 30 per 1000 a year, and the rate in

1964 was rather high in the context of the new mortality regime, in which it is not difficult to find death rates as low as 8 or 9 per 1000. Even so, the contrast is striking. In Figure 5.1, note the area between the two survival curves, each showing the portion of a stable population of 100 000 remaining alive at each age. Turning from the measure of males remaining alive (1_x) to the measure of years lived (L_x), we see the issue better still for we see it in terms of quantities of years lived:

1964 population	6 856 617 years lived
1861	4 047 024
difference	2 809 593

The 1964 population lived 41 per cent more years. If we examined the experience of females rather than males, the difference would be greater still because the life expectancy of women has increased more than that of men. This is a telling way of presenting the contrast between the two mortality regimes. It shows quickly and efficiently that when we measure health by death rates, as we usually have done, we arrive at an unambiguous conclusion: in the past, especially the more distant past, ill health typified popular experience.

In the eras of the high and the intermediate mortality regimes, which persisted until 1870, the health of the people who lived in Europe was wretched. We extract this impression not merely from high death rates but also from the imposing list of diseases prevailing in those times, from the awesome and repetitive qualities of many of those diseases, from stories of people seen to be disabled and marked by disease, and from common sense. The environment in which many infants failed to survive to maturity, in which disease was common, was surely also an environment in which sickness was commonplace and sickness rates were as much higher over today's sickness rates as today's mortality rates are lower than mortality rates then.

This is the impression we extract from biographies, autobiographies, and diaries which, if they dwell on health, dwell on ill health rather than good. We know that Isaac Newton's mother often felt despair as her frail son repeatedly fell ill and seemed threatened by death; that Alexander Pope, who acquired a hunchback deformity after suffering a childhood case of tuberculosis of the bone, complained repeatedly of his illnesses through a life of 56 years; that James Boswell recorded nineteen attacks of gonorrhea between the ages of 20 and 50 (not to mention his other maladies); and that Ralph

Josselin mentioned 148 episodes of ill health experienced by his wife Jane in the course of forty years, mostly during pregnancy and childbirth.[3] We believe that pain and suffering, deformity, and disability were common and accepted.[4] People resigned themselves to these things because they lacked medical remedies, and because they preferred suffering to death. In the words of the medical historian Øivind Larsen, 'diseases . . . withdraw from historical examination, because they were so common that they were not noted'.[5] Once such characterizations have been applied to any historical period, they tend to be projected backward, only in aggravated form.

The comparison of historical and recent experience is further troubled by the intrusion of efficacious therapy. Consider, for example, peptic ulcers. They remain common and, if we believe that tension may induce them and that modern life is more stressful, we would suppose that their prevalence has increased. But peptic ulcers may no longer produce visible signs – haggardness – so readily because they are today treated effectively with drugs and diet. Comparing images of people on the street, we have the impression that diseases have disappeared when it is instead their symptoms that have disappeared, or their sufferers. The sick were likelier to be seen on the streets and paths of Europe before 1870 because, although the population was smaller, its hospitals were in proportion still fewer. The ill lived among the well or, at least, the visibly well. Only in the clinic, and more especially the autopsy room, might the true incidence be observed.

The realm of therapy offers another counterargument to the generalized image of ill health. One of the most popular literary forms of the seventeenth and eighteenth centuries was the treatise explaining how to reduce the chances of falling ill and treat common maladies.[6] The very plentitude of these books argues that the people who bought them believed in the efficacy of treatments recommended by physicians more than they believed in the efficacy of physicians, and that they believed that ill health could be avoided by appropriate habits of diet, exercise, and emotional behavior, such as the physician Cheyne's recommendation of a 'spare and simple Diet'. But, counterarguments notwithstanding, we carry with us the image of widespread ill health.

When the old mortality regime finally gave way to the new – when, that is, the death rate declined very close to the minimum consonant with the human life span – the result was a 'transformation of health'.[7] Modern observers claim further that 'the decline in the death rates has meant a decline in the rates of morbidity, i.e. of the incidence of disease'.[8] The general reduction in morbidity rates helped increase life expectancy.[9] In the longer run, and if we consider the earlier phase of mortality decline dating from about 1740 to about 1870 as well as its later phase after 1870, the population growth allowed by mortality decline is itself an indicator of the improvement of health.[10]

The same assertions are made and the same assumptions prevail when specific periods are under discussion. In England after 1660, the 'disease situation' was 'one of relatively high morbidity with many endemic diseases'.[11] In London in the long period from 1750 to 1909, changes in the mortality rate signaled parallel and equivalent changes in health, and the mortality decline showed the improvement of health.[12] Chronicles of disease in specific areas, such as Louis Torfs's for the Southern Netherlands, confirm the impression.[13] Epidemics occurred in one region or another of each country in nearly every year. What is lacking is a sense of the numbers affected and the numbers at risk. We know that epidemics were common, but we do not know even approximately how many additional deaths they caused. We lack a way to distinguish epidemic from non-epidemic mortality.

The belief that mortality and morbidity will be parallel in incidence and trend can be traced to the late eighteenth century and the earliest formulation of a sickness curve. Lacking a body of sickness experience to consult, the actuary Richard Price hypothesized the age curve of sickness by assuming that this curve would be closely associated with the age curve of mortality. It was in this form that the notion of a 'law of sickness' appeared, so that the law expressed an expectation that the mortality experience of a population could be used to estimate its sickness experience and, indeed, that knowing the mortality rate at any one age would allow the calculator to infer the mortality rate for all other adult ages and the sickness rate for all ages. These possibilities were stated explicitly in the 1830s by T.R Edmonds, who used them to construct hypothetical tables of sickness risk and thus insurance rates. Edmonds further distinguished between the incidence and the duration of sickness, and he suggested a fixed relationship between what is here called the risk of falling sick and the size of the population, a risk that he believed did *not* change with age.[14] This particular formulation and the distinction that Edmonds made between two sickness risks seems to have been discredited when consultations of experience showed that Edmonds's hypotheti cal values did not coincide closely with actual values. Later commentators construed the laws of sickness and mortality more often to refer to curves that were fixed by age and over time, and they set aside Edmonds's distinction between two sickness risks. Thus nineteenth-century actuaries tried to discover a putatively singular sickness curve by consulting larger and larger bodies of experience, considering ways in which populations observed in different surveys differed from one another, and elaborating techniques to smooth irregularities from one age to the next.

Another conviction arose about the same time. Whereas Edmonds believed that the risk of falling sick was, for adults at least, a function of the size of the population rather than of age, other observers noticed regularities between the numbers of people sick and those dying. The physician Gilbert Blane's report of morbidity and mortality in his hospital practice during 1784–94 and his private practice during 1794–1805 showed that the ratio between admissions or cases and deaths worked out to about 10:1. Among hospital admissions of males numbering 2406, 239 died; among females, 135 of 1429; and in the private practice, 384 people of 3816.[15] That simple ratio came to the notice of the French actuary Nicolas Hubbard, who employed it not only to propose a general rule but also to distinguish by sex and income: in 10 000 sicknesses, one can expect 1001 deaths among the well off (Blane's private patients), 993 among poor males, or 944 among poor females (the latter two based on Blane's hospital practice).[16] Other observers suggested somewhat different ways of stating the relationship but accepted the notion that a fixed proportion would be found between the incidence of sickness and the death rate. For example, after consulting English army and friendly society records, Edmonds concluded that a ratio of one death to two years sickness would prevail, and Edmonds was William Farr's source for the same inference.[17]

These expectations were no longer held by the early twentieth century, because, among other reasons, Watson's study of Odd Fellows experience during the period 1893–97 proved that the duration rate of sickness had increased substantially since 1870 and thereby put to rest the idea of finding a fixed sickness curve. Nevertheless, the belief that a parallel relationship would always obtain between mortality and morbidity rates acquired further support from early epidemiologic studies showing that the fatality and morbidity curves of given diseases tended to parallel one another. In the early decades of the twentieth century, when disease-specific morbidity and mortality curves often showed a decided downward trend, these observations buttressed the notion that the high mortality rates of the past could be assumed to signal high morbidity rates.

Notions about the history of ill health in the overall population are often stated more forthrightly still in descriptions of the part of the population we might suppose to have been the healthiest, those who worked at physically demanding tasks. Having consulted the reports of physicians and work inspectors who visited workshops in France in the late eighteenth and early nineteenth century, the historian Arlette Farge summarizes the prevailing view:

> Un corps au travail est un corps qui se dépense et se fatigue, qui accomplit une suite routinière de gestes et de déplacements dans un lieu particulier. S'il s'agit d'artisans et d'ateliers au XVIIIe siècle, on devine aisément les conditions rudes, précaires et insécures dans lesquelles s'accomplit le travail. Malaises, blessures, maladies incurables font partie du paysage quotidien, aussi habituels que le sont les salaires insuffisants, les ateliers mal aérés et l'instabilité de l'emploi.[18]

More plentiful still is testimony concerning the lot of the industrial worker of the early nineteenth century, when urban workers were crowded together and subjected to an often pitiless discipline in order to accommodate to the factory, its tools, sources of power, and taskmasters. Farr, who helped pioneer the consultation of health statistics as a way of formulating policy, believed that many people worked while ill, lame, or infirm.[19] He had in mind especially the episodes of sickness that did not incapacitate for work but that did show up in statistics when records were kept of consultations with surgeons supplied by the employer. The implication is clear. Industrialization – more specifically, the advent of large-scale factories concentrated in cities – aggravated the misery and distress of the working classes, a segment of the population of Europe already in misery and distress before the advent of factories.

What makes this testimony astonishing is parallel evidence of the physical demands of labor before and during industrial modernization. Printers and typesetters who worked in Antwerp, men who fished for cod off Newfoundland, men and women who worked on the farms and in the households of rural France, and many of the laboring people of early modern Europe worked long days, often in

TABLE 5.1   *Life expectation among males in England and Wales, 1861 and 1964*

age	1861	1964
birth	40.5 years	68.6 years
10	47.9	60.5
20	40.2	50.9
30	33.3	41.4
40	26.4	31.9
50	19.8	23.0
60	13.5	15.4

SOURCE   See Figure 5.1

circumstances in which furious activity was interspersed with mild activity or inactivity.[20] A noteworthy feature of this labor in the early modern era lies in the inability of the laborer to get a day's work into a shorter period than 14 or 16 hours. The work day expanded to what now seem punitive durations in order to allow more cycles of typesetting, inking, and printing; line baiting, dropping, and retrieval; and the myriad interdependent tasks of agricultural and household work. For the pre-factory period, we acknowledge this when we observe that work was paid not by time but by task and output in a system that induced enthusiastic work because the organization of work did not by itself admit discipline. Factories began to change this system, substituting disciplined for intermittent activity and using time more efficiently. But factory jobs, too, demanded fitness. Many people could not sustain the exertion required, and they gave their jobs up. But how far can we imagine that exhaustion dominated the lives of adults in the working classes? The life expectancy of adult males did not deteriorate with the advent of factory labor in Britain, although it did cease to increase both in regions with and regions without factories, presumably because of urbanization and its attendant crowding and filth. Nor – and this seems to be the telling point – did life expectancy increase much in the century after factory labor had become common, represented in Table 5.1 by the year 1861. No gross signs of change appear in the degree to which labor determines life expectancy even though the working day has been appreciably shortened and the requirements of labor moderated.

If those who worked in such demanding jobs are presumed to have suffered so grievously, what are we to suppose about those who could not work because their health had already deteriorated? With such images before us and remembering that many diseases were infectious and thus unlikely to respect divisions of wealth or status, it is difficult to imagine any substantial segment of pre-industrial and early industrial society free from the burden of sickness.

These beliefs and assumptions about the history of health are unequivocal: to my knowledge, no one has argued that health was good or the morbidity rate low in early modern Europe or indeed in any populations since the sparsely peopled paleolithic world. Yet the very evidence that leads us to conclude that the health of Europeans and North Americans was unrelentingly bad from at least the neolithic revolution until some time after 1870, and perhaps as late as about 1950, supplies us with reasons to be skeptical about this characterization. These reasons are implied by the evidence collected in Chapter 4. Until about 1870, we believe that most people died of infectious diseases which usually took an acute rather than a chronic course. Health status can be measured by mortality rates because 'most serious illnesses resulted from [potentially] fatal diseases of relatively short duration'.[21] We believe also that the case fatality rates of diseases and injuries were substantially higher than they are in the twentieth century and that the experience of disease was rife. If these things are so, then we should expect to find that the risk of falling sick was high. But should we expect also to find a high risk of being sick?

One of the anomalies in our view of morbidity in the past is the belief that historical populations were likelier than modern populations to be ill and to be disabled. That is, our conclusions imply that we expect the risk of being sick to have been high even though we ascribe sickness chiefly to acute infectious disease. This apparent anomaly is resolved by the suggestion that the people who survived sickness were often disfigured or disabled. Chronic disability was also a severe problem for historical populations because disease was so prevalent. People who survived disease often lost the ability to function normally, but that loss of ability did not reduce their life expectation in proportion. The life expectation of people age 20 and above has increased much less than life expectation at birth, as Table 5.1 shows for the male population of England and Wales in 1861 and 1964.[22] Furthermore, we believe that these same people were both prone to disabilities and capable of performing the physically demanding tasks of an era in which human power played a large role and jobs requiring fitness made up a large proportion of the jobs in which people engaged. The two ideas are inconsistent. It is unreasonable to suppose that people reaching the age of 20, by which age many were disabled by disease, managed at the same time to live long lives and to work at the jobs we know to have characterized economic activity.

In addition, a higher probability of death signals by itself a lower probability of sickness *among survivors*, who constitute the population whose morbidity will be measured. That is, if we insist on allowing for survival – which of course we must if we are to acknowledge the l_x and L_x values found in populations from the era of the high mortality regime – then we must admit one or some combination of the following propositions:

1) case fatality rates were much lower than has been supposed,
2) sicknesses were infrequent, or
3) sicknesses were frequent but brief.

Before trying to resolve these discrepancies, it will be useful to consult some evidence about sickness rates.

MEASURED SICKNESS

The greatest problem posed by using sick fund records to substantiate an impression of sickness experience lies in the small number of populations available for study before 1850 and especially before 1800. The individuals who belonged to sick funds always represent a part of the overall population. The part is diminished further by loss of records and by the as yet limited progress made in identifying and reconstructing sickness experience from surviving records. And sick fund members can fairly be held to represent only themselves. This feature needs to be acknowledged so that it will be clear that it is not representativeness that is alleged.

The case studies that follow have been selected. The selection has been made on grounds of the span and comprehensiveness of sources rather than the characteristics of people belonging to the funds or of the funds themselves. Further research will identify more funds for which financial accounts, rules, and other sources are still available for appreciable periods. It will eventually be possible to choose populations for comparison. In the meantime, caution argues in favor of deferring comparisons and generalizations, but it will lose out to curiosity. I will summarize what can be said about measured sickness from the experience of a few individual funds. In each case study,

attention will be focused on the issues a given fund's experience i
best calculated to illuminate, which are not always the issues we
would choose to have illuminated. From this fragmentary basis
generalizations and comparisons will be made. However tentative
these will fashion some propositions, which can then be compared te
the beliefs and assumptions we have about sickness experience.

Plantin Printery, Antwerp, 1654–89

In 1653, the employees of Balthasar II Moretus, master of the
printing firm called Plantin, fashioned their occasional fund fo
assisting colleagues in need into a regular insurance scheme, and in
the following year members began to draw benefits from thi
scheme.[23] They wrote the rules of this scheme so readily that we
recognize a tradition they had derived from experience, a tradition
governing central problems: how to set a premium-benefit ratio tha
would sustain the fund in the long run and how to guard assets agains
the persistent temptation to plunder them. The firm had been formed
in 1555, and it lasted into the nineteenth century. The fund lasted
only until 1782, at which time it still retained some assets, but the
number of Plantin employees had diminished so much that the func
no longer made any sense. By ourselves, we are all self insurers.

The part of the record that serves present needs concerns 1654–89
a period during which the firm prospered, regularly hiring new men
The attrition of personnel – deaths and departures, but mostly
deaths, replaced by new employees – and the dispersal of firs
employment dates for the charter members from 1621 to 1653 sugges
that the average age and probably also the age structure of func
members remained stable between 1654 and 1689.[24] This will have
been only approximately true, but the approximation is close
enough. Since the manuscript sources record benefit payments on a
weekly basis and by name, it is possible to follow sickness experience
at the individual level. From these data can be inferred the four
unknown quantities: the denominator – the time at risk to sicknes
and death; and three numerators – the number of episodes, the
duration of those episodes, and the number of deaths.[25] The two
series – the rate of falling sick and the rate of being sick – appear ir
Figure 5.2. Table 5.2 presents aggregate experience over the thirty
six years in several areas.

Plantin sick fund members did not miss work at a particularly high
rate. The average claim came to 1.08 weeks – not quite 6.5 days in a

scale

being sick: weeks lost per 1000 at risk (i.e., weeks per member per year $\times \frac{1000}{52}$)

falling sick: episodes per 1000 weeks

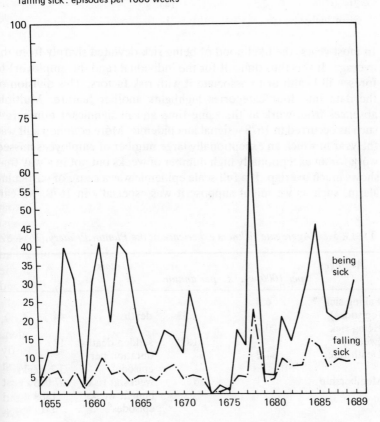

FIGURE 5.2   *Sickness at the Plantin Printery, 1654–89*

SOURCES   Plantijnsch Archief, Antwerp, Museum Plantin-Moretus, 334, 432-3, 666, 697, 772, 781 and 1168.

6-day work week – per year. But they did miss work in a strikingly variable and unpredictable way. In one year, 1673, no sickness claims were paid, but one member died suddenly. In 1678, seven members died and benefits were paid for 34 episodes and 108 weeks among 1516 weeks at risk. From Figure 5.2, we can infer that being sick rates clustered in four categories:

0–10 weeks per 1000	7 years
11–20	14
21–50	14
51 or higher	1

In most years, the likelihood of being sick deviated sharply from the average. It was thus difficult for the individual (and the employer) to foresee ill health or to associate it with risk factors. This division of the data into four categories highlights another feature. Multiple absences from work at the same time and in significant numbers – such as occurred in 1678 – signal an epidemic. More common still was the year in which an exceptionally large number of employees missed work for an exceptionally high number of weeks but not in a way that shows much overlap. If a full-scale epidemic was a cause of particular alarm, such as we might suppose it was especially in 1678, we can

TABLE 5.2   *Aggregate sickness experience at the Plantin Printery, 1654–89*

Averages	per 1000 weeks	per annum	Totals	
Falling sick (episodes)	6.4			
		.33	deaths	44
Being sick (weeks)	20.7			
		1.08	sudden deaths[a]	12
Death rate	34.0		duration per episode[b]	3.2 weeks
Membership		36	weeks at risk[c]	67 026
			benefit weeks	1389
			episodes[d]	431

Trend			
	1654–77	*1679–89*	*1654–89*
Death rate	–0.0008	–0.0045	–0.0006
Being sick	–0.5660	2.0600	0.0887
Falling sick	–0.0694	0.4036	0.1516

NOTES   a. that is, without a sickness claim in the preceding week; b. that is, 1389 weeks divided by 419 episodes, deleting sudden deaths; c. 1294.47 years, including only ten months of 1654; d. counting all occasions in which claims were not preceded, so that some individuals received benefits during more than one period within a year; including as episodes the twelve sudden deaths.

SOURCES   See Figure 5.2.

nevertheless see a statistical form of what early modern physicians may have meant when they wrote of 'sickly years'. The years 1684 and 1685 are good examples, for in those years 53 episodes of sickness accounted for 149 claims weeks, though only one member died.

The estimated average age of Plantin sick fund members in 1653 was 40, and regular turnover suggests that this average was maintained thereafter.[26] The masters preferred to hire experienced workers, meaning workers who had survived to ages at which we might expect their sicknesses to have been both acute and chronic. In fact, however, the average duration of their sicknesses was 3.2 weeks (or 4.2 weeks if half weeks are added on the falling sick and recovery sides to estimate unobserved sickness).[27] This figure is itself inflated by the exceptionally protracted sicknesses of a few employees. Fully 90 per cent of claims were for episodes lasting 26 weeks or less.

Looking only at episodes resolved in death strengthens this impression. Somewhat more than a quarter of deaths occurring from 1654 through 1689 were sudden; they were not preceded by claims in any of the four weeks before death. Among all members dying, the average duration of sickness before death totalled nearly nine weeks, but this figure is distorted by three especially protracted terminal episodes, one of which lasted nearly two and a half years. The distribution of sicknesses before death can be shown in a frequency distribution:

sudden	12	6–10 weeeks	7
1 week	6	11–20	3
2 weeks	8	21–30	0
3	1	31–40	1
4	2	41–128	2
5	1		

More than half the deaths occurred after no more than two and a half weeks of sickness. If we take out of consideration the three deaths preceded by markedly longer periods of sickness, the average episode ending in death lasted not nine but 3.7 weeks.[28]

Figure 5.2 also suggests the presence of cycles, which are brought out more clearly by the slope values given in Table 5.2. In one year, 1678, deaths and claims were markedly more numerous, and that year has been omitted from the calculations for 1654–77 and 1679–89 but not from those regarding 1654–89. The death rate remained approximately stable with the exception of a modest downward turn in 1679–89, a feature influenced by the absence of deaths in the last three years under observation. The duration rate of sickness moved downward during 1654–77 and strongly upward during 1679–89. The episode rate shows the same pattern but in milder form. Over the entire period, 1654–89, the death rate remained stable but both the being sick and the falling sick rates tended to increase.

These data lead to a characterization of sickness in the Plantin work force of which the leading features are these. First, acute sickness dominated, even in a labor force believed to have been distributed across ages from the late 20s into the 60s or higher. Chronic sicknesses appear in the Plantin manuscripts, especially after 1689, but they were prevalent only in periods in which the labor force was aged and its numbers small. Second, epidemics occurred period- ically and unpredictably, but they seem to have been overshadowed by sickly years. Fewer people fell ill in sickly years than in epidemics, but sickly years occurred far more often. Third, this was a healthy workforce. It stood at risk from death at more or less the expected rate: 34 per 1000 per annum.[29] But, among Plantin members, ill health incapacitating the individual for work was uncommon. From 1654 through 1689, claims accounted for 2 per cent of the time at risk (that is, an average of 20.7 weeks per 1000), although the workforce was actually incapacitated for work a slightly higher percentage of the time with the difference made up of uncompensated sick time on the falling sick and recovery sides of claims, and of episodes too short to earn compensation. Fourth, the ratio of episodes to deaths was approximately 10 to 1. Most sicknesses were resolved in recovery rather than death. And, fifth, mortality and morbidity experience did not parallel one another in trend. Whereas the death rate remained stable, the sickness rates showed downward and upward trends that are especially marked in the measurement of sickness duration (that is, being sick).

Ashford Female Friendly Society, 1789–1833

Many friendly societies were organized among people close to one another in age with the expectation that recruits would be added over time. As the charter members grew older, the age profile of the entire society would come to approximate that of working people in gen- eral. If this plan evolved in a steady way, the average age of members

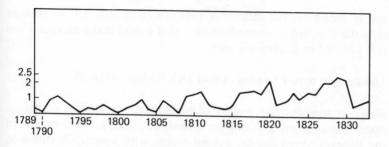

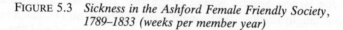

FIGURE 5.3   *Sickness in the Ashford Female Friendly Society,*
            1789–1833 (weeks per member year)

SOURCE   Derbyshire Record Office, Matlock, D747A/PZ1/1.

would rise gradually during the first 15 to 20 years of the society's experience, then level off. Although the surviving record is incomplete, notably in the absence of age or date of birth information for early members and of rules specifying terms of the contract, the Ashford Female Friendly Society of Ashford, Derbyshire, appears to give an example of this manner of development.[30] Figure 5.3 depicts annual crude sickness rates, again drawing on a small population (averaging 62 members). For its first 20 years, this society exhibits both a rising sickness rate, which can probably be explained as the consequence of the aging of charter members, and a variable rate. From such a pattern, it is easy to understand why the members of this society were able to accumulate a reserve fund lent out at interest and why they treated themselves to an annual feast.

The continued variability of sickness rates also sheds light on the attitude an individual might take when considering insurance for wages forgone because of sickness and on the appeal of sick funds to working people. The average portion of wages lost because of sickness amounted, in the case of the Ashford Society from 1789 to 1833, to less than 1.1 weeks per member per year, a quantity too small to constitute a serious threat to impoverishment even in a class of people able to pay contributions no greater than six pence a month. What made membership attractive, besides fellowship, was both the unpredictability of sickness experience and the prospect of assistance in old age. In the Ashford Society, the annual rate varied from as little as 0.1 to as much as 2.5 weeks. Since both figures are averages for all members, the difference between them still fails to capture fully the element of unpredictability that would make an individual feel justified in joining a society.

The Bennett Street Sunday School Sick Society, 1816–35

Many of the working youths of Manchester, a leading center of textile manufacturing during the British industrial revolution, joined the Bennett Street Sunday School which, with some 2500 students, was the largest Sunday school in the city. It offered religious education, taught reading, and sought to inculcate certain values, chiefly submission and docility. Many girls and boys also joined the sick society organized by the Sunday school teachers in 1811 and opened to students in 1814. The humanitarian managers of the sick fund believed that 'cessation of labor, and other comforts in seasons of sickness and languor, are especially needful to the Children of the Poor'. By contributing small sums each week, students could support an insurance fund that encouraged the independence of the working poor, that is, independence from publicly funded relief. Members included children working in Manchester factories, domestic servants, children working for tradesmen, and some children living at home.[31]

During the period in which it flourished, from 1815 to about 1850, the Bennett Street Sick Society admitted children age 11, 12, or 13 and older, and found that most left when they reached the age at which adult sick clubs accepted members, usually 18. A few adults belonged, apparently because they joined the Sunday school classes where reading was taught, and students who became teachers in the Sunday school sometimes remained members after age 18. Judging from the rules and recorded ages at death, the overwhelming majority of members were ages 12 to 26 and most were ages 12 to 18, periods of life in which the sickness risk is low.[32] Since the information that survives about individual members is incomplete, it is not possible to separate time at risk and sick time for members younger than 26 or younger than 18 years old. It is also difficult to measure time at risk accurately. The manuscripts reveal what appear to be end-of-year membership totals, which means that they include initiates not yet eligible for benefits. Turnover was high because this sick fund served a narrow age band and perhaps even more because of its association with Sunday school attendance.[33]

Figure 5.4 shows the limited results that can reliably be drawn from

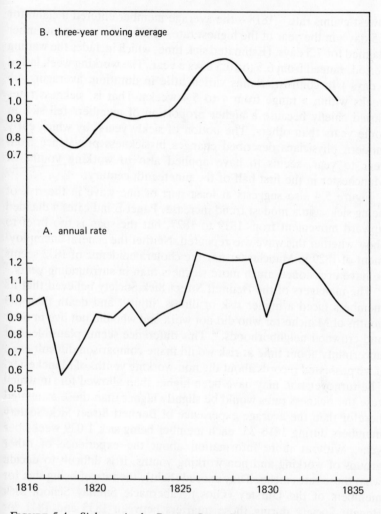

FIGURE 5.4 *Sickness in the Bennett Street Sunday School Sick Society, 1816–35*

SOURCE Manchester Central Library, Archives Department, Bennett Street Sunday School Sick and Funeral Society, M103/10.

this data set. Although the Bennett Street Sick Society enrolled a large number of people within a narrow age band (from 441 to 867 members mostly from ages 12 to 26), its records, too, reveal striking fluctuations in the sickness rate from year to year. In the year of the lowest claims rate – 1818 – the average member entered a claim for 3.5 days; in the year of the highest rate – 1826 – the average member claimed for 7.5 days. (Estimated sick time, which includes the waiting period, ranged from 6.5 to 10.5 days a year. The working week lasted 6 days.) In contrast, claims varied little in duration, averaging 4.5 weeks within a range from 4 to 5.4 weeks. That is, sickness rates varied chiefly because a higher proportion of members fell sick in some years than others. The notion of sickly years, by which early modern physicians described changes in sickness prevalence from year to year, seems to have applied also to working youths in Manchester in the first half of the nineteenth century.

Figure 5.4 also suggests at least part of one wave in the risk of being sick, and a modest trend increase. Panel B indicates a decided upward movement from 1819 to 1827, but the span is too brief to show whether this wave was repeated. Neither the general unemployment of 1829 in Manchester nor the cholera epidemic of 1832 seems to have occasioned much more sickness than in surrounding years.

The managers of the Bennett Street Sick Society believed that its members faced a higher risk of illness, injury, and death than the youths of Manchester who did not work and who did not live in poor and crowded neighborhoods.[34] This difference seems plausible, but uncertainty about time at risk would make comparison difficult even if we possessed records about the non-working youths of Manchester. The turnover rate may have been higher than allowed for, in which case the sickness rates would be slightly higher than those estimated here or than the average experience of Bennett Street Sick Society members during 1816–35: each member being sick 1.029 weeks per year. Without more information about the experience of other groups of working and non-working youths, it is difficult to decide what these rates mean. They exceed slightly the rate of being sick for members of the Dursley (Glos.) Tabernacle Sunday School Sick Benefit Society during those quarters between 1833 and 1841 for which the necessary information is available. In that population, like working youths of Manchester in age but perhaps unlike them in other respects, the being sick rate was 0.962 weeks per member per year.[35] One of the physicians who testified in the 1834 parliamentary Factories Inquiry, Bisset Hawkins, reported that in 1833 he had examined 115 factory youths age 18 or younger from Preston. He found 84 of them (73 per cent) in good health, 25 (22 per cent) in 'middling' health, and 6 (5 per cent) in bad health.[36] Hawkins knew about the Bennett Street Sick Society records, and he used a sample from 1830–32 to estimate the rate of falling sick among working children. Farr, who studied evidence given the Factories Inquiry Commission, believed that these figures indicated that poor youths in ill health nevertheless worked, as did poor adults in ill health.[37] Both the Bennett Street and Dursley Tabernacle records show that Farr was correct, although those were cases in which youths did not work when their health incapacitated them because they belonged to sick funds. Even so, without bases for comparing Hawkins's findings with other groups at the same time or youths in other times, and especially without some idea of what Hawkins meant by 'middling' health, it is difficult to decide what this distribution means. Does it signify a worse health distribution than would be expected among all youths or among youths not working? Does it signify a health distribution that had deteriorated since Manchester had become an industrial city or that would improve when working youths were taken out of their factories (but not out of poverty)?

Scottish Friendly Societies, 1750–1821 and 1831–42

In Chapter 3, large data sets from the experience of friendly societies show how sickness risks are associated with age. These data pertain to the second half of the nineteenth century, and we shall encounter some of them again in the following chapter. They are mentioned now as a reminder about the importance of inferring sickness rates from sources that deal with large numbers of people whose ages are known, two requirements not met by the preceding case studies. The earliest known body of age-specific morbidity data derives from some Scottish friendly societies, surveyed in the early 1820s regarding claims experience during 1750–1821. Scottish friendlies were examined once more in the early 1840s by Francis G.P. Neison, Sr, with the study considering claims experience during 1831–42. Comparing the two results, we learn less about the trend of sickness between 1750–1821 and 1831–42 than about its distribution by age in the two periods and about some intriguing questions that the Committee and Neison put for the first time.[38]

The space between curves A and B in Figure 5.5 implies that the age-specific sickness rate increased from 1750–1821 to 1831–42. But some of the difference may be attributable to changing rules. During 1750–1821, some societies surveyed by the Highland Committee shifted from a practice under which members entered claims only if both sick and destitute to a practice in which claims related only to

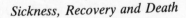

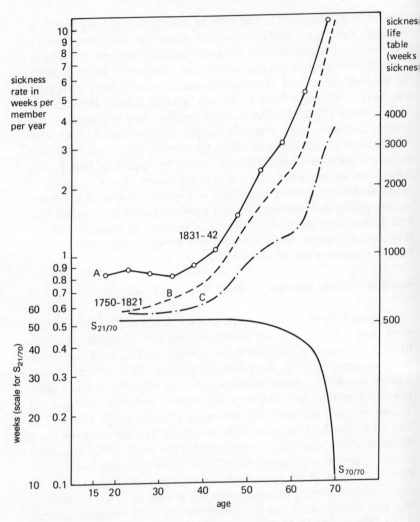

FIGURE 5.5 *Sickness in some Scottish friendly societies, 1750–1821*

SOURCE Committee of the Highland Society of Scotland, *Report on Friendly or Benefit Societies, Exhibiting the Laws of Sickness . . .* (Edinburgh, 1824).

health. The Committee knew this and adjusted the raw data it received, but it may still have underestimated the effect of this shift. The sickness rate probably increased, but the increase may be overstated in Figure 5.5.

Both curves nevertheless show that the sickness rate should be expected to increase with age in pre-1870 populations, as the figures in Chapter 3 have already shown applies to populations after 1870. Why, then, are the crude sickness rates reported above for the Plantin men and the Ashford women – 1 to 1.1 weeks a year – so low? Using the 1831–42 curve (curve B) in Figure 5.5 as a guide, we can see a leading part of the answer. The overall average sickness rate was low because the median age of sick fund members and of the entire adult population in seventeenth- and eighteenth-century Europe was low. Members under the age of 50 were sufficiently more numerous than members aged over 50 to make up for the sharply different gradients of sickness risk curves before and after 50. The Plantin men and the Ashford women recorded a low average rate of sickness because so much of the experience of their members concerned sickness in early adulthood and early middle age and so little of it concerned sickness after middle age. Acute episodes dominated because of the age structure of the population. Older people in the membership probably suffered chronic sicknesses in a way similar to their counterparts in more recent populations.

The members of the Highland Society's Committee, chaired by Charles Oliphant, calculated a life table and used it together with their graduated sickness schedule to construct the first known sickness life table. Out of 1000 members belonging to these Scottish friendly societies at the age of 21.5 years, mortality evidence indicated that 800 would survive to age 40, 528 to age 60, and 336 to age 70. Sickness liabilities would diminish as members died, and indeed the financial survival of the societies depended on these deaths. If everyone in the hypothetical 1000, or even a larger proportion than one-third, lived to the age of 70, when sickness claims were much higher, then the societies must fail. The Committee chose to express this relationship among age, sickness rate, and death rate by multiplying the age-specific sickness rates by numbers surviving out of the hypothetical 1000. Thus while age 21, the hypothetical 1000 would experience 575 weeks of sickness (1000 x .575). By age 40, this figure would have increased to 606 weeks, and it would have risen because the increase in the duration of sicknesses outpaced the decrease in the number of survivors. By 60, it would total 1239 weeks and by 70, 3596 weeks. Although only 336 men would be expected to survive to the middle of their 70th year of age, each of those would on average experience nearly 11 weeks of sickness. This is curve C in Figure 5.5; its vertical axis appears on the right side of the figure.

The Committee's calculations guide us toward another way of

expressing sickness risk, one analogous to the concept of life expectation. Rather than asking how long the members of each age group could expect to live, let us ask how much time they could expect to spend in sickness. This *sickness expectation* shows how much time lost from work would occur, assuming that each age group would, as it aged, have health experiences similar to those of people at those higher ages during the survey period. In this instance, a sickness expectation can be inferred only for ages 21–70 because the Highland Committee did not report work loss at higher ages. The Scots worked at higher ages, but members of these friendly societies were not numerous enough at ages above 70 to persuade the Committee that their experience was representative.

The fourth curve in Figure 5.5 is marked $s_{21/70}$ to $s_{70/70}$; its scale appears on the far left side ranging downward from 60 to 10 weeks. The letter 's' stands for sickness expectation, and the subscripts denote the ages to which the expectation applies. At age 21, Scottish friendly society members in 1750–1821 could expect 52.7 weeks of sickness through age 70. Virtually the same expectation would prevail until age 50. This is another way of saying that, between age 21 and 50, the size of each age group would shrink through deaths at about the same pace that the risk of being sick increased. Only after age 50 would the sickness expectation change noticeably, declining until about age 65 at a moderate pace and afterwards at a much more rapid pace. At age 70, the sickness expectation – 10.7 weeks of ill health while aged 70 – would equal the sickness rate. The sickness expectation curve identifies an important measure but it provides an incomplete example of it. The complete sickness expectation of Scottish friendly society members – that is, the expectation extending to death rather than age 70 – will not have decreased sharply after age 65 because their health experience, like their survival, did not stop at age 70. Even in incomplete form, however, the measure underscores how age composition affected the sickness experience of pre-1850 populations.

Sickness expectation can also be stated inversely, as health time or, in this case, future life time free of incapacitating sickness. In that form the expectation will include time in health, time in ill health but not incapacity, and a small body of time in uncompensated ill health (that is, the waiting periods). This limited version expresses a positive *health expectation* for some ages between 21 and 70 (h_{21-70}, h_{25-70} . . .); it appears in Table 5.3.[39] At age 21 members of these Scottish friendly societies could expect to live 35.5 of the 49 years to age 70,

TABLE 5.3   *Health expectation in the Highland Societies, 1750–1821*

Age	Life expectation	Health expectation
21–70	35.46 years	34.45 years
25–70	32.85	31.84
30–70	29.51	28.50
35–70	26.16	25.16
40–70	22.80	21.80
45–70	19.44	18.44
50–70	16.05	15.06
55–70	12.57	11.63
60–70	8.99	8.12
65–70	5.19	4.46

SOURCE   See Figure 5.5.

and to live 34.4 of those years in health. At age 50 they could expect to live 16.1 of the 20 years to age 70, 15.1 in health.

Neison's survey of experience in some Scottish societies from 1831 to 1842 provides another perspective on the issue of age composition as well as some new information. A man of strong opinions, Neison also had an intense curiosity. He asked not only how long the average sickness episode lasted at each age but also distinguished sicknesses ending in recovery from those ending in death. Table 5.4 reproduces some of his findings.[40]

If we use each column of figures in Table 5.4 to sketch in our mind's eye a picture of changing risk, it will be apparent that the progression is not always smooth. Although this survey dealt with more than 70 000 aggregate years of experience, the number of people in each age group in columns 2 and 3 was not always large. Even so, the results suggest clear patterns. The average duration of episodes rose with age. The risk of being sick was influenced more by age than any other known characteristic distinguishing members from one another. But the average length of episodes ending in recovery did not change much until the age group 51–55, when it more than doubled the average at 46–50. And the average length of episodes immediately before death sketched yet another curve, descending from ages 16–20 to 41–45 and then rising. In this population, long sicknesses struck especially the aged and *youths and young adults who died*. Lacking information about individual members, we cannot determine exactly how these protracted sicknesses ending in death were distributed among young adults. Certainly some died during

TABLE 5.4   *Durations of sickness in some Scottish friendly societies, 1831–42 (in weeks per year)*

Age	Average duration of each episode	Average duration of episodes resolved in recovery	Average duration of episodes resolved immediately in death
	(1)	*(2)*	*(3)*
16–20	3.6	5.6	19.0
21–25	3.9	4.1	10.9
26–30	4.2	4.8	17.3
31–35	4.4	4.0	14.6
36–40	4.9	5.0	8.5
41–45	5.9	5.3	6.0
46–50	6.9	5.1	22.2
51–55	8.5	11.6	25.1
56–60	10.9	11.9	44.2
61–65	15.2	21.5	83.8
66–70	24.2	47.9	60.0
71–75	32.6	84.0	134.7

SOURCE   Neison, *Contributions to Vital Statistics*, pp. 160–2.

acute infections. According to the survey in Figure 4.2 (p. 111) of the fatality curve in some diseases, deaths from acute infections are usually concentrated at the beginning of the episode. The extended episodes reported in Table 5.4 therefore suggest that some of the youths and young adults died after exceptionally long sicknesses, sicknesses so long that their lengths brought the overall average for these ages to the high figures given in column 3. That is, young adult sicknesses resolved in death seem to have fallen into two modes, one consisting of acute infections and the other of episodes more or less as protracted as those of people aged over 50.

GENERALIZATIONS

The case studies are few in number and deal with populations removed from one another in space and time. Some reveal more than others. These are important limitations, but they are not sufficient to paralyze curiosity. What are the common themes?

First, the studies that report sickness experience over time suggest that the compelling feature of ill health among sick fund members was not its persistence but its unpredictability. The sickness risk luctuated from year to year, in short waves, and in longer cycles. Even when the mortality risk was uniformly high, as it was in the Plantin fund throughout 1654–89 and in the Ashford fund after its youthful initiates attained middle age, the morbidity risk remained unpredictable.

Second, these studies indicate that working adults and youths lost relatively little worktime to sickness. In three cases – the Plantin males, the Ashford females, and the Bennett Street youths – the overall average was about one week a year, or about 2 per cent of potential working time. These rates understate actual sickness, because they count only compensated sickness, but they are too low to support an argument that, in the long run, ill health in the workplace was rife. However, sharp year-to-year fluctuations in sick time and the repeated reappearance of sickly years show that sickness among workers was episodically rife.

Third, the death rate does not appear to be a good predictor of the sickness rate, construed as either the risk of falling or the risk of being sick. In the Plantin work force, both duration and episode sickness rates described marked trends for the entire period and for subperiods within it, while the death rate remained stable. Experience in British friendly societies during the nineteenth century indicates that the risk of being sick rose with age along a curve quite similar to the risk of death. But even in the period before 1850, the sickness risk was dominated by episodes ending in recovery, and it is by no means apparent that fixed ratios prevailed across time.

Fourth, most episodes were comparatively brief. Among Plantin employees, the average claim lasted 3.2 weeks, and the average sickness warranting compensation was therefore 4.2 weeks (adding separate half weeks for uncompensated sick time on the beginning and recovery sides). Bennett Street Sick Society members entered claims lasting, on average, 4.5 weeks, these signifying 5 to 5.5 weeks of actual sickness per episode. Even though some sick fund members were sick for months or years at a time, the overall average remained within the realm of acute sicknesses as specified in the previous chapter. In some instances, these spells will have been relapses of chronic diseases, such as rheumatism, gout, or syphilis. This is a likely explanation for intermittent claims made by the same person, for example in the Plantin records. Those, too, constitute a minority of claims and episodes, so that the typical sickness took the form of a single episode lasting 4 to 5 weeks or less and occurring every 4 or 5 years.

More significant still, age did not dominate the duration of sickness in the way it would after 1850 because the aged made up such a small proportion of the adult population of the memberships. Bennett Street Sick Society members may all have been younger than any member of the Plantin fund, but their sicknesses did not last a markedly shorter time than those of Plantin workers. Acute sickness remained characteristic even as workers matured. The risk of falling sick continued to dominate sickness experience even in that part of life – age 45 and above – which, in later times, chronic sicknesses and the risk of being sick would dominate. This was so even though individuals who joined the workforce when young remained in the sick fund after they were disabled. To a substantial degree, the overall domination of acute episodes can be explained as an artifact of the age structure. Even though ages in the 1654 Plantin workforce are estimated to have ranged up to 61 or more, the average age was 40. At any given time through 1689, most members must have been in their 30s. Acute episodes dominated not so much because chronic sicknesses were absent – clearly they were not – as because sick fund members in these case studies were overwhelmingly youthful. At the same time, however, Neison's survey of experience in Scottish friendly societies during 1831–42 suggests that sickness lengths differed markedly between youths and young adults who would die and those who would recover. It also suggests that those who died included some who died only after extended sicknesses. Chronic sickness occurred at all ages, but it was concentrated in two parts of the population that were relatively small: a few youths and young adults who suffered extended sickness before dying, and the aged.

Fifth, the way the Highland Committee analyzed experience in some Scottish friendly societies from 1750 to 1821 guides us toward a new formulation: how much future ill health can we expect at each age? The information the Committee supplied allows only one form of the calculation: how much ill-health time could be expected from age 21 to age 70? The answer provides further insight into the ways in which age, mortality, and sickness risks worked together to influence sickness expectation. The sickness expectation of this one population remained stable from age 21 to age 50, which suggests again the degree to which sickness rates extracted from sick fund records from the seventeenth into the nineteenth century reflect the experience of young adults. Since sickness expectation is the inverse form of health expectation – how much health time could be expected? – the

Highland Committee's tables furnish the information required for a new vital statistic. Values given for this statistic in Table 5.3 have limited meaning, however, since they refer to ages 21-70 and to a particular form of this vital statistic.

Other generalizations find less support, either because the case studies disagree with one another or because there is no corroboration. Points for which no corroboration is available are most numerous in the Plantin experience, for which more complete records survive. In that population sudden deaths accounted for more than a quarter of the total. The falling sick rate amounted to about a third (31 per cent) of the being sick rate. And, regarding the odds of recovery, nine out of ten episodes ended in recovery rather than death. That is, even though the standard of judgment is the comparatively strict one of incapacity to work, and even though Antwerp remained open to the full array of seventeenth-century diseases, including plague, sickness typically ended in the resumption of work. Most of the printers and typesetters who fell sick could expect with some confidence to recover.

Finally, each case study is internally consistent, to the point at which it is reasonable to infer sickness rates from one year to the next, such as has been done for Figures 5.2 to 5.4. But the case studies are not mutually consistent; the sickness rates from one cannot be set against those from another to reveal a trend over time. Considering each one separately, it is apparent that trend appears to be an important feature. All of the case studies undermine the expectation of nineteenth-century actuaries, which was to discover a fixed age-specific sickness curve. We cannot see clearly what the overall trend of the risk of falling or being sick may have been, but we can compare the amount of variance in the case studies to determine whether there was a trend in the variance. The technique is to calculate coefficients of variation, which express the standard deviation of each series as a percentage of the arithmetic mean of each series. These calculations produce the following results:

Antwerp printers, 1654–89	73 per cent
Ashford women, 1791–1833	60 per cent
Bennett Street youths, 1816–35	18 per cent

The figures suggest a downward trend. Over time, the amount of variance declined, although the degree of decline is exaggerated by the reference to one group – Bennett Street youths – with a built-in tendency to less variance than the other groups because they belonged to a narrow age band.

CONCLUSION

Oft-repeated beliefs and assumptions assure us that ill health was characteristic of the general, and more especially of the working, population of Europe in the early modern era and during the early stages of industrial modernization. But this characterization conflicts with some of the features of the medical and demographic regimes of Europe between about 1600 and 1870, and with case study findings about sickness. It is inconsistent to expect high case fatality rates, frequent but short illnesses, high mortality, and widespread ill health in the surviving population. The measurement of ill health in a few small populations of working people suggests that the abiding characteristic was not poor health but variability in the threat of sickness. Clearly, we know too little about the history of sickness in the period before 1870 to draw firm conclusions. But we know enough to formulate some questions that need to be answered and in that way to influence the search for further understanding.

To admit the value of distinguishing between the risk of being sick and the risk of falling sick is to see at once some ways in which high mortality rates signal that the surviving population grew healthier as it aged. That is, the case fatality rates that are associated with the leading causes of death in seventeenth, eighteenth, and early nineteenth-century Europe are themselves evidence of the degree to which people who fell ill would die rather than recover. Each cohort faced a series of epidemics beginning perhaps with dysentery in infancy and extending through smallpox, measles, diphtheria, and other childhood diseases to typhoid fever in adolescence and typhus in late adolescence. By the age of 20, the cohort did not closely resemble its counterpart at birth precisely because it was made up of survivors. The sicknesses of the people who died do not show that ill health prevailed among the people who survived.

These observations lead us to expect a certain pattern in morbidity rates. First, regarding childhood and youth, we may suppose that the risk of falling sick was high if only because the frequency of exposure to infection was high. But the risk of being sick was low. Although illnesses were common, they did not long incapacitate the sufferer because they were for the most part infections with a short clinical course. Second, regarding adulthood, we may suppose that both risks were low to the degree that diseases with a short clinical course continued to dominate. Only the Plantin series speaks precisely to this point. The average duration of sicknesses in that population – 4.2 weeks including unobserved sickness time – still suggests a profile of mostly acute infections, a characterization reinforced by the high rate at which Plantin workers died suddenly (12 deaths in 44). Third, among the aged, who are poorly represented, we may suppose a stronger effect from chronic sicknesses, one resembling the pattern of Figure 3.1 (p. 70). Chronic sickness was clearly present among Plantin men and Ashford women and in the Scottish friendly societies, and chronic diseases made up a part of any physician's practice. But the aged were not numerous.

It is also significant that all the direct evidence at our disposal reports the experience of people with jobs. Their sickness rates will understate sickness in the overall population to the degree that people without jobs are likelier to have been disabled and to have suffered the chronic illnesses and disabilities that outside observers so often noticed. The health of working people was surely better than the health of people of the same age who did not work, even though some did not work because they were comparatively wealthy and may, for that reason, have had different health and mortality histories. Of people who worked but did not have formal jobs, such as women working at home and self-employed men and women, the evidence is suggestive but not revealing.

Finally, it is already apparent how difficult it will be to link case studies to one another in order to present a long-run historical trend. Although sickness was defined in much the same way in sick funds across Europe and from century to century, the characteristics of populations belonging to funds differed markedly. Most funds were small, which reduces the confidence we can have in the generalization of findings based on their data. The environment of work and of sickness has changed so radically over time that we must also suspect changes in the definition of sickness. Such changes will have been modest and gradual in the experience of any one group, but they may distort comparisons between groups. For this reason, the search must be directed not only toward inferring average sickness and mortality rates but also toward finding measurements that warrant comparison. Several have been suggested here – the coefficient of variation, the percentage of worktime lost, the health (or the sickness) expectation, the average duration of claims, the relationship between the risk of falling sick and the risk of being sick, and the odds of recovery – and they will reappear. If we cannot always link measured sickness rates directly, in the way that mortality rates are compared over time, we can nevertheless find indirect indexes that bear comparison over time.

6 Sickness in the Second Half of the Nineteenth Century

> So far as care of the body goes, it
> concerns a man more to know his
> risks of the fifty illnesses that
> may throw him on his back, than the
> possible date of the one death that
> must come.[1]

To enter the second half of the nineteenth century is to confront a choice. The volume of information about morbidity is much greater and extends through the European and Europeanized world, from Scandinavia to New Zealand. The record becomes richer in detail, revealing more about the individuals insured and more also about their sicknesses. Suddenly, the questions that might be answered exceed the space and resources available. My response will be to focus on the part of the world about which the most detailed information is available – Britain, especially England and Wales – and on questions attractive for their broad implications and for the degree to which they prepare us to understand twentieth-century sickness experience.

Before 1850 or so, it appears that short-run variations in morbidity overshadowed long-run trends. After 1850, however, the age-specific sickness rate established a certain trend at the same time that short-run variations continued to diminish in scale. A transition occurred, but it consisted neither of a shift in the leading causes of death nor of the epidemiologic transition, which is a shift from a mortality regime dominated by infections to a regime dominated by degenerative disease. It consisted instead of a shift toward recovery. The proportion of sickness episodes resolved in death in the short run declined, and the quantity of sickness, especially protracted sickness, increased at every age.

The emergence of a trend, and especially this trend, makes it more important still to distinguish the risk of falling sick from the risk of being sick and to devise ways of measuring the effects of each. Some of the methods are obvious. It will be important to calculate the average duration of sickness episodes, or of acute and chronic episodes. If that cannot be done directly, it must be done indirectly. The previous chapter introduced the notion of a sickness expectation: with a given body of sickness and mortality experience, how much ill-health time should be forecast? This chapter will expand that measure by distinguishing an expectation of falling sick from an expectation of being sick: how many episodes of sickness should be forecast? It is important to remember that the health expectation applies only to the population whose sickness and mortality experience will be measured. But this more detailed analysis will prepare us for another way of considering the relationship between sickness and death.

Records from the sick funds shed light on the sickness experience of people who lived in the past not because they measure ill health in the entire population but because they measure it in the central ranks of the working population and in ways that remain consistent over time. Late in the nineteenth century on the continent and early in the twentieth century in the United Kingdom, the terms of measurement shifted. The same basic test – capacity to work – remained central, but incapacity came to be divided into certain parts: the incapacity of job-related injuries, of old age, and of chronic disability. Each division removed exposure and sickness experience from the record, narrowing the definition of sickness applied in the sick funds. Thus began a profound and complex series of adaptations that made sickness increasingly difficult to measure in a consistent manner. In this chapter, the exploration of these issues will take up some ways in which economic factors influence sickness rates, some differences between insured and general populations, and the decomposition of sickness into illness and injury.

TREND

The second half of the nineteenth century is the first period in which it is possible to examine the sickness and mortality experience of large populations in which age is known, and in which locale of residence and occupation appear also in periodic surveys or censuses. The populations consist of the members of two familiar friendly societies that operated chiefly in England and Wales. The Independent Order of Odd Fellows Manchester Unity and the Ancient Order of Foresters enrolled large numbers of working males, and they invested in surveying sickness and mortality experience among their members the better to set premium and benefit levels for the future. Among the Odd Fellows, the surveys considered experience during the periods 1846–48, 1856–60, 1866–70, and 1893–97. Among the Foresters, surveys considered 1850–52 and 1871–75. The Odd Fellows implemented sickness tables constructed from the 1893–97 survey in 1912 and continued to use those tables until 1970, when they adopted modified tables. Other friendly societies concluded that the Odd Fellows tables were a sufficient guide and could be adjusted in simple ways for any differences between Odd Fellows experience and actuarial reports about their own experience. With some exceptions, notably the Rechabites, who required that their members abstain from alcohol, other friendly societies did not see the need to invest in their own surveys.

Odd Fellows or sometimes Foresters tables could be used by other societies not because they achieved the goal of nineteenth-century actuaries, which was to discover the law of sickness, but because they showed that sickness rates vary over time in certain patterns. These patterns were the subject of Chapter 3, which showed that the most important factor influencing the sickness rate, like the mortality rate, is age. Sickness and mortality rates are also influenced by gender, occupation, residence, health status, unemployment, and other factors. Some of these factors can be observed directly from actuarial reports or other sources, and some cannot.

In Figure 6.1, age-specific sickness rates have been plotted for the four Odd Fellows surveys. If we look only at the first three lines, concerning experience during 1846–48, 1856–60, and 1866–70, it is difficult to see any trend. The three lines cross one another; studying them, one can see why the actuaries expected to discover a fixed age-specific curve (the 'law of sickness') and why, as survey succeeded survey, they came to believe they had succeeded. When the Odd Fellows actuary Henry Ratcliffe published the results of the 1856–60 survey in 1862, most authorities believed that it so closely approximated the law that further investigation could turn to subtle points. When Ratcliffe completed his third and last survey, in 1872, it appeared as a *Supplementary Report* published in a few copies.[2]

But when we shift our gaze from the first three surveys to the fourth, it is clear that a trend had established itself. The sickness rate – here the rate of being sick – had increased substantially at every age. In

Figure 6.1, the increase consists of the gap between the 1893–97 curve and the earlier three. The curve of the risk of being sick had not changed shape, but it had shifted upward on the scale.

When did the trend increase begin, and did it continue after 1897? Case studies presented in the last chapter suggest that sickness rates had moved in waves or cycles before 1850 in individual sick funds with stable age structures. They had fluctuated over time in a way that might by itself explain the small deviations among curves from the first three Odd Fellows surveys. But those case studies leave us unprepared for a persistent trend, and they leave us unprepared for a trend emerging as the coefficient of variation narrowed. Waves or trends apparent in seventeenth-, eighteenth-, and early nineteenth-century sources can be attributed to fluctuations from year to year in the intensity of the sickness risk. In the second half of the nineteenth century, however, these fluctuations became muted and the sickness risk was no longer dominated by acute infections and epidemics.

The Foresters surveys show that sickness rates were higher in 1871–75 than 1850–52, and the Foresters were similar enough to the Odd Fellows to allow us to suppose that this indication can be applied to interpret the Odd Fellows surveys.[3] That is, the increase began before 1871–75, but after 1856–60. Timing on the other end is more difficult to fix because I am unaware of any other surveys in either organization after 1897, because the government began to compel employers to compensate employees for on-the-job injuries, and because a national insurance plan was introduced in 1911. Each modification changed the rules of the game, making it more difficult to determine the trend of sickness *as measured in the 1893–97 survey*.

The increase of sickness rates from 1866–70 to 1893–97 and perhaps beyond has striking implications. Those were decades in which mortality in England and Wales declined and per capita income and wages increased. They are also the period of the first phase of the epidemiologic transition, so called because the acute and infectious diseases that had dominated cause-of-death registers began to give way to chronic and degenerative diseases. In other words, the Odd Fellows experience suggests that morbidity increased at a time when mortality and the incidence of acute infections were declining and income was rising. Since this will seem counterintuitive to many people, it is necessary first to examine the four trends, especially the sickness trend sketched by the Odd Fellows surveys, to see how each trend has been detected and measured and, second, to consider whether the result is indeed counterintuitive.

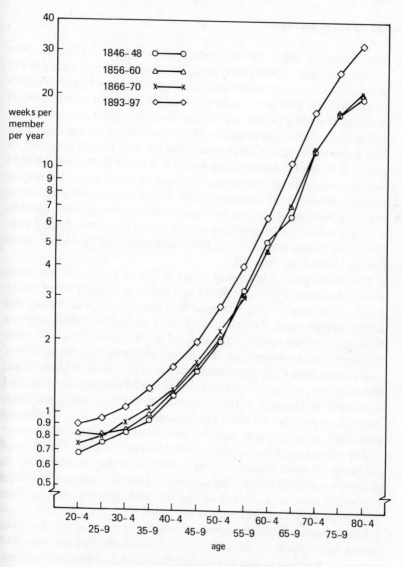

FIGURE 6.1   *Odd Fellows sickness rates, 1846–97*

SOURCE   Alfred W. Watson, *An Account of an Investigation of the Sickness and Mortality Experience of the I.O.O.F. Manchester Unity . . . 1893–1897* (Manchester, 1903), pp. 18–19.

Did Sickness Increase?

The testimony from the actuaries is unambiguous. Sickness rates among the Odd Fellows increased, and they increased because the average sickness episode became more protracted. The Odd Fellows resembled other friendly societies closely enough for other societies to apply Watson's tables to calculate their own premium schedules, and at the government's request Watson's tables were used to calculate expected sickness rates and costs for the British program of national insurance inaugurated in 1911. The 1893–97 Odd Fellows survey seemed such convincing evidence because several other inquiries pointed in the same direction. Besides the increase shown in the Foresters surveys, Sutton's extended report on some friendly societies providing 1876–80 experience to the Registrar showed sickness rates higher than those in Ratcliffe's survey of the Odd Fellows during 1856–60 or 1866–70.[4]

This is compelling testimony that the risk of being sick was rising among friendly society members and rising in every part of adulthood. Over time, these organizations found they had to pay out longer claims, and the minutes of their meetings reflect conflicts between their members, who resisted higher premiums, and their managers, who reported on the annual accounts and the actuaries' conclusions about the implications of those accounts. What is more, the actuaries considered whether the increased sickness rate might be attributed to changes in the composition of the friendly societies. Watson, a member of the Odd Fellows actuarial office, reviewed Ratcliffe's tables, which included breakdowns by both occupation and residence, and found that the Odd Fellows of 1893–97 remained similar to those of earlier surveys in the trades they followed and in geographical distribution. He concluded that the increase could be explained only as a change in the average duration of episodes: sicknesses were more protracted in 1893–97.[5]

Much rests on Watson's investigation, but it is not always a simple matter to interpret his findings. He found that the sickness rate had increased because sicknesses among the Odd Fellows had become more protracted rather than because there had been any change in the risk of falling sick. But he reported the number of claims by treating each year in his five-year-long survey as a new claims period. Episodes continuing into a second year were counted as a second claim, a procedure that inflated the number of claims. When Watson computed the average duration of claims, he reported figures that fo most ages barely exceed Neison's figures on the Foresters during 1871–75, even though the Odd Fellows sickness rate in 1893–97 was much higher than the Foresters rate in 1871–75.[6] Nevertheless, Watson's conclusion – that the risk of being sick had increased – was sound. That sicknesses became more protracted is apparent when the proportions of claims for different durations are compared. Between 1866–70 and 1893–97, claims lasting from 27 to 260 weeks increased by 26 per cent, and from 105 to 260 weeks by 82 per cent.[7] Protracted claims increased in every age group but most sharply among young adults, and at longer durations.

Although the finding that the risk of being sick increased while the risk of falling sick remained approximately stable may also seem counterintuitive, it is in fact central to the explanation of why sickness increased in the demographic and economic circumstances prevailing in England and Wales, and among the Odd Fellows, in the last three decades of the nineteenth century. To explain this, let us consider first the relationship between the Odd Fellows, or friendly society members in general, and the overall population.

The Odd Fellows Order represented what is often called a select part of the population. Use of this label runs the risk of creating confusion because 'select' has a specialized meaning in insurance investigation and a general and different meaning in ordinary usage. In terms of insurance, 'selection' refers to attempts to reduce risk by allowing some applicants to obtain coverage and denying coverage to others. The process is contentious, if only because the grounds for selection have usually been established before evidence was accumulated to show they were appropriate, and because, once in place, selection denies the insurer access to data on people with undesired characteristics whose experience might be compared to that of applicants who obtained coverage. (Some observers also maintain that political or human rights override the insurer's right to discriminate among applicants.) Whereas it is manifest that some people live much longer than others, it is also, as we saw in Chapter 1, manifestly difficult to decide in advance who is most likely to be long-lived. This is the selection issue that faces life insurers. It is troubled enough in the late twentieth century, after decades of intensive investigation into the mortality experience of insureds and the general public. It was more troubled still in the nineteenth century when few such investigations had yet been undertaken.

For the friendly societies, the issue was very complex. From the perspective of the friendly society's financial well-being, the optimal

candidate for insurance was someone who would live a long life
without sickness. Friendly society actuaries noticed, however, that
this was a self-contradictory hope. The longer an average member
lived, thereby deferring the society's payment of burial benefits, the
likelier it became that the society would pay out heavy sickness
claims. That is, the friendly societies could not select people for
characteristics believed to be identified with long life without also
selecting people who seemed likelier to require the much higher
sickness compensation of the aged. The response of the friendly
societies to this dilemma was straightforward. Applicants would be
examined about their health status and history, and individuals with
serious health problems would be denied admission. Since the typical
applicant was a young person aged 18 to 25 with a job, the rejection
rate was low, much lower, for example, than rejection rates for
military recruits. Nineteenth-century actuaries who compared the
claims experience of new members with established members of the
same ages found that the selection effect in this form was insignificant
after one or two years.[8] Some members soon developed traits that
would have been grounds for refusing admission, but the societies did
not expel members because they became unhealthy (and rarely
denied claims even when there was reason to suspect a fraudulent
characterization of health at application). In short, friendly society
members were 'select' lives in the sense understood by insurers, but
selection in this form had little bearing.

The more important features of selection relate to the way this
word is used in general parlance and to a process of selection that
began before application and continued after admission. The friendly
societies served people threatened by the loss of their wages during
illness and injury. That is, they served people with jobs, mostly jobs
requiring physical labor and paying modest wages. Friendly societies
often enrolled the upper strata of the working class, which Eric
Hobsbawm designated the 'labour aristocracy'.[9] But they also enrolled ordinary skilled workers, farm laborers, domestic servants,
and people following many other occupations. A majority of the
working classes belonged to friendly societies and, among these
people, more belonged to the Odd Fellows than to any other society.
From 1866 to 1870 the Odd Fellows enrolled some 262 000 men,
about 4.5 per cent of the male population of appropriate ages and a
higher part of the population with regular employment. That proportion had increased by 1893–97.

The friendly societies did not serve the rich, who were obvious but not numerous in England and Wales in the second half of the nineteenth century, and they did not serve the poor and unemployed, who were obvious and numerous. The ranks of applicants were therefore thinned by social and economic processes which ensured that many members of the 'working classes' would not obtain the regular employment that made it reasonable to contemplate paying weekly, monthly, or quarterly premiums, or to feel apprehension about the effects sickness might have on their wages. They did not have regular wage incomes. The same form of selection operated after admission. Members who lost their jobs lost the ability to pay premiums and, strictly speaking, the need for insurance against the loss of wages which they no longer earned. Most people who seceded from the friendly societies, and secession was a regular feature of friendly society experience, did so by failing to pay premiums. Sometimes this lapse was associated with migration or with a decision that the costs of belonging outweighed the benefits. Given the job insecurity and levels of unemployment and underemployment that prevailed in nineteenth-century Britain, as well as the recurrence of business cycles, secessions must be linked also to jobs lost.

In this form, selection by attrition was important, for it meant that the friendly societies distanced themselves from the people served by Britain's poor laws. Members who lost their jobs would be carried on the books for some months, even a year or longer, so that they could resume paying premiums when they reacquired jobs. But the individual who remained unemployed for a long period, or who fell into destitution before becoming disabled, would no longer be assisted. These people depended on poor relief, and the friendly societies successfully resisted efforts by local authorities to force them to contribute to the relief of former members.

This brief discussion shows important ways in which the experience of Odd Fellows, Foresters, and members of other friendly societies will have failed to resemble that of the overall population. Among adult males, the people whose health and mortality is unobserved consisted of the poor, the unemployed, and the elite. The poor and the unemployed outnumbered the elite, and it is reasonable to suppose that they had higher sickness and mortality rates than did friendly society members. Thus sickness rates drawn from friendly society experience probably understate the rates of being and falling sick in the unobserved and in the overall population at any given time. But the sickness *trend* prevailing among friendly society members should capture the trend prevailing in the society as a whole. The characteristics of the observed population – friendly society members – remained stable through the period in question, and the Odd Fellows lived amongst the people whose health experience we can no longer reconstruct. That is, of course, something that defies proof, simply because we cannot reconstruct the health experience of the unobserved part of the population. For this reason, I prefer to focus on the Odd Fellows themselves and their counterparts, people in the central ranks of the working population, in considering the conjunction among morbidity, mortality, income, and epidemiologic patterns.

Conjuncture

The key period is 1870 to 1900, and the key segment of the population consists of the central ranks and central ages of the working population. Among males in England and Wales and among the Odd Fellows, mortality declined in the age groups 20–24 to 45–54 and remained stable at ages 55–64 (as appears in Figure 6.2). Among the Odd Fellows, the sickness rate increased in all age groups but at a somewhat higher pace among older than younger members. However, the incidence of protracted sickness, especially of very protracted sickness, increased most among younger members. Protracted sickness had already been common among aged members; it became more common among them and appeared as a prominent feature of sickness in young adults.

Odd Fellow mortality began the three decades at lower levels than mortality in the general population, and it remained lower through 1893–97. The difference can be attributed to selection, more especially under the second, general meaning of the term. Compared to the entire population of adult males, but especially to the poor, Odd Fellows were regularly employed and adequately housed, fed, and clothed. For most of them, moreover, work meant exercise and fitness.

Over the same period, average weekly wage earnings rose while retail prices declined (also Figure 6.2), signifying substantial gains in real wages. These measures of material well-being do not speak specifically to Odd Fellows, but they are shaded toward the central ranks of the working population, the kind of people who made up most of the Odd Fellows membership, because most sources on wages speak only to that part of the labor force.

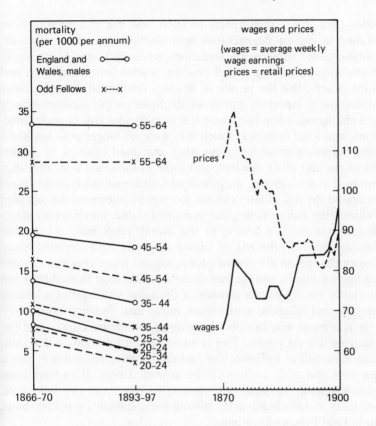

FIGURE 6.2 *Demographic and economic trends, 1870–1900*

SOURCES B.R. Mitchell and Phyllis Deane, *Abstract of British Historical Statistics* (Cambridge, 1971), pp. 38–9; Watson, *Manchester Unity*, pp. 18–19; C.H. Feinstein, *Statistical Tables of National Income, Expenditure and Output of the U.K., 1855–1965* (Cambridge, 1976), T140–T141.

The epidemiologic transition is more difficult to date and to characterize quantitatively.[10] Although it appears in the cause-of-death registers as a shift from infectious, mostly acute, to chronic, often degenerative diseases, the difficulty lies in deciding how much significance this shift possesses by itself. The age structure of the population changed with the profile of diseases causing death, and much of the changing cause-of-death profile can be attributed to the shifting age structure. Males who died in England and Wales in 1901 were older than their counterparts in 1871, and for that reason alone likelier to die of degenerative and chronic than acute diseases. Undoubtedly, some acute infections were declining as causes of death. Into this category fell cholera, scarlet fever, smallpox, and some others. But the profile of diseases contracted did not change substantially, especially among adults. More people survived infancy and childhood, when they were still at particular risk to acute infections, and lived to ages at which they were no longer at so marked a risk. Surviving acute infections, they remained exposed to chronic infections and other diseases, and some of the acute infections they survived (for example, streptococcal infections and typhoid fever) increased the risk of later chronic disease. Furthermore, among Odd Fellows, the risk of falling sick remained stable, and it seems plausible to transfer this finding to the overall adult male population. Among children, the risk of falling sick may have declined, since known changes in the disease profile suggest fewer episodes of some leading infections. But the best-documented change in morbidity and mortality among youths consists of declining virulence of a leading streptococcal infection, scarlet fever, rather than declining morbidity.[11]

It is unclear whether the changing age structure outweighed the changing disease profile. This is an important question, with significant implications for historians and epidemiologists, but it is also a question that does not need to be answered here. Both transitions were underway at once and, working together, the two influenced mortality and morbidity in the overall population in a way that shows up in Odd Fellows experience.

About the same proportion of each adult age group in the Odd Fellows fell sick in 1893–97 as in 1866–70, but those who fell sick were sick for longer periods. They died later in each specific episode or recovered later, or both. Such outcomes would be expected if medical therapies improved, and there are some reasons to suppose that they did. Injuries and surgical cases were treated more successfully at the end of those three decades as antisepsis and asepsis reduced case fatality rates. Although Odd Fellows consulted physicians in order to obtain claims at the beginning as well as the end of this period, the advice they received may have changed. Physicians may have begun to recommend rest – time off from work – at an earlier stage in certain diseases – for example, tuberculosis. Such a regimen might not influence the outcome, but it would lengthen sickness claims. In short, therapy may have played some role in the prolongation of sickness, especially in increasing the proportion of episodes in which leath was deferred or avoided. This is another instance in which qualitative sources – physicians' records – must be consulted in order o resolve questions unanswered by quantitative sources. Public health reforms and the improving standard of living may also have contributed. These, too, are complex issues that cannot be settled here, nor do they require settlement in order to see why morbidity increased while mortality diminished.

Comparing the Odd Fellows of 1893–97 to their counterparts in earlier surveys, Watson observed that they remained unchanged in terms of occupation and residence. Increased sickness could not be attributed to shifts toward more hazardous occupations, to migration toward unhealthier locales, or to changes in age structure. But he did not consider how declining mortality should be expected to influence sickness rates, and this is the key. The composition of the Odd Fellows population had not changed in the ways Watson suspected it might have. But it had changed: a smaller proportion of members died at each age. This alteration in the mortality regime influenced the sickness regime. To see how it did so, consider again the discussion about insult accumulation in Chapter 2. Mortality declined not because the risk of falling sick declined – that is, not because the Odd Fellows were exposed to fewer diseases – but because the sicknesses they did experience were resolved less frequently in death. The pace at which insults accumulated remained unchanged, but the outcome did not. Each successive age group contained members who lived longer lives and, on balance, the new survivors were people who had experienced more rather than less illness and injury. Morbidity increased because mortality decreased. The composition of the Odd Fellows changed toward people who had accumulated more insults because they had survived longer.

The Epidemiologic Transition Redefined

Without losing its character as a shift in leading causes of death away from infectious toward degenerative diseases, the epidemiologic transition needs to acquire two further characterizations. First, it was also, and perhaps more profoundly, a sign of change in the age structure of the population which in turn brought changes in the disease profile. These changes were related to age prevalence. Although high fertility reduced the average age of the population, more people in late nineteenth-century Britain died of chronic and degenerative diseases because more people lived through the ages in which acute infectious diseases were the leading causes of death into ages at which degenerative and chronic infectious diseases had been and remained the leading causes of death. This aspect of the transition is not especially marked in the comparison between 1870 and 1900 because relatively little change occurred in age structure in those three decades. But it is marked when the age structure of eighteenth-century populations is compared with that of late nineteenth-century populations.

Second, the transition consisted of longer lives, and the longer lives meant that more people lived into the right-hand side of the morbidity curve, and especially into its sharpest upward angle. More survivals into advanced ages increased the overall quantity of sickness in the population in a revolutionary manner. The curve of the risk of being sick as sickness was measured in the friendly societies resembled the curve of the mortality risk, as we have seen above. But the risk was no longer as evenly spaced across the ages to which people lived as it had been in earlier populations. By the late nineteenth century, it was coming to be dominated by people who lived toward its highest rather than its lowest points.

What is more, the decline of mortality without any compensating decline in the risk of falling sick signals that, among the Odd Fellows at least, people who survived in the new mortality regime but who would not have survived in the old had already experienced more sickness and were on those grounds still likelier than the average member of their age group to experience additional sickness. They were 'impaired lives' in the limited sense that survival of earlier sickness meant, at the population level at least, an accumulation of insults and therefore greater risk of future sickness, especially protracted sickness. The composition of each successive age group was shifting toward a higher average propensity to be sick. Earlier discussion (in Chapter 3) suggested reasons to suspect that this higher propensity was composed of the average of two quite different groups. One group may have been made up of people who had experienced little sickness and who therefore carried with them a lower risk of subsequent sickness. The other was made up of people who had experienced more sickness *but had survived*; they carried a higher risk of subsequent sickness. The second group had always existed, but now they were a sizeable part of the population. Their share was growing. And it was already large enough to drive the overall average of each age group's sickness to a higher level.

Among the Odd Fellows, the aggregate sickness rate may have increased less sharply than it did in the overall adult male population to the degree that the overall population had been winnowed more radically by higher mortality rates. A sharper decline in overall population mortality seems consistent with a sharper increase in morbidity, as the overall population shifted in composition toward a larger proportion who had survived more ill-health episodes.

SICKNESS, THE WAGE LEVEL, AND UNEMPLOYMENT

The phenomenon under observation in insurance sources was and is not sickness itself but the submission of claims. To be paid, claims required evidence of illness or injury compelling enough to persuade a physician or another third party that the claimant was incapacitated for work. Nineteenth-century observers understood that claims and sickness did not overlap exactly.[12] For one thing, the same level of incapacity had different effects depending on the job a friendly society member held. A clerk could work with disabilities that would incapacitate a miner. Thus the occupational composition of a friendly society's membership might influence sickness rates if the composition shifted toward or away from more hazardous or more physically demanding jobs. Furthermore, economic cycles influenced sickness rates even if the direction of influence was and is not always clear. A surge in unemployment might persuade some workers to report to work even when sick in order to protect their jobs, and it might persuade other workers to feign sickness in order to collect compensation in lieu of unemployment benefits. Higher real wages might lower the threshold of what workers considered incapacity by bringing workers to a target income sooner, or higher real wages might induce workers to raise the threshold of what they considered incapacity in order to spend more time at work earning the higher wages. These problems are central to the understanding of how labor markets operate, and they are unresolved. They cannot be resolved here, but we can examine the impact these choices had on sickness rates in late nineteenth-century Britain. If sickness rates were chiefly or even to an important degree produced by economic rather than health considerations, that distortion can be expected to show up when economic indicators and sickness experience are compared.

The Odd Fellows and Foresters usually collected information in the form of five-year surveys and reported findings as averages over the five years. These surveys cannot be used to probe associations between sickness rates in the friendly societies and wage, income, and unemployment levels in the overall working population. Only one large-scale longitudinal survey of a society with a broadly dispersed membership has come to light. The actuary Ralph Price Hardy studied experience in the Hearts of Oak Benefit Society over the period 1884–91 and reported his findings in the 1894 *Journal of the Institute of Actuaries*, giving annual as well as aggregate values.[13] Established in 1842, the Hearts of Oak had enrolled 153 595 members by the end of Hardy's survey, a membership large enough to provide reliable estimates of sickness experience for the age groups 20–24 to 55–59. In Figure 6.3, its annual sickness rates appear together with curves plotting three measures of economic performance: the unemployment percentage, the per capita gross domestic product at constant prices, and index numbers of average weekly wage earnings deflated by means of a retail price series.[14] To the side of each plotted line appear the results of a calculation about the direction of change, given in the form of a slope value. Large positive or negative values indicate a marked trend, and this procedure makes it possible to estimate the degree of association between two variables by comparing their change over time. (It would be preferable to estimate association by means of coefficients of correlation, but the time series is not long enough to produce coefficients that warrant much confidence.) A large positive slope value, such as appears for the wage index, indicates sharp upward movement: workers in the United Kingdom enjoyed sharply rising real wages from 1884 to 1891. A large negative slope, such as appears for the unemployment rate, indicates sharp downward movement: unemployment among skilled workers, the only group measured in this period, declined.

The important conclusions to be drawn from Figure 6.3 are these three. First, age-specific sickness rates fluctuated little. Last year's rate was a good predictor of next year's rate in each age group. Second, each economic variable established a strong trend, and unemployment, the factor to which we would expect sickness claims to have been most sensitive, fluctuated sharply. Third, from appearances, it is difficult to detect associations within the several series. Sickness rates peaked together with unemployment in 1886, but they did not fall uniformly thereafter as unemployment declined. They did rise uniformly between 1890 and 1891, when unemployment increased. Sickness rates increased as real wages and per capita income rose but at a much weaker rate.

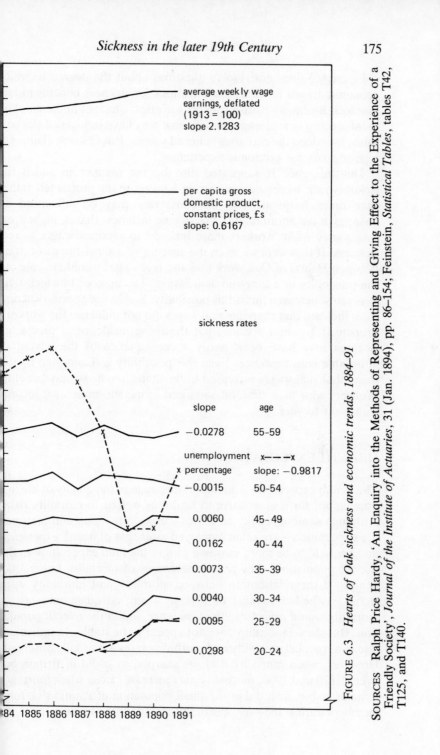

average weekly wage
earnings, deflated
(1913 = 100)
slope 2.1283

per capita gross
domestic product,
constant prices, £s
slope: 0.6167

sickness rates

slope	age
−0.0278	55–59
unemployment	
percentage slope: −0.9817	
−0.0015	50–54
0.0060	45–49
0.0162	40–44
0.0073	35–39
0.0040	30–34
0.0095	25–29
0.0298	20–24

'84 1885 1886 1887 1888 1889 1890 1891

FIGURE 6.3 *Hearts of Oak sickness and economic trends, 1884–91*

SOURCES Ralph Price Hardy, 'An Enquiry into the Methods of Representing and Giving Effect to the Experience of a Friendly Society', *Journal of the Institute of Actuaries*, 31 (Jan. 1894), pp. 86–154; Feinstein, *Statistical Tables*, tables T42, T125, and T140.

Figure 6.3 does not resolve questions about the degree to which economic trends influenced applications for sickness benefits in late nineteenth-century British friendly societies. Changes in the employment level or in real wages and income may have influenced sickness rates, as indeed the actuaries believed was so. But sickness claims are a poor proxy for economic experience.

This inference is supported also by the manner in which the sickness rate increased: sicknesses became more protracted rather than more frequent. The work-loss rate may be influenced by changes in the affordability of sacrificing income – that is, higher real wages may make workers more inclined to sacrifice wages to real sickness. If that were so, even the absence of a short-run association between Hearts of Oak work loss and real wages would not rule out the possibility of a long-run association. The manner in which sickness rates increased limits this possibility. Stable age-specific sickness rates indicate that changing real wages did not influence the worker's propensity to enter a claim, but the rising incidence of protracted sickness may have been partly a consequence of the advent of affordable convalescence. Even this possibility is diminished by noticing that real wages increased faster than friendly society benefits. Workers who took time off sacrificed more and more real income from year to year.

HEALTH EXPECTATION

The health expectation is an important gauge of the quality of life in a population, for it is sensitive to health as well as to mortality risks. Although some mortality measures – especially infant and maternal life expectation – are often employed as gauges of health experience and are held to be more sensitive gauges than life expectation in the overall population, they remain measures of mortality rather than health. If the relationship between mortality and morbidity were stable – whether parallel or inverse – any adequate measure of mortality would reflect health at each age and in the overall population. But the relationship does not appear to be stable. In individual diseases, parallel mortality and morbidity rates are usually observed. However, when mortality declines sharply, as it did in Britain between 1870 and 1900, morbidity may increase. Even when mortality remains stable, as it did in the small population of Plantin sick fund members during 1654–89, morbidity may describe its own trend. In the aggregate and over time, the relationship between these two measures is uncertain and demands further exploration.

Health expectations provide additional information and in a form analogous to the measure of life expectation itself. Like the calculation of a life expectation, the health expectation relies on the life table and the assessment it presents of the risk of death at each age. From that point, however, the two techniques depart. The life table is a basis for obtaining the sum of years lived at all subsequent ages in the population under study, thereby to arrive at a life expectation for each age. For the health expectation, the life table serves as a basis for calculating either the sum of ill-health time at future ages and a value that can be designated the *expectation of being sick*, or the sum of ill-health episodes at future ages and a value that can be designated the *expectation of falling sick*. Each series draws on its counterpart risk, using the age-specific risk of being sick or falling sick rather than the death rate as a second basis for calculation. The health expectation relates the amount of remaining life that will, according to these data, be spent in good health.[15] In sum, three versions of the expectation have now been introduced:

(1) the sickness expectation (or the expectation of being sick), represented in Figure 5.5 for Scottish friendly society members from 1750 to 1821, which is a statement about future *ill-health* time;

(2) the health expectation, which is a statement about future *health* time; and

(3) the expectation of falling sick, which is a statement about the number of future ill-health events.

Neison's survey of experience in the Ancient Order of Foresters from 1871 to 1875 permits a calculation of the three expectations. They appear in Figure 6.4 together with two additional curves, life expectation and sickness expectation at ages 18–70. At age 18, when men were first admitted to the Foresters, they could expect to live nearly 42 years, which is to say they could expect to die at about age 60. The second additional curve reports a sickness expectation limited to ages 18–70; it is useful for comparing the experience of the Foresters to that in the Highland Societies, encountered in the last chapter in Figure 5.5 (p. 148).

Each curve in Figure 6.4 is distinctive; each measures a different kind of experience. The sickness expectation, which is a measure of the cumulative duration of future ill-health time, rose gradually with age among the Foresters. At 18, the future time of incapacitation for work totalled 2.4 years. At its peak, during ages 72–73, this measure

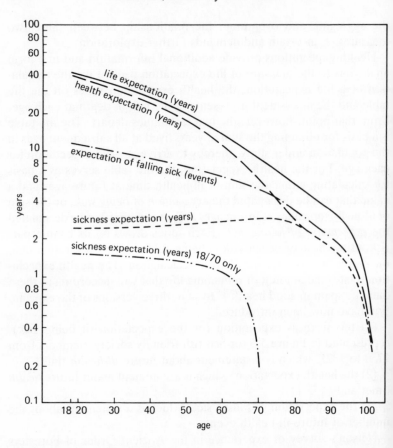

FIGURE 6.4   *Life and sickness/health expectations among the Foresters*

SOURCE   Francis G.P. Neison, Jr, *The Rates of Mortality and Sickness According to the Experience for the Five Years, 1871–1875, of the Ancient Order of Foresters Friendly Society . . .* (London, 1882), pp. 35–6 and 53–6.

reached 2.85 years. In old age, it declined. The expectation of falling sick, which is a measure of the number of ill-health events to be expected, shows that the 18-year-old Forester could expect an average of nearly 12 episodes of incapacitation through the remainder of life.[16] From that point forward, the Forester aged somewhat more rapidly than he lost life expectation, so that, at age 60, he retained an expectation of living 13.5 years more. He also aged more rapidly than he shed expected sickness episodes. At 60, he could anticipate somewhat more than six further ill-health episodes. Finally there is the health expectation curve, the positive version of the sickness expectation which here, as in the case of Scottish friendly society members, has a limited meaning.[17] It shows a health expectation beginning close to the life expectation but declining more rapidly with rising age until this curve converges with the sickness expectation curve at age 82.[18]

Only 'order of magnitude' conclusions are warranted, but the Foresters living in England during 1871–75 experienced longer if not also more frequent sicknesses than had Scottish friendly society members from 1750 to 1821. When nineteenth-century actuaries compared Highland experience to that of English and Welsh workers in the 1820s and afterwards, they were surprised to discover lower age-specific sickness rates among the Scots. They tried to explain that by finding reasons why some sicknesses might have been overlooked. We approach the same comparison from a perspective different in two ways. First, the prior experience we have observed suggests that age-specific sickness rates were probably more variable in earlier periods but were also lower. Highland society members with an average age of nearly 39 lost 1.117 weeks per year, which is more than Plantin workers during 1654–89 with about the same or a slightly higher average age. Second, we have discovered reasons to expect that morbidity rates may increase in periods in which the mortality rate was declining. The committee gathering Scottish experience investigated a period during which (as we know but they did not) the crude mortality rate was declining.[19] That is, we encounter Scottish sickness rates from 1750 to 1821 having reasons to expect that they will be intermediate between earlier and later observations, and that they will have tended to rise, rather than expecting, as the actuaries did, that later sickness rates would be equal to or lower than earlier rates. Living a half century and more after their Scots counterparts, the Foresters of 1871–75 could anticipate higher life expectations and could expect to live more years between ages 18 and 70. But they could also anticipate longer periods of ill health.[20]

ILLNESS AND INJURY

Sick funds in general and friendly societies in particular counted sickness as incapacity to work caused by illness or injury. Toward the end of the nineteenth century, the states of Western Europe began to require that employers compensate employees for industrial accidents.. This legislation introduced a distinct category of sickness, one composed initially of job-related injuries that would eventually grow to include job-related illnesses. Only a portion of all injuries would be covered by such legislation, which excluded accidents away from the workplace. Nevertheless, the legislation calls attention to distinctions that may be made between illness and injury, to the place of each in sickness rates, and to the question whether determinants of injury or illness risk may be distinctive. The transition from an era free of legislation or possessing only ineffectual laws toward an era of effective regulation provides some opportunities to consider these issues.

What part of earlier sickness claims should be assigned to illness and what part to injuries? Because the sick funds elected to treat sickness as a problem of function rather than diagnosis, the evidence on this point is comparatively fragmentary. From British sources, it consists of case studies, which may leave unnoticed certain features (such as whether the ratio between these two risks changed over time), impressions derived from experience but unsupported by statistical findings, and statistical studies of occupation-specific sickness rates. These sources suggest two things. First, people following different occupations were to some degree subject to illnesses peculiar to their occupations, but those tended to balance one another. What was left unbalanced was the risk of injury, which differed markedly between non-hazardous and hazardous occupations. Occupation-specific sickness rates varied chiefly because of differences in the risk of job-related injury.[21] Second, the leading hazardous occupations were mining, quarrying, iron and steel manufacturing, seafaring, and heavy outdoor labor. People following those trades entered significantly more sickness claims, to the point that some friendly societies refused to admit them.

Figure 6.5 shows how different regimes of injury risk affect sickness curves by contrasting experience among the Odd Fellows as a whole with the experience of non-hazardous occupations (categories A, H, and J) and the most hazardous large-scale occupation, mining (category G), among the Odd Fellows.[22] The important point is not irregularity in the curves (especially the two curves for miners, which are based on comparatively small numbers) but the manner in which injury hazards affect overall shape. In the extreme form represented by miners, the injury risk could alter the sickness curve. In the risk of

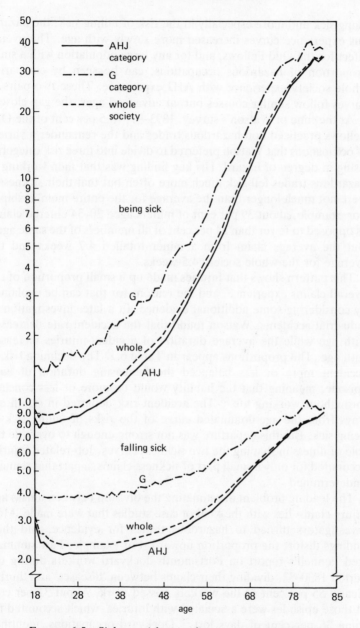

FIGURE 6.5 *Sickness risk according to occupational hazard*

SOURCE Watson, *Manchester Unity*, pp. 138–41, 176–83, and 200–13.

being sick and more especially in the risk of falling sick, the hazardous experience curves increased more slowly with age. The overall
effect for the Odd Fellows, and for any large population with a small
proportion of hazardous occupations, can be seen by comparing
whole society experience with AHJ experience. These two pairs of
curves follow similar courses but, at advanced ages, the gap closes.

At the time of Watson's survey, 1893–97, 78.5 per cent of the Odd
Fellows practiced non-hazardous trades and the remainder a variety
of occupations that Watson preferred to divide into three risk categories
rising in degree of hazard. His key finding was that men working in
hazardous trades fell sick much more often but that their sicknesses
were not much longer than the average for the entire membership.[23]
For example, about 39 per cent of miners aged 30–34 entered claims
as opposed to fewer than 24 per cent of all members of the same ages.
But the average claim from a miner totalled 4.7 weeks and the
average for the whole society 4.5 weeks.

This pattern shows that injuries made up a small proportion of the
overall claims experience, and the reasons for that can be explained
by considering some additional evidence. In a later investigation of
industrial accidents, Watson found that the accident rate decreased
with age while the average duration of accident-injuries increased
with age. The proportions appear in Table 6.1. The declining risk of
accident more or less balanced the increasing duration of each
episode, meaning that the liability would be more or less constant
throughout working life.[24] The accident risk departed in significant
ways from the age-dominated curve of the risks of falling sick or
being sick. But this departure was not strong enough to override the
role of illness in shaping the two sickness curves. Job-related injuries
accounted for only a small part of sickness claims, a part that remains
undetermined.

The leading problem in estimating the division between illness and
injury claims lies with the kind of case studies that were made. Most
investigators turned to hazardous trades for evidence, and their
findings distort the proportion upward. For example, Farr summarized Pennell's report on Portsmouth dockyard workers during the
period 1830–32, dividing their claims between 'diseases' and 'hurts'.
Nearly 55 per cent of the workers missed work. About 31 per cent
of those episodes were associated with injuries, which accounted for
some 36 per cent of days lost.[25] Dockyard occupations, identified
later in the century as hazardous, posed a serious risk of injury.
Another survey, Walter Dickson's study of Custom House officers in

TABLE 6.1 *Accident claims by age*

Age	Accident rate	Average duration per claim
Under 20	16 per cent	2.6 weeks
20–29	15	3.7
30–39	14	4.0
40–49	14	6.2
50–59	10	7.1
60 and over	6	7.0

SOURCE Adapted from Alfred W. Watson, 'Some Points of Interest in the Operations of Friendly Societies, Railway Benefit Societies, and Collecting Societies', *Journal of the Institute of Actuaries*, 44 (Apr. 1910), p. 211.

London and Gravesend from 1854 to 1874, found much lower accident rates. About 10 per cent of all episodes were attributable to accidental injuries and external violence', a category broader than job-related injury, and those injuries accounted for 11 per cent of time lost from work.[26]

The part of sickness claims that can be assigned to injury rather than illness will depend on occupations followed in the population under consideration and on whether the category of injuries is meant to exclude those not associated with work. No fixed ratio between illness and injury should be expected. Except when hazardous trades dominate, illnesses should be expected to override injuries in economic circumstances like those prevailing in nineteenth-century Britain. Shifting attention from that place and period, however, it appears also that the injury risk has distinctive characteristics, the more so as legislation influences the identification and counting of accidents. We cannot yet see clearly the ways in which employer liability for job-related injuries would reshape sickness insurance, but we can see that employer liability refashioned the measurement of sickness in an important way.

1893–97 AND BEYOND

The terms of reference have suddenly shifted in several ways. First, certain injuries have been taken out of consideration. The friendly societies no longer needed to pay claims for job-related injuries, although in practice British societies adjusted gradually rather than abruptly to the provisions of the Workmans Compensation Act of 1897, which required employers to pay half the wages forgone because of employment-related injuries, and to later legislation.[27] Watson had divided Odd Fellows experience into four occupational categories in order to show that, age and gender aside, the sickness rate was influenced more by occupation than any other variable. He prepared those tables at a moment when the experience of individuals at little or no risk to job-related injuries became dramatically more important for, with employer compensation, the AHJ tables rather than the whole society tables could provide the basis for estimating future sickness rates.

A second way in which the terms of reference shifted suddenly in Britain and elsewhere lay in the inauguration of retirement.[28] Among the working classes of the nineteenth century, work had generally continued as long as the individual remained capable. The friendly societies provided reduced compensation – sometimes as little as one-quarter of wages – for long-term disability and thereby created the chance of relinquishing employment without going on poor relief. But they did not make the practice of retirement general, and they did not settle the question of when retirement should occur. In Britain those issues were settled by the Old Age Pensions Act of 1908, which furnished a state-funded pension to all workers at age 70 (later 65).[29] Like employer liability, the generalization of retirement, and specifically its generalization among manual workers, required the intervention of government and the replacement of worker-funded savings by publicly funded transfer programs. Labor force participation by men age 70 and over declined sharply.

A third shift in the terms of reference occurred with the National Insurance Act of 1911. This measure made friendly society benefits compulsory for certain categories of workers (mainly weekly wage and small salary earners), using existing societies to manage the expanded program. At its outset, the people newly insured under the act included only those currently employed and therefore no one completely disabled.[30] Although Odd Fellows experience provided the basis for estimating sickness rates under the act, the two bodies of experience were not directly comparable and would never be so again. In 1946, compensation was extended to most of the populace. After 1911, and especially after 1946, friendly society coverage of work loss came to be regarded as supplementary to the subsistence level coverage of the national insurance benefit.[31]

The net effect of these and other innovations has been to detach sickness compensation for certain segments of the employed population: manual workers injured on the job, people age 65 and over and, more recently, people with protracted and disabling illnesses and injuries however acquired. Thus the population at risk has changed. When in 1911 friendly society sickness compensation was extended from wage and small salary earning members to all wage and small salary earners, no significant changes were expected in sickness rates (except regarding the initial acceptance of only people with jobs and changes associated with rule differences). The part of the population previously covered closely resembled the population newly covered (except that there was no medical selection under the 1911 act).[32] In the longer run, however, the population at risk did change, as workers with disabling illnesses and injuries found compensation from other sources and withdrew from those whose experience was counted on either side of the fraction: episode (or time) divided by people at risk.

Sometimes called the 'healthy worker effect', this change in the population at risk profoundly influences both the morbidity trend and the morbidity curve observed among employed people.[33] Regarding trend, this effect may lead to a situation in which an increase in age-specific morbidity in the overall population is masked by a decrease in age-specific morbidity in the employed population. Permanent or protracted disablement for work at any time before retirement is lost from sight in morbidity statistics concerning currently employed people, whereas it remains under observation in the friendly society series. Hence friendly society sickness curves rise more steeply with age than curves inferred from the experience of the currently (that is, presently and recently) employed alone.

On the one hand, we might expect sickness rates among the Odd Fellows, as among other beneficiaries of the first National Insurance Act, to have declined merely because of the redistribution of some experience, especially protracted sickness, to other programs. That is, we might expect a step-like series of reductions in the age-specific sickness rate if sickness were defined and measured in the same way after 1893–97 merely because blocks of the sick were transferred to other programs. On the other hand, we might expect age-specific rates actually to have diminished if we believe that twentieth-century medical innovations reduced either the incidence or the duration of ill-health episodes, or that other changes contributed to the creation of a healthier population.

There are other reasons, too, why it is difficult to determine the trend of sickness in Britain after 1893–97. Changing the rules in as many ways as they have been altered since 1897 means a still more complex shift in the area of motives and inducements. Each change both alters the terms of any trade-off between income and leisure (here considering sickness as one form of leisure) and adds fresh combinations to the statistical problem of measuring this trade-off. Although I am unaware of any compelling grounds to do so, we tend to believe that the capacity for change grows as proximity to the present nears. For example, observers of sickness experience are prone to suggest that workers have recently altered the threshold between capacity and incapacity, usually by lowering it. However, the same observers are willing to believe that in the more distant past the threshold was fixed, usually at an ideal state at which workers worked even when they were sick.[34] And, finally, a shift from five-year survey periods (with the years selected for periods in which economic, epidemiologic, and other distortions were likely to balance) to year-to-year assessments means that what actuaries call 'subjective factors' may once again bear heavily. In this instance, they are notably important, for the five decades after 1897 contained a series of shocks: legislative innovations, world wars, severe business cycles, and the influenza epidemic of 1918. The confusion produced by these shocks is apparent in learned commentary on British sickness rates and their trend between the 1920s and 1950s.[35]

In short, a fine scholarly problem is posed: untangle the confusion that contemporary observers felt about the sickness trend. Until this puzzle has been worked out, any estimate remains tentative. The most compelling tentative estimate is this: the trend observed between 1866–70 and 1893–97 continued thereafter, but it continued haltingly and in a fashion influenced to an increasing degree by factors previously of little importance. Before 1900, the most important factors to work out in valuing friendly societies were age and occupation. After 1900, these were joined by what amount to rule changes, that is, changes in the complex of incentives and disincentives influencing employees, employers, physicians, and public authorities in decisions about whether to enter, accept, tolerate, or pay for sickness claims. These forces can be illustrated by returning to experience in the Guild of St George Friendly Society, organized in Carrington, near Chester, around 1837.

Surviving records tell the story of sicknesses among the men and women who belonged from 1873 through 1946 excepting only one year, 1885.[36] This experience is summarized in Figure 6.6, which

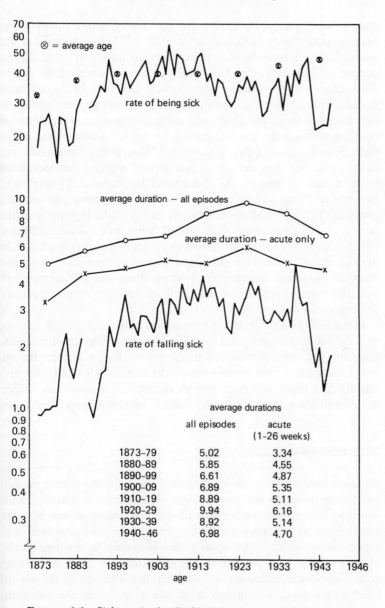

FIGURE 6.6 *Sickness in the Guild of St George Friendly Society,
1873–1946.*

SOURCE   Cheshire Record Office, Chester, DDX 186.

shows three points. First, the average age of Guild members in creased until about 1893 and again after 1923. On grounds of age alone, sickness rates would be expected to have increased slightly during 1873–93 and after 1923 but to have remained stable during 1893–1923. Second, the rate of being sick increased in the last three decades of the nineteenth century, and at a faster rate than is likely to be accounted for by the small increase in average age. It continued to increase through the pre-war period, as did the sickness rate of the Odd Fellows. During the First World War, claims diminished be cause some members were in service and the military shouldered the costs of their sicknesses. As in National Insurance Act experience the rate of being sick increased from 1921 (the early post-war de pression) to 1927. It declined sharply in 1929 (the beginning of the later post-war depression). The rate of falling sick followed a similar trend. Third, sicknesses continued to become more protracted. The average duration of all episodes increased more than did the average duration of acute episodes even when these are distinguished as episodes lasting up to 26 weeks. Until the 1940s the spread between the two measures widened.

In the Guild of St George the transition into and the early decades of the twentieth century did not diminish the incidence of sickness. Even though the mortality of its members declined, even though other authorities took over some of the claims that the Guild pre viously had paid, and even though therapeutic innovations helped build confidence in medicine, the sickness rate continued to increase.

THE DEFERRAL OF DEATH

Sickness became more protracted after 1870. In the earlier period, insofar as fragmentary sources inform us, most sicknesses were resolved in recovery rather than death, and most sicknesses were brief. Even at advanced ages, the typical episode lasted less than eight weeks, which is an appropriate boundary to distinguish the clinical course of representative acute infections from the longer course of chronic infections and degenerative diseases. In the overall adult population, and therefore all the more so in the complete population, sicknesses were short because such a small part of the population survived to the ages at which chronic disease was common as well as because acute episodes continued to occur at older ages.

These characterizations emerge from reviewing information presented above.[37]

After 1870, the death rate declined – which is to say that the
average case fatality rate of all illnesses and injuries fell. Recoveries
became still more numerous in proportion to deaths. It is clear that
the likelihood of dying while sick diminished but it is not apparent
that the likelihood of falling sick declined. Formerly, death had been
associated chiefly with brief illnesses and had often been the sudden
aftermath of a sickness too brief to be recorded as a claim. Before the
1870s, however, death in adulthood in Britain had come to be
associated with extended sickness, and by the 1870s the association
was blatant (Table 3.4). It would develop further thereafter. Yet it is
one of the most puzzling of findings, for the appearance and development of deaths preceded by protracted sickness seems to be a sign of
definite influence over the timing of death. In some aspect of epidemiology, medicine, or self-care, the sick patient acquired the
capacity to defer death. But the acquisition preceded the 'medical
revolution' of the 1930s. It occurred in the earliest stages of sanitary
and public health reforms, which in any case seem an unlikely arena
for explanation. And it occurred apparently in the early rather than
the late stages of rapid growth in real personal income.

Although several authorities have offered explanations for the way
in which mortality changed after 1870, the explanations disagree with
one another.[38] To add morbidity experience further complicates the
problem and elevates the importance of the discussion.

CONCLUSION

Much rests on knowing the trend of sickness over the last century or
so. In truth, determining this trend will be more difficult than I have
suggested. Consider the evidence from Carrington once more. The
sickness risk declined during each world war and during two de-
pressions. That is, it declined when times were good (full employment and rising wages) and when times were bad (unemployment
and falling wages). There is no particular logic to this pattern. The
reverse might just as readily be expected. The economic theory that
informs analyses of lost work time suggests that more unemployment
may cause workers to do whatever they can to hold on to their jobs or
to turn to alternative sources of income, such as feigned sickness.

Likewise it suggests that higher wages may either increase or diminish the wage earner's propensity to take time off from work. Nearly everyone has an opinion about the direction in which the labor supply curve shifts. The opinions seem to be biased toward the view that workers value leisure over income, but the doctrine of universal consent was dismissed already in the eighteenth century as ground for accepting the validity of an hypothesis. On the basis of the small sample consulted here, it is not apparent that the labor supply curve shifts in a consistent direction.

Seemingly contradictory options appear also in medical theory. Therapeutic innovations that diminish the risk of dying may have little influence on the risk of falling sick, and they may promote an increase in the risk of being sick. In the aggregate, anything that promotes an aging of the population also promotes an increase in the sickness risk. In every circumstance, age remains the leading factor influencing the sickness risk, and in both of its forms, but especially in sickness duration, that risk rises rapidly with age. Moreover, there remains the vexing issue of threshold. Do communities raise or lower the threshold at which, on average, their members count themselves incapacitated for work in ways that are not associated with factors already identified? We can see that this threshold will shift as the mixture of jobs changes. It will be lower when more people work at physically demanding jobs bearing a high risk of injury and will be higher when more people work in less demanding and less hazardous jobs.

Much depends on knowing the sickness trend, because we cannot decide the significance of any present-day health measurement without knowing whether it is something higher or something lower than past measurements. Now, on the verge of examining recent experience, what facts and reasonable inferences can we marshal about the longer historical trend? First, until the latter part of the nineteenth century, sickness appears to have moved in waves. Although additional series may show pronounced trends, especially during early periods of declining mortality risk, *long-run* stability is a remarkable feature of age-specific and age-adjusted series up to about 1870. Another remarkable feature is short-run instability. The sickness risk fluctuated from year to year, often violently, and much more sharply than did the mortality risk.

Second, the two forms of the sickness risk – falling and being sick – describe distinctive patterns and expectations. To live in a regime in which the risk of falling sick is high and coincides with significant case fatality rates is to live in a regime in which the risk of being sick must be diminished except among those people who have natural or acquired resistance to common diseases. Considered as a risk of falling sick, the sickness expectation would rise sharply in childhood, *because* survivors acquire the prospect of subsequent illnesses, and decline in adolescence and adulthood, as acquired immunity diminishes the proportion of the profile of diseases to which people remain susceptible. That is, at birth the individual is projected to fall sick but a few times, and this expectation holds *because* the case fatality rate is high and resistance and acquired immunity are low. Considered as a risk of being sick, in contrast, the sum of the time the individual can expect to spend in ill health rises for a much longer period. The Foresters experience speaks to a later and different population but it can be compared with the sickness expectation of members of Scottish friendly societies during 1750–1821. The Scottish experience suggests lower annual sickness rates, which appear to be plausible but may be unduly low. And it has been curtailed at age 70 whereas Foresters experience has been estimated through the life course as well as for ages 18–70. If we suppose that the risk of being sick had been lower in the early nineteenth century and before (as seems to be true on the basis of other case studies), we see nevertheless that the expectation of being sick will have increased for a much longer part of the life cycle, until perhaps age 70 or so. Survivorship carried with it the opportunity of more ill-health time, and more ill-health time from one year of age to the next.

Another way to illustrate this point is to compare Guild of St George experience with earlier measures of dispersion in sickness rates. It is, of course, undesirable to make a great deal from small sets of data. But this particular measure depends on small case studies because by substantially enlarging the body of experience we move automatically to lower coefficients of variation. Considering once again only the period of stability in average age, 1893–1923, the coefficient of variation for the Guild of St George is 18 per cent. The lower level manifest in the narrow age band of Bennett Street Sunday School Sick Society members during 1816–35 has appeared now in a group of adults. From year to year, both the risk of falling sick and the risk of being sick remained more nearly stable and therefore predictable. The situation has reversed itself. Sharp short-run variations within a stable long-run risk have given way to short-run stability within a pronounced long-run trend.

Third, the ill health gained by longer average lives consisted chiefly

of more protracted rather than new episodes of sickness. The more
life expectation gained, the more the aggregate risk of being sick
increased. Since we know that age is the dominant factor influencing
the sickness rate, this relationship is not surprising. What is more
unsettling is the discovery that the expectation of being sick increased
at every adult age in England and Wales between 1870 and 1900.
During a period in which mortality declined sharply and the risk of
falling sick remained approximately stable at each age, the risk of
being sick increased. Years added to life meant that the expectation
of being sick increased in these years. But we are now in possession
of evidence indicating that it increased more rapidly still because the
amount of sickness increased *at each age.*

These trends created certain consequences for the future: still
longer lives and continued increases in sickness rates at each age. The
continued increase could be masked by deletions from the sicknesses
that would be counted, deletions taking the form especially of protracted episodes transferred from the friendly society experience that
had served as the basis for estimating rates to other agencies and
organizations. The evidence at our disposal suggests not only that the
age-specific sickness rate continued to increase after 1897 but that it
also increased more than the figures provided in this chapter will
show. The increase of life expectation at each age coincided with an
increase in the expected amount of sickness at each age, and the
amount of sickness would continue to increase as long as the life
expectation also increased.

There was a transition between 1850 and 1900. It was a transition
from an age of death to an age of sickness.

7 Sickness and Death in the Twentieth Century

Illness became chronic and degenerative.[1]

Twentieth-century observers sometimes express puzzlement about what seems to be a paradox in health demography: as the death rate shrinks toward the minimum consistent with the human life span, ill-health rates and health spending rise rather than decline. But there is no paradox. Even if we set aside other reasons why health spending might increase in real terms – such as greater access to physicians and health facilities, a shift from less to more costly health problems, the earlier or more comprehensive discovery of health problems, and greater awareness of health problems – reasons why ill-health rates and health spending should be expected to increase are apparent. They follow from increased numbers of the aged in the population, the prevalence and duration of ill health among the aged, and the intractability of many sicknesses of the aged. They follow also from changes in the composition of the population that occur *because* of the decline in the death rate. And they follow because the decline of death rates is a sign that health conditions are improving, but not that health itself is improving. Focusing on the mortality and morbidity experience of males in the United States since about 1880, this chapter will show that it is possible to take away from and add to factors determining health. Following male experience makes it easier to compare this part of the record with earlier periods, in which male experience is better known than female.

Three models inform us about ways in which the sickness risk changes over the life course. First, the senescence model (discussed in Chapter 2) attributes health status to endogenous processes that remain inadequately understood but manifest themselves in the obvious signs of what we call aging. The endogenous processes cannot be avoided or reversed, although some researchers hold that they can be slowed. It is inescapable that an aging population will require more health services and an aged population more still. The requirement may go unmet, and there is room for argument about the adequacy with which it has been met at any time and place. From

193

an historian's perspective, what is striking is that health personnel and facilities have expanded in the last century even more rapidly than the population.

The second model about changes in the sickness risk over the life course attributes health status to the combination of prior ill-health experience and present health risks. According to insult accumulation theory (also discussed in Chapter 2), individuals and cohorts experiencing more ill health early in life are likely to experience more ill health later in life also. Some prior insults are endogenized and become part of a complex that influences whether future sickness will occur, especially in forms noticed clinically. This theory suggests that a population is always divided in two ways. Some cohorts experience more ill health than others, and they carry that experience through their life course. Some individuals within a cohort experience more ill health than others, and this division tends to polarize the cohort: its members gravitate toward future ill-health rates either above or below the average but not toward the average itself.

The third model concerns not the life course so much as the profile of illness and injury risks faced in a given period and region, that is, the health environment. It was introduced in Chapter 4 and discussed in terms of some representative diseases confronting seventeenth- and eighteenth-century Europeans. The sickness experience that we can measure over time consists, however, not of specific diseases so much as of episodes. Although we can learn something about the diseases said by lay and medical observers to have been leading causes of death in a given place and time, we lack reliable statistical sources about the diseases causing illness but not death and about the incidence of those diseases. Due to the limits of the sources we possess, the disease-specific model has been pushed into the background here: it is a profile known well enough in terms of the identity of some major diseases but, until the middle of the twentieth century known poorly or not at all in terms of disease-specific morbidity rates. Here health is distinguished from ill health by means of evidence about functional impairment rather than by diagnosis. The standard by which functional impairment is ascertained must either remain constant or come to us with sufficient information to allow its standardization in order to identify trends. It is also important that the impairment of function is closely associated with age, in a manner similar to the way in which age influences the kinds of diseases that will be suffered. But the leading feature of this third model consists of the reoccurrence of sickness risk over the life course and over time

In terms of present needs, the third model reminds us that many risks are neither endogenous nor endogenized but consist instead of fresh insults.

In the long historical frame of reference, it is apparent that the *age* of the population is an important determinant of health status and ill-health rates, and also that the tendency of *aging* to push ill health rates and health spending upward is limited. The most important limiting factor is the human life span. Unless the life span is found to be manipulatable, aging must encounter a ceiling. In recent discussion, the ceiling has come to be thought of in terms of a rectangularized survival curve–a situation in which nearly everyone born survives to the modal age of death. Since that situation is being approached in some countries, it follows that a transformation has been underway in those countries.

The transformation has two aspects. First, there has been a long period of declining death rates. In that period, which in many parts of Western and Central Europe began around 1740, was suspended from about 1820 to 1870, and renewed after 1870, the composition of the population changed continuously because declining death rates altered the characteristics of survivors in every higher age group and in the overall population. This part of the transformation has not been completed, but the latitude for further change is bounded by the human life span, the unlikelihood of eliminating all existing causes of death at ages below the limits of this span, and the likelihood that political, cultural, and behavioral causes of death will continue to evade medical or scientific remedies.

Second, the transformation can be thought of in terms of the mean or median age of the population located on a curve of the risk of being sick, or still more effectively in terms of the aggregate expectation of being sick – the expectation of an entire population and the expectation of cohorts within a population. The value of these expectations is at once a function of the distribution of people by age and their prior health experience. Cohorts that have experienced more ill-health episodes will continue to experience more ill health as they age (because the portion of the cohort whose health status has been compromised will be larger than in cohorts that experienced less ill health). If, over time, the risk of falling sick also declines, then it follows that the pace of insult accumulation will turn downward. Cohorts that experience more sickness in childhood will carry that experience to their extinction. But if they are followed by cohorts that experience markedly less sickness, the subsequent cohorts should be expected to suffer less ill health later in life insofar as insult accumulation in this specific form influences the risk of falling or of being sick. Reducing ill health rates at lower ages should be expected to reduce ill health rates when the cohorts affected arrive at all higher ages.

Such an effect might be forecast for the American baby boom cohorts, people born from 1946 to 1964. While it is not clear whether the key risk in insult accumulation consists of falling or being sick, the baby boomers enjoyed lower risks in both forms. Their births coincided with the introduction of immunizations that saved many of them from experience with common infectious diseases that had compromised health in prior cohorts. The baby boomers also grew up with chemotherapies far more effective in limiting the severity and duration of illnesses still experienced than any available to predecessors. The baby boomers cannot escape aging, and they have not escaped all exogenous health hazards. If the sum of their insult accumulation experience consisted of diseases avoided by immunization or reduced in severity or duration by new drugs, then the baby boomers would already display a marked advantage in mortality and morbidity rates over people from earlier cohorts at the same ages. There are signs of such an advantage, as this chapter will show. But there are signs also of compensating morbidity and mortality risks which leave in doubt the net effects of health experience in cohorts born since 1946.

With this chapter the focus shifts from Britain to the United States. The shift follows a principle articulated earlier in this book: sickness and death will be examined where the sources are strongest. Mortality data for the US are not, compared to several European countries, notably reliable before the 1930s. But morbidity experience has been surveyed for a longer continuous period in the US than in any other Western country.

MORTALITY AND MORBIDITY IN THE UNITED STATES SINCE 1880

Mortality Trends

'The period from 1850 to 1915 [especially after 1880] witnessed unprecedented improvements in the health of Americans.'[2] This is the impression Edward Meeker obtained after investigating life expectancy, mortality, and cause of death records. Although sources about sickness experience in the nineteenth-century US – counterparts to the friendly society records from Britain – remain to be uncovered, Meeker's judgment should be refined. The risk of death – especially the risk of death in childhood from infectious disease – declined sharply, as he observed. The causes and circumstances of this decline were sufficiently similar to those prevailing in Britain from the 1870s forward to indicate that in the United States, too, the risk of being sick increased in the aggregate among adult males, and increased in each age group as well. The US cause-of-death data alone are evidence of this. The risk of dying decreased in combination with a shift in causes of death from acute infections to the chronic diseases that by 1900 led the list of causes. Together the two trends signal longer average episodes of sickness, at least among those dying.

The American population began to age, and it began to do so earlier and more rapidly than the British population because in the US fertility declined earlier than in Britain. An older population required more and different health services, and it intensified concern about making economic provision for old age. Understood vaguely rather than well, these shifts prompted a search for additional information about the death rate, life expectation, and ill health, and about insurance and pension programs in force in other countries where similar changes were underway. Census authorities attempted, beginning in 1880, to discover the number of Americans age 15 and above unable to work because they were sick or disabled. Between 1880 and 1933, the US death registration area – the region in which vital statistics were gathered on a regular basis – was expanded from a small part of the country (Massachusetts, New Jersey, the District of Columbia, and several large cities) to all the states. William Franklin Willoughby investigated sickness and other insurance programs in force in Western and Central Europe, aiming to advise private and public authorities in the US about useful precedents. An actuary for the Travelers Insurance Company published the first table of sickness experience in the US. Irving Fisher addressed the Association of Life Insurance Presidents on 'Economic Aspects of Lengthening Human Life', and argued that the life insurance companies could promote still greater gains in life expectation by supporting public health reforms. Lee Frankel and Louis Dublin inaugurated sickness surveys in Boston, Pittsburgh, North Carolina, and other sites, using agents of the Metropolitan Life Insurance Company as canvassers.[3] This search for information and understanding – of which these are but a few examples – provided the United States for the first time with detailed vital statistics, which are the basis for an investigation of sickness and mortality experience.

The first events to be counted accurately – deaths – form the subject of Figure 7.1, which provides crude and age-specific death rates for the male population from 1900 to 1985.[4] The comparison of lines in this figure shows the extent to which age has influenced changes in the death rate. In general, the rate of decline has been inverse to age, highest in the low age groups and lowest among the aged. The influenza epidemic of 1918 and the four wars in which the US has engaged all appear in some age groups but not in others.[5] In the long historical framework, the noteworthy feature of this diagram is, however, the infrequency rather than the frequency of mortality peaks, especially of peaks caused by epidemics. Although local epidemics are likely to be left obscure by national experience covering such a large territory and population, it is obvious that epidemics have lost considerable importance.[6]

To be understood in the way required here, Figure 7.1 should be examined for some factors relating more especially to periods and others relating more especially to cohorts. To prepare for this, it is useful to review what the figure shows about changes in the death rate as different cohorts passed through each age category. For example, the cohort born between 1900 and 1904 appears first in the age groups 0–1 and 1–4 and then moves gradually through all other age groups with the passage of calendar years, attaining the group '85 and over' in 1985 and thereafter. Consider the information in Figure 7.1 in terms of trends within each age category:

0–1 more or less continuous decline at a similar rate (a feature that shows up because the scale is semi-logarithmic)

1–4 a rapid decline prevailed throughout, but the rate of decline was more rapid between 1935–39 and 1950–54 than before or after

5–14 similar to 1–4 but lower on the scale (that is, the decline began from a lower starting point)

15–24 decline prevailed until about 1950; disregarding the influenza epidemic of 1918 and additional casualties associated with war, the rate of decline was greater from 1935–39 to 1945–49 than earlier; after 1945–49 the trend stabilized (although the death rate was somewhat higher during the late 1960s and 1970s than during the 1950s and early 1960s)

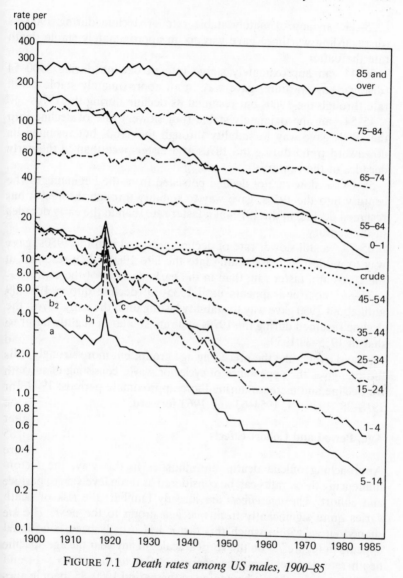

FIGURE 7.1 *Death rates among US males, 1900–85*

SOURCES US, Department of Commerce, *Historical Statistics of the United States: Colonial Times to 1970* (Washington, 1975), pt. 1, 61; US, National Center for Health Statistics, *Vital Statistics of the United States: 1981*, DHHS Pub. no. 85–1101 (Washington, 1986), II, part A, 3 and 36–48; and US, National Center for Health Statistics, *Monthly Vital Statistics Report*, 34, no. 13 (19 Sept. 1986), 15.

25–34   an approximately stable rate of decline during 1900–54 (disregarding wartime) gave way to an approximately stable death rate thereafter

35–44   an approximately stable rate of decline during 1900–54 (disregarding wartime) gave way to an approximately stable death rate through the 1960s but resumed its decline during the 1970s

45–54   an approximately stable (but slower) rate of decline into the 1950s gave way to stability through the 1960s but resumed its downward trend during the 1970s at a faster pace than in the early decades of the century

55–64   a slow rate of decline persisted from the beginning of the century into the 1950s, gave way to stability through the 1960s, but resumed decline in the 1970s at a faster rate than in the early decades of the century

65–74   a still slower rate of decline persisted into the 1950s, gave way to modest increase lasting into the late 1960s, then resumed in the 1970s at a faster rate than in the early decades of the century

75–84   no trend appears until 1935–39; decline during 1935–39 until about 1950 gave way to stability lasting until the early 1970s; the decline resumed during the 1970s at a rate similar or slightly faster to that of 1935–39/1950

85 and over   like the preceding age group, but more strongly still, this one gives the appearance of cycles or waves consisting of successive decline and increase during these approximate periods: 1900–18, 1918–28, 1928–54, 1954–63 and 1963 forward.

Age, Period and Cohort Effects

Approaching official death rate statistics in this way, the factors influencing those rates can be considered at three levels: age, period, and cohort. The *age effects* are already familiar: the risk of death varies quite significantly from one age group to the next. The U-shaped curve within which this factor has usually been considered appears in Figure 7.1 on the vertical scale: in any year the age-specific death rate declines from the age group 0–1 to the group 5–14 and then rises again. At the beginning of the period 1900–85, people ages 0–1 were at about the same risk of death as people ages 85 and over; by the end of it, that risk had fallen sharply and infants faced a lower risk of death than people ages 55–64. That is, the largest gains in life expectation continued throughout to occur among infants.

In considering the second factor, *period effects*, one effect occupies a long background position, three are identifiable with specific years, and a fifth is to be added further on:

(1) *Circa 1850–1970*. A secular improvement in the standard of living began around the middle of the nineteenth century and continued into the 1960s. It was characterized by rising real income per capita and the acquisition within the central ranks of the adult population, the working classes, of added discretionary spending (that is, the option of buying goods and services not required for subsistence). In the long run, discretionary income paid for more spacious housing; medical services; superior public services, including sewage systems, water purification, public assistance for the poor that improved their nutrition, housing, and access to medical services; and other benefits. Most authorities believe that these changes explain a significant part of the mortality decline that began later in the nineteenth century, but it is difficult to attribute specific parts of the decline to specific elements in the overall improvement of the living standard.

(2) *1935–54*. Especially for the age groups 1–4 and 5–14, the death rate declined more rapidly during the period 1935–54 than before or after. There seems to have been a mild acceleration in the rate of decline of the death rate during those 20 years for some other age groups (15–24 to 45–54, 75–84, and 85 and over), but it is difficult to distinguish this period effect in the age groups 55–64 and 65–74. The effect identified in this way was an immunological and chemotherapeutic revolution, meaning the introduction and dissemination of immunization against many prevalent childhood infections and the use of sulfa drugs and antibiotics that suddenly and sharply increased the efficacy of medical care.[7] Before 1935, medical texts acknowledged that physicians could do little to treat many common infectious diseases; by the 1950s, the clinical course of diseases subject to treatment with new drugs had been curtailed.[8] The effect of new immunizations and drug therapies was felt most sharply in children, among whom immunity acquired through vaccination diminished the risk of falling sick at the same time that new drugs shortened the clinical course of may illnesses still experienced. The revolution had less impact on people from ages 15–54 to the extent that they already possessed immunity to common childhood diseases or, having matured to higher ages, no longer stood at risk to childhood diseases to the same degree. It had little or no effect on death rates in the age groups 55–74. But, because some of the new drugs were especially effective at deferring death from some chronic diseases that were

leading causes of death among the aged (for instance, pneumonia), death rates also declined in the age groups 75–84 and 85 and over during this period. The revolution in therapies did not stop in the middle of the 1950s, but its capacity to lower death rates within the overall population approached exhaustion.

The introduction of drugs that shortened the clinical course of many diseases and injuries also shortened the average duration of many disease and injury episodes. All other things being equal, the risk of being sick would be expected to have declined.

This period effect has dominated thinking about health and life expectation in the mid and late twentieth century. So impressed have observers and beneficiaries been with the conquest of infectious disease that it has become axiomatic to claim, as the American Surgeon General did in 1979, that 'the health of the American people has never been better'.[9] The improvement in health is undeniable in many forms. But the claim is also generalized too broadly, as this chapter will show.

(3) *The 1960s*. During this decade the death rate stabilized among the age groups 1–14 and 35–84 while it increased in the age groups 15–24 and 25–34. Overall (as the line in Figure 7.1 for the crude death rate shows), there was no change. This transient stabilization awaits satisfactory explanation; some of the leading factors behind it seem to be increased motor vehicle mortality, homicides, and suicides, especially among young men, and a lull between exhaustion of the immediate effect of therapeutic innovations during 1935–54 and the introduction of a new series of innovations with a fresh capacity to diminish death rates further.

(4) *The 1970s and early 1980s*. The decline of death rates resumed during the 1970s in every age group (although it is plausible to argue that there was no net trend for the 1960s and afterwards for ages 15–24 and 25–34). The resumption has been attributed to the earlier diagnosis and treatment of chronic disease, especially in life-threatening rather than seldom-fatal chronic disorders, and to improved awareness of some health risks, notably cigarette smoking and hypertension, that led to changes in lifestyle.[10] Medical and self-surveillance improved. Medical personnel detected life-threatening illnesses earlier and people at higher risk to some life-threatening illnesses perceived the risks better and acted to reduce them.[11] Such innovations might increase the being sick rate – if earlier diagnosis led to convalescences beginning at an earlier point within sickness – but would not alter the falling sick rate. Better

surveillance of this kind detected some illnesses earlier but not more often. This decline seems to have been interrupted in the middle 1980s; in most age groups, death rates of males appear to have leveled off again after 1983.

While period effects, like age effects, are evident on the vertical scale of Figure 7.1, cohort effects appear in two other ways. In one form they show up along the diagonal traced by following males born in one year or group of years throughout life. Two *cohort effects* of this sort stand out, and the first of these points to a *fifth period effect*.

If we follow the age 5–14 cohort in 1900–09 through age 75–84 in the 1970s, we notice a stability or mild decline in its death rates in each decade. (Follow this cohort in Figure 7.1 by tracing its mortality experience from one decade/column to the next – for example a to b_1 to c – and by comparing the cohort's mortality experience in each decade/column to the preceding decade/column for the same age group – for instance, b_1 to b_2.) If we follow the age 15–24 cohort in 1900–09 through age 85 and over in 1970–79, we notice declines that are at once more numerous and more rapid. Tracing older cohorts – people age 25–34 and above during 1900–09 along their diagonals – supplies little evidence of changing mortality rates. But it appears that some cohorts obtain more favorable mortality risks early in life and carry those throughout their lives. In this instance, the favored cohorts were composed of people born between 1885 and 1899 and aged 0–14 at the beginning of the twentieth century. This cohort effect in turn points to a period effect: something happened during 1885–99 that reduced the risk of dying for people born in those years. This *fifth period effect* consists of public health reforms – especially water purification and sewage disposal – inaugurated in US cities in the 1880s and thereafter. Those reforms reduced the risk of death especially among children and young adults by diminishing exposure to diseases carried by contaminated food and water, and they worked in harmony with an improving standard of living whose effects are more difficult to date or to assign to particular age groups.

The persistence of stable or declining mortality rates in these cohorts through the remainder of their lives, and the absence of such an effect in older cohorts, suggests that the public health reforms reduced the risk of falling sick *among children* but not among adults. At least in cities, adults had for the most part already suffered the diseases (for instance, typhoid and bovine or milk-transmitted tuberculosis) that public health brought under control. According to insult accumulation theory, the cohorts born from 1885 to 1899 died at

declining rates through the remainder of their lives because they had
suffered less damage early in life. This is a classic example of the
effect the medical physicist Jones believed he found by comparing
cohort experience: a period effect transmitted along the cohort
diagonal. Members of the favored cohort lived longer because they
possessed what Jones called lower physiologic age.[12]

Another period effect transmitted along the cohort diagonal would
be expected to follow from the revolution in immunoprophylaxis and
chemotherapy of approximately the years 1935–54. It appears in
Figure 7.1 in the form of declining mortality rates carried forward in
time. The cohorts most clearly affected consist of individuals then
ages 0–4, 5–14, and 15–24. The health of each group changed in a
striking manner but to a diminishing degree from younger to older
cohorts depending on whether the revolution delivered immunizations and efficacious drugs or chiefly efficacious drugs. The scale of
the effect remains inconclusive because we are unable to follow the
mortality experience of cohorts born after 1935 into the higher ages
where a lasting reduction in hazard will show up: they are not yet old
enough.[13]

New Hazards

According to Jones's formulation of insult accumulation theory, a
reduction in insult risks has more value if it occurs in childhood than
in young adulthood and less value if it occurs after age 30. This
formulation suits a version of the theory stressing acute infectious
diseases most likely to occur in childhood – for example, those that
increase the risk of artery or valve damage and later heart disease –
better than it does the broader version of the theory developed here,
a version which holds that stresses and insults of all types may
concentrate in other age groups, too, and influence later health and
the timing of death.

To see the potential effect of stresses and insults in other forms, we
can consider cohort risks in another manner. Some increases and
decreases in health hazards can be located not by the period of years
in which they occurred but by the life stage at which they were
focused. In US experience since 1900, three 'life stage cohort' risks
can be identified. First, the US engaged in four wars that were fought
chiefly by young men ages 18–34. Figure 7.1 records deaths occurring
in US territory, which includes only some war casualties. But those
are numerous enough to show the effects of these wars on the death

rate of young men during the periods 1917–19, 1943–45, 1952–53, and 1965–71.[14] Wartime deaths occurred chiefly on foreign territory, but wounds were far more numerous than deaths in each conflict, and the men who suffered them were repatriated. In the First World War, 117 000 US soldiers died and 204 000 more were wounded, a ratio of about 1 to 2; in the Vietnam War, 47 000 died (during the years 1965–71) and 304 000 more were wounded, a ratio of 1 to 6.[15] New survivors with war wounds and injuries became numerous in some cohorts.

Second, the twentieth century brought an important change in tobacco use. In 1900, comparatively few men used tobacco in a significant volume, and those who did mostly chewed it. By the 1920s, more men used tobacco, and they used it by smoking cigarettes, a mode that heightened the risk of disease and death. By 1955, between one-half and two-thirds of men age 21–54 smoked. The higher disease and mortality risks are chiefly a function of the rate at which cigarettes are consumed and the length of time over which they are used, something measured in 'pack/years'. Consumption above the threshold at which these factors combine causes a lasting increase in the risk of some cancers, heart disease, emphysema, and other diseases. Although, quite clearly, the risks to health are not associated with only one stage in life, they are aggravated when smoking begins early and continues through life. In the US, males who smoked often started smoking at ages 15–24. Although smoking prevalence declined after about 1968 in the overall population, it did not decline among teenagers.[16]

Smoking is also a metaphor, in this case for a variety of life-long practices and habits that may cause lasting damage to health. Attitudes and habits about diet, alcohol use, exercise, and other elements that influence health in the long run are also often adopted in young adulthood, chiefly ages 15–44.[17] For present purposes, the leading difference between cigarette smoking and these other practices is that widespread cigarette use is a recent innovation. Within this realm can also be distinguished several factors known or suspected to influence health and mortality risks but of which the historical trend is undetermined. For example, epidemiologists have linked rapid social and cultural change to morbidity and mortality risks and have attributed higher risks to such factors as social isolation. 'People who report having few friends and relatives and/or who see them infrequently have higher mortality rates than those people who have many friends and relatives and see them frequently.'[18] The causal direction of this effect is difficult to determine, leaving open the possibility that social isolation is both a consequence *and* a cause of higher mortality and morbidity risk. More problematic still is the direction of historical change. While it is usually said that the pace of social and cultural change and the likelihood of social stress or isolation have increased, it is rare to encounter even a nod toward evidence showing that trend. And if the trend has been one of increase, the problem remains of measuring the amount of additional change, stress, or isolation.

Smoking is a metaphor, too, for health risks of which the individual or society may be unaware and that may, like cigarette smoking, be latent and partial rather than immediate and complete. These further hazards fill a long inventory not yet well known; they extend from substances linked unambiguously to ill health in humans or plausible animal models (such as polychlorinated biphenyls in soil and ground water) to substances in which a link has been proposed but the evidence is ambiguous or uncollected. In many cases, the incubation period – the period between exposure to hazards that may cause disease and the appearance of symptoms – is long, lasting even decades, a circumstance that seriously complicates the issue of specifying cause. Many observers maintain that the variety and intensity of environmental hazards increased with industrialization, population growth, and environmental pollution, and there is some support for this view, largely from experiments with laboratory animals. For example, automobile transport has increased the risk of injury in accidents and added to air pollution from carbon monoxide, which is believed to heighten the likelihood that someone already ill from cardiac disease will die and is suspected of other negative health effects.[19] But death rates have declined as environmental pollution is said to have increased, making it difficult to evaluate the effect of environmental hazards as latent health risks.

Third, the leading causes of ill health and death among young adults have changed during the twentieth century. At its opening, sicknesses and deaths between ages 15 and 34 occurred chiefly because of infectious disease. Since 1900 the health condition of those age groups benefited from an improving living standard, public health reforms, a less easily explained change in exposure to tuberculosis, and drugs introduced during the 1930s and thereafter. By the 1980s, the leading causes of death and sickness in 1900 had virtually disappeared, but the death rate had not fallen as far or as rapidly as the history of the diseases successfully treated by the new drugs

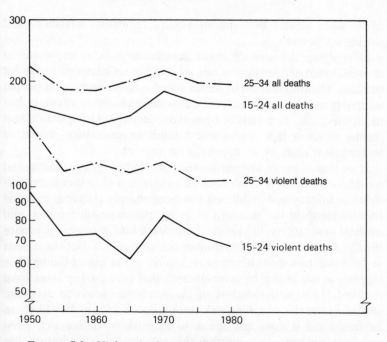

FIGURE 7.2 *Violent deaths and all deaths, ages 15–24 and 25–34*
(deaths per 100 000)

SOURCES See Figure 7.1.

would lead us to expect. René Dubos noticed that respiratory and digestive diseases were increasing in incidence (or at least in rate of detection and treatment), that infection remained a major cause of ill health, that drug-resistant forms of bacteria and new pathogen strains were appearing, and that many diseases remained impervious to either public health or chemical means of prevention and treatment.[20] Louis Weinstein detected the increased incidence of venereal diseases, especially gonorrhea, syphilis, and genital herpes; subacute bacterial endocarditis; and other infections.[21] Novel hazards appeared, especially after the Second World War. Foremost among them were motor vehicle accidents, which joined accidents in other circumstances to make up the leading cause of death, plus increases in homicide and suicide.[22] The effect of these factors in mortality appears in Figure 7.2, which enlarges a part of Figure 7.1 and sketches the trend of the death rate for the age groups 15–24 and

25–34 when deaths from motor vehicle accidents, homicide, and suicide are deleted.

In applying the idea of insult accumulation, it is important to recognize that neither deaths nor injuries are an adequate proxy for sickness. Deaths from these causes signal a larger number of people injured in motor vehicle accidents, assaults, and suicide attempts, but in injuries, too, case fatality rates have declined. Using data about deaths to show this cohort effect tends to understate it and to understate it more as we approach the present.

If we search for an impressionistic balance between beneficial and harmful effects, using death rates as a guide, it is clear that the risk of dying in infancy and childhood has been sharply reduced, and that improvements in the standard of living, public health reforms, and medical innovations that lowered the death rate in these age groups benefited infants, children, and other age groups, too. But the decline in the death rate tends to overstate change in the risk of falling ill or injured, as we notice by remembering that case fatality rates have declined. That is, the decline of the death rate tends to overstate decline in the risk of falling sick from illnesses and injuries likely to be fatal, and it does not speak to the risk of falling sick from non-fatal illnesses and injuries. Moreover, risk substitution has occurred on a significant scale, especially in the emergence or growth of risks associated with youths and young adults. The balance that needs to be struck requires an acknowledgment of this substitution and its three levels: age (from infancy and childhood toward adolescence and young adulthood), category (from acute infections toward injuries), and form (from immediate to deferred effects).

Being Sick and Falling Sick Reinterpreted

During the twentieth century, the risk of falling sick (i.e., illness plus injury) has both decreased and increased. In insult accumulation theory, changes in this risk are held to be important in the short and the long run. In the short run, a *decrease in the risk of falling sick* means a reduced risk of dying or of being sick. In the long run, it means a reduced risk of dying at each later age, but those effects may result in a higher risk of being sick in the aggregate and at each age. The risk of dying may decline rapidly enough to increase the risk of being sick at each age because the composition of the population has changed. In the short run, an *increase in the risk of falling sick* augments the risk of dying and being sick. In the long run, it means a heightened risk of being sick or dying in each cohort that shares the experience of a higher risk. These countervailing tendencies shape expectations about sickness in the US population in general and among males in particular.

Considering age, period, and cohort factors together, several leading effects emerge. First, a decline in the adult death rate began in the US in the 1880s and led to a higher being sick rate among survivors who were already adults in the 1880s. The rate of being sick increased because the composition of the population changed to include more new survivors whose capacity to resist future sickness had been compromised in childhood but who had, because of an improving standard of living and perhaps for other reasons, too, begun to survive longer as adults. This period effect should be distinguished from a second period effect occurring at the same time but focusing on infants and children and attributable chiefly to public health reforms. Cohorts born during 1885–99 died at lower rates than cohorts born earlier, and they died at lower rates from birth and throughout their lives. Their longer lives included more sickness in the aggregate, but it is unclear how their age-specific sickness rates compared with those in earlier cohorts. Theoretically, public health reforms and other innovations reduced the risk of falling sick in a manner similar to the way they reduced the risk of dying, and that reduction of risk was carried forward through life in the form of lower subsequent risks of falling or being sick. It was partially counterbalanced by new risks (for example, cigarette smoking) and by the changing composition of this cohort in comparison to its predecessors. The actual sickness experience of these cohorts has not yet been measured.

Third, another decline in the risk of falling sick occurred during 1935–54 but was less highly age-specific. It diminished the risk of falling sick and of dying most sharply among people ages 0–14 during 1935–49, but it also caused somewhat lower death rates and a lower risk of falling sick for people ages 15–44. These cohorts carried the lower mortality risk forward, enjoying declining mortality rates at subsequent ages, but they too encountered higher risks from war, accidents and violence, and lifestyle. Fourth, especially marked countervailing mortality risks appeared in the 1960s. They were sufficient to offset forces tending to reduce the death rate in the age groups 15–24/35–44. Fifth, another decline in the risk of dying occurred during the 1970s and early 1980s. People susceptible to life-threatening chronic diseases, especially heart disease, survived longer, and it may also be that changes in lifestyle reduced current and future health hazards among young adults. After 1973, death rates in young adult age groups (15–24 and 25–34) regained levels prevailing around 1960 but do not give evidence of trend movement.

In this complicated way, we see that any profile of the population at a given date is a story of simultaneous change in three risks: falling sick, being sick, and dying. Each change has both immediate and delayed effects. The effects sometimes harmonize, so that one or more risks may decline at the same time or over time in the same cohort, but they also sometimes conflict, so that one risk may rise because another has declined. The discussion of Figure 7.1 calls attention to these simultaneous risks by using age-specific mortality rates to locate periods and age groups in which the risk of falling sick changed or, in the case of cigarette smoking, in which the change consisted of an alteration of lifestyle that had deferred effects.

In general, the persistent decline of mortality since 1900 should be expected, according to the argument developed here, to have promoted a persistent rise in the risk of being sick, a rise attributable to changes in the composition of the population that would continue as long as the death rate declined and that would occur in the cohorts experiencing decline. However, the risk of being sick is also a function of the risk of falling sick. This relationship is immediate (a decline in the risk of falling sick shows up as less time spent in sickness) as well as deferred (a decline in the risk of falling sick reduces the subsequent likelihood of falling *and* being sick). Thus the tendency of a decline in the death rate to augment the being sick rate may itself be countermanded by subsequent changes in the risk of falling sick. Sudden reductions in exposure to pathogens – for example, water purification that reduces diarrheal disease, immunizations that evade infectious diseases, or less smoking that lowers susceptibility to chronic disease – may show up immediately in lower death rates and lower falling sick rates in at least some age groups, and they may show up later as lower rates in those areas plus a lower risk of being sick.

To make these several distinctions is to recognize that age-specific mortality and morbidity rates may move in opposite directions in different versions and with different intensities. Health experience in the US since the 1880s has been a history of more one-sided and more modest period effects than those prevailing in earlier times. Periods in which the risk of falling sick declined outweigh periods in which the risk increased, not because these periods were more numerous but because they were sustained longer and affected a larger group of people. These effects were also more modest, something that can be appreciated by contrasting the sharp short-term changes in life expectation common in the era of epidemics with the muted changes of the twentieth-century US. For example, epidemic spasms in mortality, such as occurred in three nineteenth-century cholera epidemics and the influenza epidemic in 1918, caused sudden plunges in life expectation and contributed to lower long-run life expectation values. Life expectation is higher in the twentieth century in part because of the absence of such spasms. Nevertheless, the history that needs reconstruction and the projections that need to be made require an equation complex enough to allow for all the combinations so far identified. The objective of the equation is to predict future risks of death, falling sick, and being sick in circumstances in which each of those is held to be a function of past rates of death, falling sick, and being sick plus future changes in the risk of falling sick.

Sickness Trends

Twentieth-century US health experience has been monitored by a variety of public and private observers using non-standardized identities of sickness, varying means of measurement, and changing sampling techniques. Here the leading problem is not to identify surveys but to find data sets that will bear direct comparison over time or that can be adjusted so that they represent sickness over time in similar terms. The most satisfactory time series is provided by the National Health Survey, begun in 1957 and more recently known as the National Health Interview Survey (NHIS). It can be linked to earlier measures of sickness experience. Although the way in which the survey has been conducted has changed since 1957, the changes do not appear to have undermined confidence in health trends revealed by the survey.

In turning to the NHIS, we turn to a source differing in many ways from sick fund and friendly society records and to measured levels of sickness that cannot be compared to levels derived from sick fund records without adjustments that have not been attempted here. The NHIS is a stratified random survey of the civilian non-institutionalized population. Ill health is distinguished from health by the respondents in two basic forms: the restriction of activity and the presence of acute or chronic conditions.[23]

A good way to illustrate the marked difference in the way ill health is identified and measured between this source and sick fund records is to point to one of the most important age curves derived from NHIS data. In the friendly society approach, acute sickness was a sub-category distinguished by time since onset and usually distinguished by the omission of episodes lasting three to six days or less. Even sicknesses that would last longer than three months appear in the measure of short sicknesses whenever they began during a survey. The actuaries also simplified by counting discrete episodes experienced by the same person within one year as continuous, so that they derived a statement about the risk that work incapacitation would occur at least once within a year. This approach produced age curves of sickness risks resembling a misshapen W and a measurement in which the sickness risk increased with age from childhood to first employment, diminished slightly, and then increased again until old age. Both the risk of falling and being sick described W curves, and the two differed chiefly in the slope of the curve at advanced ages.

By contrast, in the NHIS approach, acute sickness is a distinct category covering only conditions *unlikely* to last longer than three months. Conditions that began less than three months before the reference date but are likely to last longer than three months, such as heart disease, are transferred to the category of chronic disorders. What is more, in the NHIS, different episodes are counted separately rather than continuously. The result is a measure of the risk of acute sickness in which the risk declines from childhood to adulthood. The NHIS approach recognizes that the risk of falling sick *for a short period* declines with age even though the risk of falling sick *for any cause* rises. It cannot be said that one approach is correct and the other not; the two simply measure different varieties of risk, and they measure those different varieties in different ways.

The difference in the two approaches is illustrated by Figure 7.3, which adds a dimension to the forms of sickness risk identified in Chapter 3 and which contrasts different ways of measuring sickness by converting all values to index numbers.[24] The new dimension focuses on the kinds of sickness most prevalent among children and young people in the seventeenth century and since but observable in early records only for the deaths they caused. If the NHIS approach toward measuring the risk of acute sickness could be applied to earlier populations, we would expect age curves to have a similar shape. In the comparison, however, they differ. Among the Foresters, the risk of falling sick (solid line) rose after the mid-30s because

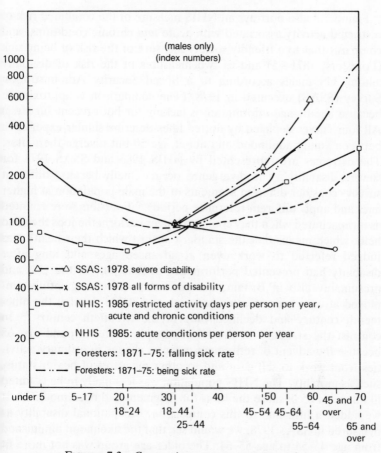

FIGURE 7.3 *Contrasting ways to measure sickness*

SOURCES   Francis G.P. Neison, *The Rates of Mortality and Sickness According to the Experience for the Five Years, 1871–1875, of the Ancient Order of Foresters Friendly Society . . .* (London, 1882), pp. 35-6; US, National Center for Health Statistics, Current Estimates from the National Health Interview Survey, 1985, *Vital and Health Statistics*, Series 10, no. 160 (Washington , 1986), pp. 14 and 110; US, Social Security Administration, Mordechai E. Lando, Richard R. Cutler, and Edward Gamber, *Data Book: 1978 Survey of Disability and Work* (Washington, 1982), pp. 3 and 200-1.

all sicknesses were counted, but in the NHIS sample, the risk of an acute condition declined after ages 18–44 because older groups experienced fewer acute conditions.

Figure 7.3 also portrays an NHIS measure of the combined risk of restricted activity associated with acute *and* chronic conditions, and compares that to a friendly society measure of the risk of being sick (Foresters, 1871–75) and to two measures of the risk of disability among US males according to a Social Security Administration Survey (SSAS) executed in 1978. (The comparison is approximate because age-by-age information is lacking for both recent surveys.) All four curves depicted by dotted lines describe similar experience between young adulthood and about age 50 but diverge thereafter. The extremes are represented by NHIS 1985 and SSAS 1978 for 'severe disability'. The divergence occurs chiefly because different surveys consider different segments of the male population at higher ages and apply different reference periods.[25] Foresters were counted as incapacitated when they could no longer perform the jobs they had held, which means that the standard against which their health was judged referred to work even at advanced ages and long after disability had prevented performance of that job. In the US, and presumably also in Britain, the percentage of men gainfully employed at ages over 65 remained high and stable through the nineteenth century and declined only in the twentieth century.[26] In contrast the standard in the NHIS sample shifted around age 65 because the advent of retirement meant a change in ordinary activities from work to self care and to other measures of health status, such as mobility. The NHIS population was less likely to be counted ill after age 65 because the basis for judgment had been modified. If we added a fifth line to this comparison, occupational disability as measured in SSAS 1978, we would see that the likelihood diminished from age 45–54 to age 55–64. The older age group was not more fit for work. Instead, its members unable to work had previously withdrawn from the labor force, which is an illustration of the 'healthy worker effect' which was mentioned above. In short, the risk of being sick is a function of age, but its relationship to age is likely to be understated to varying degrees by differences in the proportion of the population considered or changes in the standard by which ill health or disability is distinguished. All the being sick curves in Figure 7.3 understate the curve that would apply if all survivors continued to be evaluated at each age according to the standard applied in early adulthood.

The trend of US experience since 1957 has been scrutinized carefully by specialists from many fields, including health economics, epidemiology, demography, gerontology, and medical sociology. Although nearly every authority acknowledges that it is difficult to establish the exact rate of change in ill-health risk, certain trends are clear. These trends amount to a restatement of the paradox identified in the opening sentence of this chapter: why has the decline of the death rate coincided with increased health spending and higher ill-health rates? The intuitive proposition, a proposition restated confidently by specialists into the 1970s and still sometimes repeated, is that the decline of the death rate is evidence of an improvement in health that should show up in lower morbidity rates. What is actually observed, however, is that both the aggregate and the age-specific rate of being sick have increased during the period of the NHIS survey. Most authorities believe that the increase began before 1957.[27] The increase has been observed also in other countries where continuous or regular health surveys are conducted.[28] All authorities worry about how much of the trend increase is 'real' – that is, associated with actual disability and ill health – and how much is an accommodation to social, economic, or other changes.[29] For instance, the threshold at which people identify activity restriction may have shifted upward, resulting in more *reported* activity restriction time but not necessarily more *actual* time. The point is not to distinguish each component affecting actual or reported rates of impairment but to acknowledge two inferences. First, health surveys indicate a strong trend increase in morbidity across societies and periods with substantially different health regimes and health services but with similar mortality experience. Second, the trend increase in morbidity may be mostly 'real' or mostly the product of more comprehensive reporting or definition. In either event, it has occurred. People are using health services more and are reporting more health problems.

An increase in the *aggregate* sickness rate is not, for reasons made clear earlier, counterintuitive. Longer life spans mean more time at risk to ill health, and when the additional time is composed chiefly of years lived at advanced ages, when the sickness risk is particularly high, the additional sickness time will grow disproportionately. This is the situation identified in the sickness expectation based on being sick rates in Figure 6.4: even among the Foresters of the 1870s, living in a society with a much smaller portion of aged people than the US in the late twentieth century, the risk grew until about age 70. When the proportion of the aged is greater, this version of the expectation will grow for a longer period still.

What may seem counterintuitive is the proposition that the *age-specific* sickness risk should increase. To restate the hypothesis formulated here, the sickness risk should be distinguished in two forms, falling sick and being sick. The age-specific risk of being sick should be expected to rise when the death rate declines because the people who do not die at each age under the new mortality regime bear a higher risk of being sick than the average in their age group under the old mortality regime. The new survivors are not distributed uniformly across a cohort but tend to cluster into a group with a higher risk of being sick. This tendency is underscored by the idea that their present and future health is influenced by their previous health.

Trends in US health experience since 1957 have been examined recently in separate essays by Thomas Chirikos and Lois Verbrugge.[30] Both note male and female rates and point out difficulties in deriving consistent measurements of female experience owing to changes in female labor force participation.

Combining NHIS reports with earlier Social Security Administration surveys, Chirikos detects a trend rise in work disability beginning before 1950 and continuing through 1982. (More recent NHIS reports indicate continuation since 1982). His findings differ from earlier reports in that Chirikos adjusted rates for the proportion of workers disabled by chronic conditions by correcting for changes in age structure within the broad age groups in which NHIS findings have been published. The adjustment, which corrects for the aging of the US population, confirms that work disability has increased.[31]

Verbrugge's analysis deals with the period 1958–81, appraises trends in several indexes, and considers how specific acute and chronic conditions reported by respondents influence the interpretation.[32] Her findings, which concern persons 45 and older, can be summarized as follows:

First, the incidence of acute conditions (that is, the number of conditions per 100 persons per year) declined among males, but the restricted activity associated with these acute conditions increased in the same population. 'Men and women aged 45 and older are experiencing fewer acute conditions . . . but they are reducing activities for each acute condition more.'[33] Second, considering acute and chronic conditions, restricted activity increased, and the increase occurred chiefly after 1970, when the death rate was declining in these age groups at the most rapid pace observed among them in the twentieth century (Figure 7.1). Third, the percentage of the population whose ordinary activity is limited by chronic condition(s) increased, especially after 1970.

These trends are summarized in the four diagrams in Figure 7.4 using an arithmetic rather than the by now more familiar logarithmic

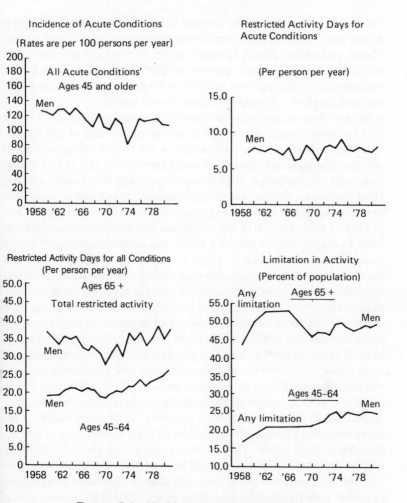

FIGURE 7.4 *Health trends in the US, 1958–81*

SOURCE: Lois M. Verbrugge, 'Longer Life but Worsening Health? Trends in Health and Mortality of Middle-Aged and Older Persons', *Milbank Memorial Fund Quarterly/Health and Society*, 62, no. 3 (Summer 1984), 478–9 and 482–4.

scale. Verbrugge attributes this configuration to 'earlier diagnosis, lower population mortality rates, and, possibly, earlier accommodations for disease' (that is, restriction of activity at an earlier stage in the illness episode).[34] That is, she believes that the decline of the death rate has promoted the survival of individuals prone to ill health at the same time that the population, or at least people age 45 and above, recognized illness episodes earlier in their course. Increased health spending – the proportion of the GNP devoted to health increased from 3.5 per cent in 1929 to 7.6 per cent in 1970 and 10.6 per cent in 1984 – coincided with increased need.[35]

In the terms of the interpretation being developed here, Chirikos and Verbrugge point to a trend decrease in the risk of falling sick from acute illnesses, a trend increase in the risk of falling sick from chronic illnesses and injuries, a trend increase in the risk of being sick, and the influence of period and perhaps also cohort effects. (Unfortunately, the age groups for which the incidence of acute and chronic conditions and activity restricted because of ill health are published from the NHIS are too broad and the period covered too brief to clarify cohort effects.) While the combinatorial problem is now complicated enough to admit of a number of possibilities, this particular grouping is a plausible outcome of what would be expected from the analysis of mortality and the hypotheses concerning sickness risks given above. First, a trend increase in the risk of being sick should be expected because of the trend decrease in mortality that persisted into the 1980s, and it should be expected to be strongest in periods (such as the 1970s) when the decrease in the death rate was most rapid. Second, a trend decrease in the risk of falling sick from acute conditions should be expected because of the continuing effect of public health, immunologic, and chemotherapeutic innovations, an effect felt directly in reduced exposure to diseases likely to be short-lived and perhaps also indirectly in greater resistance owing to less illness early in life. Third, a trend increase in the risk of falling sick from chronic conditions should be expected even though the rate of insult accumulation associated with disease slowed in comparison to earlier cohorts reaching age 45 or above. This is so because older age groups continue to be made up chiefly of people who benefited from the public health innovations of 1885–99 but much less so from the chemotherapeutic revolution of 1935–54 (they were too old). These older age groups suffered from three periods of exposure to injuries – two world wars and the Korean conflict – and they may also have experienced higher rates of insult accumulation associated with lifestyle.

CONCLUSION

In the twentieth century – which for the convenience of the moment will be held to have begun in the 1880s – striking changes occurred in the disease risks confronting infants and children. These risks declined dramatically before a broad improvement in living standards and in two specific periods. In one (1885–1900), public health reforms reduced the exposure of infants and children to diseases borne by contaminated food and water. In the other (1935–54), new immunizations and chemotherapies protected children against common diseases and controlled or curtailed the clinical course of many diseases still experienced. The risk of dying declined and, while we lack a separate measure of sickness risk before age 15, it seems impossible to avoid the conclusion that the risk of falling sick also declined. It was the century of the child.

But it was not the century of the adolescent and the young adult, especially not for males. The risk of dying also declined for every other age group in the twentieth century. But the sickness risk did not. Even though measurements of sickness narrowed their focus – excluding some injuries, disability resolved by retirement, and clinical levels of sickness no longer experienced because of new chemotherapies – the risk of being sick increased at every age, and at least in some periods it increased more rapidly among young adults than among old people. Part of the increase may be owing to more complete and earlier diagnosis, but that part appears to be small: the risk of being sick advanced when measured by function as well as by diagnosed condition. Two factors appear to take a leading role in explaining why morbidity increased while mortality decreased. The first, which applies to populations in general, is that mortality decline altered the composition of the population. The new survivors, people who did not die in each successive improvement of the mortality regime, carried a higher propensity to be sick, and their sicknesses heightened the sickness risk in every adult age group. The second applies more specifically to males and may apply more to males in the United States than some other countries. It consisted of a trend increase in the likelihood of falling injured, especially in the age groups 15–24 and 25–34. Four wars were fought by people of those ages after 1900. To a growing degree, they were fought in an era in which the war casualty became not a dead professional soldier but a wounded civilian soldier who, repaired, returned to civilian life. In the twentieth century, motor vehicles were first built; by the late 1940s their use in the US had become general. Drivers and passengers, especially when young adult males, directed them with a taste for risk. It was a century also in which more efficient means were devised for using tobacco, and those means allowed cigarette smoking, measured in pack/years, to become a serious health hazard. And it may have been a century in which the standard of living both improved and deteriorated. No one seems inclined to doubt the proposition that higher real incomes allowed people to buy better housing, nutrition, medical services, and public services that improved survival prospects. Behind these beneficial effects lurk harmful effects, some of which are factual and some imputed without persuasive evidence about historical trend: overeating, a deterioration of physical fitness, stress and social isolation, and environmental pollution, itself a side effect of producing the goods that humankind had only recently obtained the means to acquire. At the beginning of the twentieth century, sickness had been swift and often sure. As infectious diseases were subdued, illness did not disappear but became chronic and degenerative. The incubation period of disease, first measured at the beginning of this century and measured then in days or weeks, was transformed into a period sometimes lasting years, even decades. If the twentieth century gave the child a better prospect of living through childhood and of avoiding the familiar diseases of childhood, it took some of that back from young adults, especially young men.

8 Sickness and Death in the Twenty-First Century: A Transformation toward Health?

> Most of the next century must become a story of continued increase in the need for health care.[1]

Two visions of the future emerge from this review of the past, and the two seem at first glance to be at odds. According to one, both aggregate and age-specific morbidity rates will increase when the death rate declines. The death rate has declined during the past century, and further decline can be forecast. Therefore, the future would seem to promise more sickness. According to the other, the amount of sickness and the timing of death are influenced from four directions: genetic traits and propensities, exogenous hazards, endogenized hazards or insult accumulation, and age. During the last century, certain kinds of exogenous insults, usually infectious diseases, have been avoided or have had diminished effects on the health of some age groups, especially infants and children. Fewer ill-health episodes mean a slower rate of insult accumulation and arrival at advanced ages with better health histories. From this perspective, the future should promise less sickness.

Both forecasts are warranted, but they are warranted under quite different assumptions and predictions. The problem is to decide how to sort through these assumptions and predictions to find those best supported by the evidence assembled and reviewed here. It seems wise to begin this chapter of forecasts and projections with two reservations. First, it is easy to project the future by specifying certain historical trends and plotting them forward. Projections are useful but seldom prove to be accurate. Why? To take an historian's perspective is to acknowledge that the past does not 'teach us' what the future holds, but that it does teach us that the future will be interesting because it will blend the expected and the unexpected.

221

Acquired immune deficiency syndrome – AIDS – is a reminder of the capacity of the future to surprise. At the end of a century fruitful in innovations both beneficial and harmful to health, the surprise should consist not so much in the appearance of so unexpected a health hazard as AIDS as in the form assumed by this particular hazard. Taking this caution to heart, the course of wisdom lies in projecting a probable range of future events rather than a single sight-line.

A second reservation is required to underscore the degree to which projections about morbidity rest on an historical record only beginning to be uncovered and on theoretical models that remain uncertain or that contain large portions for which evidence is ambiguous or missing. Historical experience with morbidity adds to the evidence in important ways, especially when it provides information about ill-health experience over time and over the life course. It helps narrow the territory in which speculations must be adopted in place of assumptions with a basis in experience. And it clarifies the analytical issues. But the historical record is still thin. It adds guidance to propositions developed in biology, medicine and public health, epidemiology, medical physics, demography, and economics, but the additions still fail to allow a final selection of assumptions and a final specification of the theory required to forecast health experience.

What assumptions seem warranted? First, the likelihoods of falling sick and of being sick are both functions of age more than of any other variable. The health experience of individuals, and of cohorts fixed in place and time, varies by such factors as sex, prior health experience, residence, occupation (or income), the disease and injury profile, the composition of the population, and other factors, but age possesses more power as a basis for prediction than any other variable. Morbidity curves, like survival curves, shift up or down on the schedule over time, especially because of changes in the profile of diseases and injuries to which the population is at risk. Such shifts influence the shape of morbidity curves but in comparatively small ways. The search for a law of morbidity seems as unlikely to be fruitful as the search for a law of mortality. But morbidity risks respond closely enough to age that it is plausible to infer unknown values for a given population from a few known values, excepting only the extreme ends of the age spectrum about which the evidence is inconclusive.[2]

Second, changes in survivorship affect the composition of populations and the level of the morbidity risk schedule. Every population can be defined as a group made up of some people who would have survived in prior mortality regimes and others who would not have survived. In the seventeenth and early eighteenth centuries, disease and injury profiles shifted in striking ways in the short term. The shifts often represent epidemics, which show up in the form of sharp, short-term changes in life expectancy. In those populations, the composition changed in both directions without establishing a long-run trend. The winnowing of survivors by prior mortality regimes had sometimes been rigorous, and survivors possessed markedly better prospects for future survival than the average of their cohort. At other times, the winnowing had been more tractable, and survivors possessed markedly worsened prospects for future survival. A long-run trend toward survivorship emerged in eighteenth-century Europe, was suspended between about 1820 and 1870, and reappeared thereafter, shaping the process of winnowing and population composition in a certain way that remains influential today. In those periods of declining mortality risks and rising life expectancy, each cohort included a growing proportion of people who would not have survived in the previous mortality regime. Each new survivor added to the years of life measured to calculate life expectancy, but each also increased the average mortality risk of the cohort. The years added to the denominator exceeded the risk added to the numerator, so that life expectancy increased. This is the 'survivorship effect' of change in population composition. Less rigorous winnowing meant increasing life expectancy. The morbidity form of this effect preserves the element of increasing life expectancy but has an additional feature consisting of the higher level of the morbidity curve on the risk schedule. In measuring morbidity, one finds that each survivor added more time-at-risk than risk, but the difference between the two was narrower. The morbidity form of the effect shows up with particular force when considering the risk of being sick and more especially still in the risk of being sick in middle age or older.

As long as 'old' survivors and 'new' survivors accumulated disease and injury insults at a significant level, the age-specific risk of being sick increased as mortality decreased. Each successive period brought more sickness (measured by duration) in the aggregate population and at each age. Such a trend was observed in England and Wales between 1870 and 1900. It was still to be seen in the US population between 1975 and 1980.[3] Although the notion may be difficult to accept because it seems counterintuitive, the mortality decline has meant increasing morbidity. In the circumstances prevailing in the twentieth century, defined still as the hundred years before 1980, the association between mortality and morbidity was inverse.

Third, given the insult accumulation theory in its broad form – in which environmental hazards of many kinds have lasting effects on the vitality of the organism and its propensity to ill health – the inverse association appears to be a temporary rather than a lasting phenomenon. Further declines in mortality continue to add new survivors with higher morbidity risks than the average prevailing in the old mortality regime, holding everything else equal. But the risk of falling sick or being sick is an element in the risk of dying, and the association between sickness and death is also positive. That is, a reduction in mortality risks implies, in most circumstances, a reduction in the risk of falling sick. The group of people who do not die in each successive mortality regime are not composed only of people who fall sick and recover from the diseases that previously caused death but include some people who escape those diseases altogether. In the seventeenth century, people who escaped disease in infancy and childhood also failed to acquire immunity and therefore, like the smallpox victim Louis XV, stood at risk into adulthood. But in the twentieth century, avoidance, prevention, and protection are accomplished by several means, including immunization, and many infections that are not experienced early in life also will not occur in adulthood.

In theory, disease-specific and injury-specific case fatality rates capture the positive element of the association between morbidity and mortality but, in practice, the history of case fatality rates is too uncertain to be relied on to reconstruct trend. More impressionistic sources suggest that the risk of falling sick declined among infants and children in England and Wales (and elsewhere) in the last decades of the nineteenth century, and among infants, children, and young adults in many countries after 1935. At least as regards disease alone, it should be expected that the risk of falling sick declined in those periods and segments of the population, and that insult accumulation increased less rapidly.

This effect does not show up in friendly society experience because the morbidity rates from that experience deal with adults, and because it is not possible to follow the same population after 1900, when the children of 1870–1900 became adults. It also does not show up with particular force in twentieth-century US experience, which I attribute to insult substitution and to shortcomings in data. While it seems obvious that the risk of falling ill declined in the US after 1935, the risk of falling injured was increasing from an earlier date, especially among adolescents and young adults. The balance between the two requires further exploration, and the exploration requires better data about health risks. According to my assumption, it is nevertheless plausible to expect future insult accumulation indexes to be lower than past indexes, something that would partially or completely redress the effect of winnowing on survivorship and the morbidity risk. The inverse association between morbidity and mortality can be expected to rupture at this unmeasured point, which will be specific to cohorts rather than to a period.

Fourth, the relative importance of the two forms of sickness risk has shifted over time. During the seventeenth century, acute sicknesses, infectious diseases for the most part, dominated morbidity. By the late nineteenth century, chronic sickness was dominant, and protracted sickness was increasing in importance in younger age groups. During the seventeenth century, the mortality risk may have been a satisfactory proxy for the morbidity risk to the degree that sickness hazards consisted of diseases with case fatality rates that changed over time but within certain boundaries. That is, a crude mortality rate of 30 per 1000 per annum implies a certain morbidity risk for a population with the age distribution prevailing then. By the late nineteenth century, that association had been shed. Case fatality rates had become mutable and manipulatable, and an increasing portion of the population survived infections in infancy and childhood only to die of chronic diseases in middle age. More and more the measurement of sickness required a measurement of duration rather than incidence.

These assumptions underscore the degree to which projections of future health experience should be based on expected survivorship and age-specific ill-health rates. And they point up the need to distinguish between the quantity of ill-health time forecast for the aggregate and age-specific ill health will increase because mortality will decline more rapidly than insult accumulation indexes will shift downward. More sick time will be recorded because the average age of the population will rise, and because each age group will manifest higher sickness rates. According to a second forecast, aggregate ill health may continue to rise in the foreseeable future because the average age of the population will rise. But the age-specific risk of being sick may decline if insult accumulation proceeds as a slower

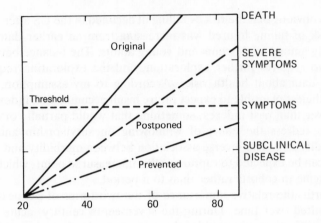

FIGURE 8.1 *Postponement of terminal disease and a rectangularized*
survival curve

SOURCE James F. Fries and Lawrence M. Crapo, *Vitality and Aging:*
Implications of the Rectangular Curve (San Francisco, 1981), p. 82. *Re-*
printed with permission. W.H. Freeman and company.

pace than the survivorship effect. And, according to a third forecast,
both aggregate and age-specific ill health may decline. Such a development is plausible if it can be assumed that the insult accumulation index is in decline and will henceforth decline more rapidly still,
rapidly enough to overcome the effect of a rising average age on
sickness risk. These are the prospects to be explored. The exploration will draw on the four assumptions just discussed, but those
assumptions themselves offer a starting point rather than a set of
fixed rules guiding future experience.

Considerable effort has been given the projection of mortality and
morbidity, and the literature of forecasts suggests reasons to expect
either an expansion or a compression of morbidity. A future reduction of morbidity has been predicted by the immunologist Fries,
encountered in Chapter 2 as the formulator of a particular version of
the idea that vitality deteriorates as the organism age. Fries's
scenario, developed in association with the endocrinologist Lawrence
Crapo, is summarized in Figure 8.1, a diagram suggesting that the
development of a clinical level of terminal chronic disease can be
postponed to a point closer to the modal age of death, estimated at
age 85, when the leading hazard is 'natural death' rather than specific

disease processes.[4] Estimating from US mortality data, Fries observes that the probability of natural death increases 'rapidly from essentially zero at age 70 to nearly 99 percent at age 100'.[5] Another feature of this argument is that aging is held to be modifiable or subject to delay. Echoing the medical physicist Jones, Fries and Crapo maintain that 'persons of the same chronological age often have very different physiological or mental ages'.[6]

The onset of terminal disease can be deferred, Fries and Crapo suggest, because the risk factors that influence the likelihood of most chronic conditions can be modified. Modification will put off the age at which most members of a cohort pass the threshold between preparation for chronic or degenerative disease and disease itself. In their view, modification depends on shifting from a medical model for dealing with health problems, in which the leading objective is to improve disease treatment, to a model stressing the responsibility the individual bears for health maintenance. Personal health habits are held to be the principal risk factors in the diseases of major importance at the end of the twentieth century, and Fries and Crapo believe that lifestyles have begun and will continue to change in ways that reduce the impact of these risk factors.[7] Specifically, Fries and Crapo recommend exercise; the avoidance of cigarettes, environmental toxins, and stress; moderate use of alcohol; and weight and diet control.[8] Although Fries and Crapo predict the compression of morbidity, the evidence they rely on deals chiefly with mortality risks.

As an argument, the case for compression presented by Fries and Crapo carries to its logical conclusion the notion that risk factors cause disease and constitute the dominant health risk of the present and immediate future. This notion is sometimes held to be contentious. Risk factors have been shown to be associated with chronic disease, including several of the leading causes of death in the US at the end of the twentieth century: arterial disease, cancer, diabetes, arthritis, emphysema, and cirrhosis. But in most of these cases, the largest category of risk remains unspecified or is specified in a tautological manner, for example, as age. Furthermore, as is often remarked, statistical association is not equivalent to causation. The association is probabilistic at the individual level but determinant at the population level: not all individuals exposed to risk will experience disease, but large groups will exhibit statistical regularities in morbidity and mortality.

More forceful still is the skepticism that comes to mind when encountering a forecast that seems to depend on changing the minds and habits of humankind. The advice Fries and Crapo offer about health maintenance has the ring of familiarity. It has been a commonplace of Western medicine since classical antiquity, but it has remained advice remarkable more for refusal than acceptance. They find grounds for optimism in noticing that mortality from arterial disease decreased in the US during the 1970s, in an anticipated decline in chronic lung disease, and in the relation of both trends to better health maintenance.

The grounds Fries and Crapo offer for a prediction that health maintenance will improve are not the only grounds that may be given. Another basis refers to the calculus of probabilities and to the banal matter of wagers. As the probability of survival to ages at which chronic diseases become manifest rises, as it has especially in the twentieth century, the putative reward for practicing health maintenance changes. The higher life expectancies attained in the twentieth century have changed the terms of the trade-off between gratification and denial in a manner analogous to the way in which superior odds enhance the appeal of a wager. They have done this by adding years of life expectation to all the ages of life and not only or even chiefly to youthful ages. Life expectation has increased for people of sufficient age – adolescence or young adulthood – to take responsibility for their own future health. At some point, the reward of superior health in middle age exceeds that of gratification of more immediate interests earlier in life. At that point, people would be expected to shift their behavior even though their judgment may be based more on intuition than mathematical calculation. That is, people are known to be able to make fine distinctions about probabilities associated with survival when they do not possess the mathematical means or evidence required to demonstrate the accuracy of the distinctions they make.[9] Whether or not such artful betting figures importantly in human behavior toward the end of the twentieth century is a matter of speculation.

In summary, Fries and Crapo forecast a compression of morbidity that will follow superior health maintenance and a general deferral of the age at which chronic diseases manifest a clinical level of symptoms. Morbidity will be reduced because terminal episodes will begin later in life. They call attention to 'organ reserve', which is a collective term representing effects divided here into four categories: birth abnormalities and propensities, the history of exogenous hazards, endogenized hazards, and senescence. And they assert that risk factors play as large a role in morbidity as in mortality. That is, Fries and Crapo believe that better health maintenance will defer the onset of chronic disease in middle age even though they acknowledge that the causes of diseases of leading concern lie earlier in life and may be quite distinct from the risk factors of middle age.

A variation on this forecast has been offered by Kenneth Manton, who argues that the modal age of death is increasing and can be expected to increase further, albeit slowly.[10] Although Manton forecasts near-term increases in age-specific and aggregate morbidity, he foresees an eventual compression in terms even broader than those expressed in Figure 8.1. By defining aging as 'a set of chronic degenerative disease processes', Manton holds out the possibility of medical innovations that will extend the life span by deferring the age at onset of degenerative disease.[11] He also expects breakthroughs in understanding the part of the aging process unrelated to disease, breakthroughs that will lead to some measure of control over aging. The long-term future may include not only a deferral of the age at onset of terminal disease but also a decline in the risk of disease at high ages.

The forecast of an at least near-term expansion rather than compression of morbidity has a large and diverse group of adherents, which falls into two segments. In one group, the argument is based on observed trend. Surveys of the incidence of ill health in the US indicate that morbidity has increased, and similar surveys in other countries attest that this trend is general in the developed countries. In the other group, the argument is based on observations about the kinds of ill health characteristic of the late twentieth century and the morbidity associated with them. The duration of terminal illnesses has increased with the transition from acute to chronic causes of death, and life expectancy has expanded more rapidly for people with disabling illnesses than for the general population.

Evidence about the morbidity trend was surveyed in Chapter 7. Although the mortality rates, on which Fries and Crapo focus attention, suggest a trend toward improvement in health, the morbidity evidence reveals that the prevalence of specific diseases and the quantity of ill-health time within the US population have increased in the aggregate and in age-specific terms. For example, the decline of heart disease mortality that began in 1964 coincided with greater prevalence of heart disease and increasing morbidity. Forecasts of further improvement in chances of survival necessarily imply deterioration in the health profile, especially at middle and older ages. While the incidence of acute diseases has declined in some periods and some age groups, these declines have been more than compensated by increases in the prevalence of chronic disease and in the overall amount of time spent in situations of restricted activity, disability, and other measures of health status. Chronic ailments, whether fatal or seldom fatal, have increased in prevalence.[12]

Gruenberg coined the phrase 'the failures of success' to describe one aspect of medical and epidemiologic progress in the twentieth century: the tools of medicine appear to prolong disease more than to diminish it. This effect is most noticeable in severe physical and mental diseases, such as senile brain disease and Down's Syndrome, and in diseases linked in the 1920s and 1930s to death from influenza and pneumonia, but it is apparent in chronic disease in general.[13] Disability rates and morbidity time increase because people with terminal and non-terminal diseases live longer and add to the sum of morbidity experience in ways that are not apparent in mortality statistics.

To choose between the two forecasts – the compression or the extension of morbidity – requires some additional evidence and a series of simulations about the plausible range of future morbidity experience. One goal, it should be remembered, is to distinguish between aggregate and age-specific experience. The technique depends on life tables and the use of life table values to forecast plausible boundaries for morbidity experience.

LIFE EXPECTANCY, 1985–2085

Most authorities expect life expectancy to continue to increase, albeit gradually, and employ projections made on that basis to forecast the numbers of people who will be alive at each age. To visualize what is expected, compare the survival curve achieved by the US population in 1979–81 with two forecasts sketched in Figure 8.2. The first forecast represents the notion Fries and Crapo have of an 'ideal' survival curve. Until age 70, the only deaths that will occur are attributable to trauma; they seem to be unavoidable according to any reasonable forecast of changes in life expectancy in the near future. After age 70, the ideal curve turns down sharply as 'natural deaths' begin and their probability rises sharply to about 50 per cent at age 85 and roughly 100 per cent at age 100. The second additional curve sketches female life expectancy projected by the Social Security

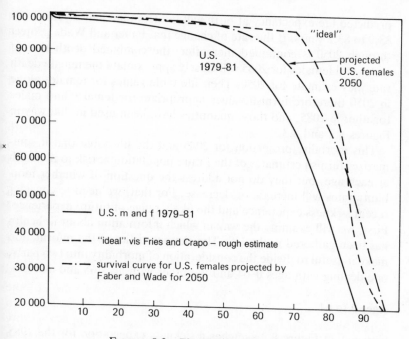

FIGURE 8.2 *The US survival curve*

SOURCES US, National Center for Health Statistics: United States Life Tables, *U.S. Decennial Life Tables for 1979–81*, vol. I, no. 1 (Washington, 1985), pp. 6–7; Fries and Crapo, *Vitality*, p. x; J. F. Faber and A. H. Wade, *Life Tables for the United States, 1900–2050*, Social Security Administration Pub. no. 11–11536 (Washington, 1983), pp. 62–4.

Administration actuaries Faber and Wade for the year 2050.[14] It embodies the basic premise that Fries and Crapo offer, which is that life expectancy at birth may rise to about 85 years. (In the Faber-Wade projection for females in 2050, life expectancy at birth is 83.9 years.) But it differs in several ways that add to its realism as a projection. Faber and Wade suppose that survival will decline gradually from about age 50, and they allow for survival after age 100. In their projection slightly more than 10 per cent of the female population of 2050 will live to age 100, and some people will live past 119. That is, Faber and Wade suppose that the life span (but not necessarily the modal age of death) may move beyond the limits observed in 1980. But they do not expect years lived at ages above 100 to be numerous. If those years are eliminated from their calculations, the predicted life expectancy at birth will fall less than half a year, from 83.9 to 83.5 years. If the rate of change that Faber and Wade project through 2050 is continued thereafter, the combined death rate of males and females for 2085 will closely approximate the female death rate they estimate for 2050. Their life table values for females alone in 2050 therefore furnish values appropriate for females and males together in 2085, and those quantities have been used in that way in Figures 8.2 and 8.3.

This mortality projection for 2085 and the life table that it summarizes furnish estimates of the future population at risk to ill health at each age, but they do not address the question of whether morbidity rates will increase or decrease. For that, we need to consider recent sickness experience and the likely range of future experience. First, we will examine the way in which information about ill health has been gathered in the US. The characteristics of the information make it useful to divide the consideration of morbidity into two parts, one dealing with ages 0–64 and the other with ages 65 and above.

Ages 0 to 64

Curve A in Figure 8.3 sketches a sickness expectation for the 1985 population at ages 0 to 64, basing survival experience on the US total population life table for 1979–81 and the morbidity risk on National Health Interview Survey (NHIS) restricted activity rates averaged for the period 1982–85. The vertical scale refers to expected future ill-health time, and the horizontal scale refers to age. This curve can serve as a basis for simulations about future experience by using 1985 mortality and sickness rates as a point of departure for forecasts. The 1985 expectation is limited to ages 0–64 because of the way ill-health data are presently collected. NHIS rates refer to six age groups: under age 5, 5–17, 18–24, 25–44, 45–64, and 65 and over. Except for the last, each has a midpoint. Although the average rate for each age group will not exactly match the rate for the midpoint age, the approximation will be close enough for present purposes. Assigning the rates to midpoint ages (2, 11, 21, 34.5, and 54.5) makes it possible to estimate values for all other ages by interpolation.[15] But the open end of the last age group, 65 and over, leaves the location of the last rate that might be used uncertain.

Another reason to distinguish experience to age 64 from that afterwards is provided by the effect of retirement on the standard that is employed to evaluate health. At age 65 and above, the ill-health

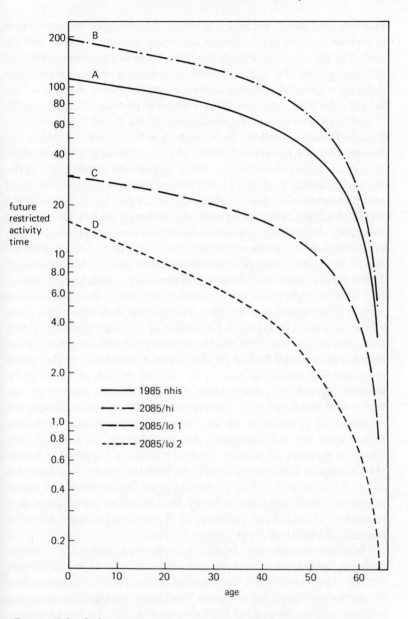

FIGURE 8.3   *Sickness expectations for the US, 1985 and 2085 (ages 0–64)*

SOURCES   See Text.

rate will tend to rise because a growing proportion of the population is unable to carry out ordinary activities, but the increase will be muted by the withdrawal from the labor force of a growing portion of the age group. To age 64, most respondents will evaluate their capacity to carry on ordinary activities by reference to work; after 65, people who have retired will use standards that are less exacting.[16]

Still another important qualification about the sickness expectations in Figure 8.3 follows from the way ill health is identified in the National Health Interview Survey. The measure adopted here – days of restricted activity because of acute and chronic conditions – is the broadest formula available in that it is intended to include both brief and protracted sicknesses. But the reference period employed in the NHIS, fourteen days, diminishes the reported rate at all ages and especially at higher ages, as does also the exclusion of people living in institutions.[17] These characteristics give a special and limited meaning to the 1985 sickness expectation curve and to simulations of future curves based on it. Once again the concept of sickness expectation is more appropriate than that of health expectation because the survey of restricted activity time omits some ill-health time. Even when the curves in Figure 8.3 measure or project the risk of being sick, they do not trace the course familiar from sickness expectation curves encountered earlier in this study. Considered in the terms given here, in which the issue is the amount of ill-health time to be forecast at each age, the sickness expectation does not rise persistently until about age 70 (as it has in previous instances), because the exclusion of episodes at 65 and above and the shorter reference period leave out the experience that would cause the curve to rise. Curve A sketches an initially gradual decline in expected ill-health time measured within these limits. At birth the expectation amounts to 113.4 weeks of ill health. From that point, it declines to 3.3 weeks at age 64. While expected ill-health time declines, the proportion it represents of time at risk increases in the expected manner, from 3.4 per cent at birth to 6.3 per cent at age 64.

The shape of each curve is more informative than specific values at each age, and the shapes of the first three curves—A, B, and C—are similar. They have been built by using the 1985 expectation as a straightforward basis for forecasts, modifying life expectancies in the gradual way recommended by Faber and Wade and modifying expected health experience between two sharply different projections of future levels, but projections that assume no radical deviation from familiar properties of health experience.[18]

The leading difference between curves B and C lies in different forecasts about future sickness risks. Curve B follows the assumption that the relationship between mortality and morbidity in the recent past will prevail until 2085. People who do not die in each successive phase of mortality decline but who would have died in earlier phases will continue to add a rising proportion of sickness experience over exposure time to the elements of the life table used to construct sickness expectations. According to this assumption, morbidity rates will increase because mortality rates will decrease, and the increase will remain proportional to the decrease. The relationship of proportionality is based on recent experience in the US. Between 1975 and 1980, the age-adjusted mortality rate declined by nearly 5 per cent (from 6.2 to 5.9 deaths per 1000) while the age-adjusted morbidity rate as measured by the NHIS increased by slightly more than 5 per cent.[19] The risk of being sick increased as the risk of dying diminished, and the increase of the one was in approximate proportion to the decrease of the other. Curve B has been built on the assumption that morbidity rates will increase by about 60 per cent over the next 100 years because the death rate is expected to decline by that proportion.[20] Curve B implies that health programs will continue to succeed in reducing the likelihood that illness will be resolved in death, that the 'failures of success' will persist.

Curve C adopts another assumption, which is that the inverse association of morbidity and mortality can be shed. Future morbidity rates will decrease (in the simulation, to an arbitrarily fixed level equal to 25 per cent of the 1982–85 rate) because unspecified ways will be found to reduce the risk of falling or being sick as the mortality risk also declines.

Curve B is a projection of the future that assumes no fundamental changes in health care; it also assumes an approximate balance in insult accumulation. That is, an inverse association between morbidity and mortality will prevail because declining disease risks in infancy and childhood will be counterbalanced by rising injury risks in adolescence and early adulthood. Curve C projects a path that might be attained if health care were improved sharply or if a substantially different projection should be made about insult accumulation. It could be deemed plausible if there were reasons to foresee the introduction of therapies capable of reducing the duration of degenerative disease to a degree similar to the way sulfa and antibiotic drugs reduced the clinical duration of many infections. It would be plausible also if most of the population should be persuaded to adopt health regimens calculated to defer the age of onset of degenerative disease, in the manner suggested by Fries and Crapo and illustrated by Figure 8.1, and if those changes in lifestyle and behavior should prove to have profound rather than limited effects on the sickness risk.

As the discussion in Chapter 1 indicated, this choice is analogous to the modification of behavior and environment achieved by transferring animals from the wild into a zoo or a laboratory. Behavioral and environmental modifications in humans are not, of course, value-free, and it is unclear that the trade-offs would be accepted.

Curve D is another vision of a future that might be attained. It assumes innovations in the treatment and prevention of degenerative diseases analogous to the drug and immune therapies introduced during 1935–54, and radical changes in the health environment. First, the element of duration has been curtailed. All ill-health episodes through age 64 that are measured by days lost within the past two weeks are assumed to last an average of one day. That is, the sickness risk has been reduced to the risk of falling sick. Second, the risk of falling sick has been redefined. In previous encounters with it, we noticed a bowl-shaped curve. The risk of falling sick from infectious disease decreased as age rose, but its decrease was always countered in adulthood by an increasing risk of falling sick from chronic disease. Curve D assumes that the risk of chronic disease can be deferred beyond age 64, so that the risk of falling sick will come to be dominated by newly encountered hazards rather than by new hazards plus hazards posed by the accumulation of prior insults. That is, curve D assumes that commonplace minor diseases and injuries will continue to occur but will, through innovations in therapy, behavior, or other areas, be deprived of the capacity to cause lasting damage. In terms of the propensity to be sick, this curve implies that the composition of the population will change in ways that reshape the age structure of morbidity. In terms of the letters U and W used previously to describe the age distribution of the risk of being sick, curve D implies a stretching of the low risk associated with ages 25–30 into middle age plus a reduction in the level of that risk. That is a substantial and apparently unprecedented departure from the age structure of morbidity observed in all historical data.

Other prospects are also possible. The insult accumulation index of the overall population might rise much more than suggested by the gap between curve A and curve B in a future involving rising rather than constant environmental hazards. Early experience with AIDS

TABLE 8.1   *Aggregate sickness time, 1985 and 2085, for ages 0–64 (rounded)*

	All years lived	Years in sickness	Per cent in sickness
1985 (curve A)	6.1 million	220 000	3.6
2085 (curve B)	6.3	366 000	5.8
2085 (curve C)	6.3	57 000	0.9
2085 (curve D)	6.3	31 000	0.05

SOURCES   See text.

suggests that the twentieth century may have been a relatively benign interlude between eras of more intense health risks rather than the harbinger of humankind's conquest of premature death. Or apprehensions about the adaptive capacity of pathogens may prove warranted, and tuberculosis, for example, might re-emerge as a leading cause of ill health and death if the mycobacteria that cause it become resistant to drugs more rapidly than new drugs can be developed. But, of course, it is possible, since only the imagination is in play, to foresee 'magic bullets' that defeat illness and injury risks altogether.

Figure 8.3 merely deals with likelier prospects. Its value lies in the contrast it sketches between the sickness expectation we have if the future holds no surprises and can best be projected from the most recent past experience, and the future we may have if ways are found to curtail the risk of being sick. Curve C, or something approaching it, seems obviously preferable to curve B, and curve D still more to be desired. Neither can be forecast without a substantial departure from the health risks of the distant and the immediate past.

Figure 8.3 also contains some information about aggregate health risks at ages 0 to 64, but that information is better seen by considering parts of the sickness expectation data on which the figure is based. In each forecast, the same assumptions have been made about survivorship in 2085. Three risks of being sick have been forecast for 2085, and those appear in Table 8.1 (together with 1985 data) as the sum of years of ill health expected at all ages from 0 through 64 under the limitations mentioned above. In each case, the figure is stated in life table terms of 100 000 live births, and each represents the aggregation of ill-health time at all future ages through 64.[21] Table 8.1 shows how much of an increase in ill-health time can be forecast under the curve B assumption of a continuing inverse association between morbidity and mortality, one in which changes in risks maintain proportionality. Only an absolute reduction in the risk of being sick, a reduction in proportion to the effect a rising average age has on morbidity, will counter this tendency.

Ages 65 and Above

Sickness experience is especially difficult to measure at higher ages and at transitions from lower to higher ages. The standard on which incapacity is determined changes not only with withdrawal from the labor force but also with other shifts in activity and outlook associated with age. Furthermore, age-specific or even age-group data have rarely been gathered. Most surveys treat people age 65 and above as a single group and focus on either the institutionalized *or* the non-institutionalized populations rather than both. For example, a segment of the 1984 NHIS was devoted to health status among people aged 65 and above and collected information about the incidence of activity limitation among non-institutionalized people at ages 65–74, 75–84, and 85 and over. For men and women together, 38.5 per cent of the survey group experienced some limitation of activity at ages 65–74, 38.7 per cent at 75–84, and 60.4 per cent at 85 and over.[22] These results suggest that people living in the community do not face a rising likelihood of being limited in their daily activities until after age 85. But the actual likelihood cannot be inferred because institutionalization itself becomes increasingly likely above age 65 (and because ideas about the desirability of institutionalization change over time, even over short periods). In 1977, the nursing home population, only part of the institutionalized population, increased from 4.8 per cent of all people age 65 and above to 21.6 per cent of people age 85 and above.[23] That is, the National Health Interview Survey does not (and was not intended to) reveal how the likelihood of limitation in activity, or disability, rises with age.

In the absence of satisfactory measurements, it is necessary to estimate. The estimates can depart from observations about the rate of disability or activity limitation at ages below 65, and draw on survey data about the likelihood at ages 65–74. Thereafter, however, there is little current evidence about the shape of the risk, even about whether the risk continues to rise. In measuring sickness and health expectation in late nineteenth-century Britain, the problem of inadequate data about men at higher ages, especially 85 and above, was solved by estimating a constant risk of falling or being sick. It can be acknowledged that the risk of dying rises to 1.0, but the risk of sickness, or at least the risk of being sick, may not reach certainty within the bounds established here, which carry the forecast to age 100 but not to the last individual living in the oldest cohort in a population. It is not clear whether the sickness risk continues to rise after age 85, nor do we know the rate at which it may increase. Thus, while there is considerable agreement among different surveys about the incidence of activity limitation or disability in the recent US population toward age 65 and between 65 and 74, the shape of the risk thereafter is uncertain.[24]

The sickness expectations given in Figure 8.4 employ this agreement about the level and slope of risk at lower ages to project two versions of risk at higher ages as of 1985. The point of departure for both is the 1977 National Health Care Expenditures Study measurement of activity limitation due to chronic health conditions, combining all categories of limitation for men and women. Curve E_1 sketches a sickness risk rising from 28.6 per cent at age 65 to 97.1 per cent at age 100.[25] Curve E_2 reports a cumulative sickness expectation as it declines from 7.4 years at age 65 to 0.8 years at age 100. At age 65 the average person could expect to live 16.5 years of which some 7.4 years would be limited in activity. Both versions of curve E should be understood as estimates of the risk of activity limitation in the *non-institutionalized* population ages 65–74 or less at higher ages. They project health risks in a certain way for people who later enter institutions and those who do not.

This estimate both overstates and understates the actual risk of ill health in several ways. Since it adopts a broad functional definition – any limitation of activity considered serious by the respondent – the reported rate may be higher than it would be if gauged by a third party, and it is certainly higher than the rate that would obtain in a survey attempting to measure the prevalence of diseases likely to result in death in the near future. There are also reasons why the reported rate will be lower than would appear in surveys based on different definitions of health. Exclusion of the institutionalized population at ages 65–74 and below understates the beginning point rate *and* the rate at which risk rises after age 65. It is also likely that the comparative position of different standards changes at higher ages. For example, people may be more likely to acknowledge some activity limitation at age 65 than they are to report health problems severe enough to limit their capacity to work. But these inclinations

240

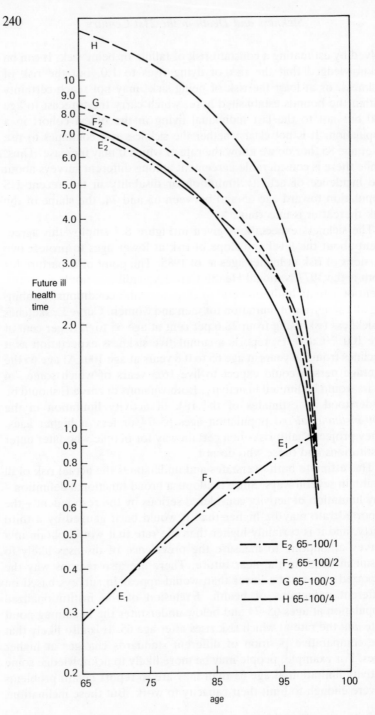

FIGURE 8.4 *Sickness expectations for the US, 1985 and 2085 (ages 65–100)*

SOURCES See text.

may change places at higher ages as people adjust to the idea that work is no longer an expected activity but still resist admitting limitations in ordinary functions, such as dressing. Some authorities believe that health problems are invariably understated at higher ages, partly because people lose memory and partly for other reasons.[26]

The F curves in Figure 8.4 follow another assumption, which is that the average risk of activity limitation levels off around age 85. Although the size of the population declines after age 85, and the risk of death rises toward 1.0, the risk of being sick may not follow this pattern. Some authorities claim that heterogeneity increases with age and is especially marked among people age 85 and over.[27] In circumstances in which the population divides itself to an increasing degree into the healthy and the unhealthy, and the size of both segments shrinks, the average risk of ill health may not rise or may rise much less gradually than is implied in curve E_1 of Figure 8.4. Curve F_1 describes one course the risk may take, adopting a more or less arbitrary estimate of the ceiling risk of activity limitation of 70 per cent for age 85 and upward.[28] In other words, curve F_1 assumes that about 30 per cent of any age group acknowledges no activity limitation that respondents consider serious from age 85 to age 100. Curve F_2 traces the cumulative sickness expectation under this assumption.

Curves E and F are intended to describe approximate boundaries for projection from 1985 experience. Curve E_1 probably understates the level and the rate of increase in the risk of activity limitation between 65 and 85 because it begins by leaving out of consideration people in institutions at ages 65–74. Curve F_1 may more closely approximate the actual risk to age 85 but understate it at higher ages. Even so, the sickness expectations (curves E_2 and F_2) do not differ a great deal. The possible biases compensate for one another. However, both the boundaries and the standards differ from those used to project the risk of being sick at ages 0–64 in several ways, of which two are most important. First, it is likely that the definition or admission of activity limitation is itself a function of age in a way that influences the projection regarding ages 65–100. In addition to reasons for changing definition mentioned above, the average number of conditions limiting activity should be expected to increase with age. In early adulthood, most respondents will think about single conditions, but at higher ages, the number of conditions may substantially exceed the number of respondents because the average number per person has risen. All the standards of measurement yet proposed seem to lose value at the highest ages. Second, the way in which ill health is defined for purposes of Figure 8.4 differs from the definition behind Figure 8.3. In place of a limited measurement of the risk of being sick – the duration of restricted activity during the last fourteen days and attributed to chronic or acute conditions – used to project the sickness expectation at ages 0–64, the projection for ages 65 and above uses estimates of the risk of being sick at a given time. The results reported in Figure 8.4 cannot simply be added to those given in Figure 8.3 because of this change in the format of measurement, a change that grows in importance after age 64. The missing values – durations falling outside the fourteen-day reference period – assume greater importance at each higher age. In the earlier figure the objective was to forecast the amount of ill-health time to be expected at each age to 64. Here the objective is to show how the probabilities of being sick at higher ages accumulate.

If the sickness risk and expectation in 1985 can be derived only by estimation, it is clear that ideas about the future trend are guided by little more than guesswork. Manton and Soldo project some decline in the age-specific disability rate on the basis of their mortality projection and an argument that mortality selection operates differently above age 85 than below.[29] Whereas below 85 the population includes a proportion of people at higher risk to morbidity that rises over time as the mortality rate declines, people age 85 and over are suspected of having triumphed over a system of rigorous selection. They will be less likely to be sick when the mortality rate declines.

Many projections of mortality rates for age 85 and over have been guided by recent experience, which seems to be moving in cycles. During the 1960s there was little improvement in life expectation at advanced ages, and observers adopted the view that the survival curve had achieved a mature form approaching a rectangle. During the 1970s, life expectation increased, especially at higher ages, and rectangularization came to be seen as a future prospect. Some commentators doubted it would emerge at all and predicted a modal age of death as high as 150 years. In the mid-1980s, male death rates leveled off again. The mortality rates and life expectancies projected by Faber and Wade seem too optimistic in the light of experience during the 1960s, too pessimistic in the light of experience during the 1970s, and again too optimistic if the leveling of death rates during 1983–85 persists. That is, they strike an approximate balance and for that reason remain useful for forecasts about sickness expectation.

For adults less than 65 years old, the insult accumulation model suggests that the sum of insults may wax and wane. Events that reduce the risk of falling sick will slow the pace of accumulation. Lower ill-health rates and superior health expectations can be forecast for 2085 when there are grounds for predicting that the insult accumulation index will decline. Around age 65, however, the relative importance of insult accumulation seems to fall and that of senescence to rise; age begins to matter more than prior health experience. The most obvious way in which this is so is apparent from considering the likelihood of multiple conditions. At higher ages the average number of conditions per person rises more rapidly than age, a circumstance that increases the probability of being sick in a way left unmeasured by the indexes used to gauge sickness risk at lower ages. For example, in 1985 the NHIS reported the following structure of selected chronic conditions:

under age 18	0.6 conditions per person
18–44	1.5
45–64	2.8
65–74	4.1
75 and over	4.6

Even with this increase, the number of conditions per person at advanced ages is understated because the NHIS deals with the non-institutionalized population.[30]

The withdrawal of a major category of insults that occur earlier in life and influence health in middle age or old age may have little effect on the sickness risk because of this multiplication of conditions. Indeed, the health risks facing the aged in the United States late in the twentieth century resemble in a certain way the risks facing children in early modern Europe. Those children survived by living through or evading a barrage of infections, a barrage so intense that removal of a single disease from the profile would have had little effect on the mortality rate estimated in its absence. The old now face a barrage consisting of accumulated insults, some risks of infection (especially pneumonia) that increase with age, and senescence. This combination of circumstances makes it unrealistic to project a sharp decline in sickness risk as one of the boundaries of likely experience in 2085. Thus the most favorable forecast adopted for Figure 8.3, a forecast in which the overall sickness risk declines to the risk of falling sick, can be set aside in predictions regarding ages 65 and above. Correspondingly, the forecast of an increase in the morbidity

TABLE 8.2   *Parameters for future morbidity rates*

| Age | 1985 | | 2085 | |
	Years lived at each age	Ill-health rate	Years lived at each age	Reduced ill-health rate (curve G)
65	76 314	.2859	88 901	.2144
66	74 683	.2990	87 948	.2243
67	72 964	.3126	86 930	.2345
68	71 150	.3265	85 854	.2449
69	69 233	.3407	84 730	.2555

SOURCES   See text.

risk is bounded by the diminishing effect of adding conditions in circumstances in which the population already, on average, bears four or more chronic conditions per person and in which the probability of being sick equals or exceeds 0.7 at the highest ages.

In the absence of any obvious guidance about how future morbidity rates should be forecast, Figure 8.4 shows two boundaries, each based on modest but equivalent changes in risk: an increase of 25 per cent (up to a probability of 1.0) and a decrease of 25 per cent. Since the sickness expectations derived from curves E_1 and F_1 are close, the forecasts are based only on E_1. They appear in Figure 8.4 as curves G and H. Both are higher than the 1985 sickness expectations because of the larger proportion of the population expected to survive to ages 65–100 by 2085. This higher survival shows up in Table 8.2 – which reproduces part of the sickness expectation tables from which Figure 8.4 was drawn – as higher values for years lived at each age. The sickness expectation is a function of both the probability of survival and the probability of activity limitation, which in Table 8.2 is estimated at a 25 per cent increase, as in curve G. As the comparison shows, the years lived at each age above 65 are expected to grow much more rapidly than can be compensated for by any plausible forecast of decline in the ill-health rate. For every 100 000 births, the number of years lived at ages 65–100 is forecast to grow from 1 271 193 in 1985 to 2 014 370 in 2085, an increase of 58 per cent. The aggregate expectation of ill health will increase.

Even a change in the definition of ill health to one that is more restrictive than activity limitation will not overturn this result. Such a change would move each curve to a lower position on the schedule, but it would have little effect on the relative positions of the curves for 1985 and the forecasts for 2085.

CONCLUSION

The future path of health remains unclear except among the aged. For the age group 0–64, the near-term future seems likely to preserve an inverse association between mortality and morbidity. Both aggregate and age-specific morbidity rates will increase because mortality will decline, and because mortality will decline more rapidly than factors contributing to ill health can be removed. Only in the longer term is a more favorable forecast plausible and, in order to be accurate, that forecast depends on substantial changes in sickness risks. To come to pass, morbidity decline seems to require major breakthroughs in the avoidance or prevention of chronic degenerative disease or in therapy. To the degree that the grounds for many degenerative diseases are prepared early in life, and the population now alive remains untreated in any apparent way, the near-term prospect for morbidity decline is limited to breakthroughs in therapy or some combination of therapeutic innovations and superior health maintenance. Only in the longer term can the younger population be expected to build better health indexes and then only if more is learned about how higher risks of chronic degenerative disease in middle age or old age are acquired early in life.

In the meantime, the health experience of people born after 1935 will draw particularly close scrutiny. These cohorts constitute special groups because they were the first human cohorts to experience a rapid and general curtailment of one of the sickness risks, the risk of falling ill, and because they include the oversized cohorts of the baby boomers. The baby boomers, born from 1946 to 1964 and ages 26–44 in 1990, will begin to reach age 65 in 2011. For the next fifty years or more after 2011, the health of these oversized cohorts will be a major determinant of the incidence and cost of ill health in the US. If the baby boomers prove to have accumulated lower ill-health indexes because they fell sick less often than preceding generations, and recovered from many illnesses more quickly, and if these gains were not offset by higher insult accumulation from the broad category of injuries, these cohorts may experience both longer lives and less morbidity as they reach those ages – 45 and above – at which morbidity and mortality risks increase. That is the best case. The worst case consists of a continuation of the inverse association between morbidity and mortality, so that ill health rates and the cost of health care rise until, between 2011 and 2050, the leading and inescapable preoccupation of the nation will be to provide adequate health care for the old. The baby boom cohorts are so large, the prediction of their health and mortality experience before and after age 65 is such an important factor in the way individuals and the nation should plan for the future, and the difficulty of compensating for any significant underprojection so great that our attention must focus on developing better means of projection.

Deferring the age at which terminal chronic diseases attain a clinical level, which is the Fries-Crapo version of a favorable forecast for future morbidity at ages below 65, would substantially reduce expected ill-health time in middle age. Without plausible reasons to expect equivalent changes in the sickness expectation at higher ages, however, more people surviving to and beyond age 65 would inevitably mean an increase in aggregate sickness among the old. That is, even a compression of morbidity at lower ages would mean an expansion of morbidity at higher ages, and perhaps in the two segments of the age spectrum together. The two have not been combined here because of the absence of appropriate measurements of health experience from lower to higher ages.

What is the most plausible overall prospect? The best sense of it can be obtained by returning to Figure 8.2 to compare the space between survival curves for the US in 1979–81 and the Faber and Wade projection at each age. Sickness has been and seems likely to remain a function of age. To add years of health to the population's expectation, it is necessary to add years of life at ages when good health is a reasonable prospect. But the comparison shows that the space of survival time is divided unevenly. Lacking a breakthrough in extension of the life span, and specifically a breakthrough that defers aging at a point when the morbidity risk is low, far fewer years are likely to be added to the survival rectangle at ages 64 and below than at ages 65 and above. Aggregate ill-health rates and aggregate ill-health time will increase because the old will live longer lives.

This history emerges as a circle, a comfortable geometric and historical form, but one leading to an uncomfortable forecast. In the earliest period yet open to reconstruction, the seventeenth and eighteenth centuries, most sicknesses were resolved swiftly and the risks of sickness and death were high. The combination of high death rates and still higher rates of falling sick produced a comparatively low risk of being sick in a mortality regime in which few members of any cohort survived the many disease hazards of earlier life to suffer protracted ill health in middle or old age. Chronic degenerative diseases were not absent, but their effects were muted by the rapid depletion of each cohort between ages 0 and 20. In the nineteenth century, a third option forced its way between the two – recovery and death – that had been dominant. Protracted sickness became common. It moved down the scale of age. The risk of being sick emerged as an important element in health, and sickness and mortality acquired a strong inverse association. This association and the inverse trend of morbidity and mortality still dominate patterns of sickness and death toward the end of the twentieth century in the United States.

Insult accumulation theory describes health risks as a function of past health experience and suggests that the rate at which insults accumulate can be manipulated by reducing the number or limiting the severity or duration of illness and injury episodes and of behavioral insults. The historical record identifies periods and cohorts in which sickness risks have changed. Up to the present, the changes that have occurred have tended to increase the risk of being sick more than to reduce the risk of falling sick, resulting in the continued force of an inverse association between morbidity and mortality. But the theory suggests that the association can be broken, that the path to lower morbidity rates lies in a reduction in the sickness risk of present and future cohorts at those years of life in which insults accumulate.

There seems, however, to be a threshold age at which even the most successful campaign against insult accumulation will have limited effect. This threshold is an individual matter, and when it is expressed as an average we must remember that the average occurs at an age at which variance in health status is high and may be rising. That threshold is not likely to be age 65, a division adopted here more because of the age structure of the evidence than because there is a compelling reason to believe age surpasses insult accumulation at that age on the average. Probably the average age is higher than 65, and it may itself be manipulatable in a rather modest way. But so far aging inescapably emerges as the dominant cause of ill health, and ill-health conditions multiply with age. Superior health maintenance earlier in life seems likely to reduce the average number of chronic and acute conditions suffered by the old, but less likely to reduce the proportion of the cohort reporting ill health.

To have reached an era in which people live still longer lives but should expect to live them partly in ill health rather than always in health is a remarkable achievement. The task that humankind set itself was, after all, not to preserve health but to preserve life through the span available to the species. Many things may still be done to avoid or prevent sickness, to defer the onset of degenerative disease, and to improve the quality of health at every age. These things warrant the expense they will require because they will reduce suffering and because they should also reduce the costs of health care. But, on the whole, we must be prepared to spend more on health care. Barring breakthroughs in the key areas of preventing or avoiding degenerative sickness, breakthroughs that counter the effects of aging and sharply reduce the risk of ill health among the old, most of the next century must become a story of continued increase in the need for health care. If the bad news is that our society faces a mounting aggregate burden of ill health, the good news is that this is the outcome of a long and only recently successful campaign to extend survivorship, and that the campaign has begun to be won at a time when material prosperity is great enough to afford the financial costs of ill health.

Notes

Introduction

1. Arthur E. Imhof and Øivind Larsen, *Sozialgeschichte und Medizin: Probleme der quantifizierenden Quellenbearbeitung in der Sozial- und Medizingeschichte* (Oslo, 1976), pp. 180ff.

1 The Boundary of Survival

1. The census overstates the number of centenarians, especially those over 107, so that life tables based on census data will show more people alive and more years lived around age 110 than actually occur – Gregory Spencer, 'The Characteristics of Centenarians in the 1980 Census' (abstract), *Population Index*, 52, no. 3 (Fall 1986), 443.
2. Sherwood L. Washburn, 'Longevity in Primates', in James L. McGaugh and Sara B. Kiesler, eds, *Aging: Biology and Behavior* (New York, 1981), p. 16; Morris Rockstein, Jeffrey A. Chesky, and Marvin L. Sussman, 'Comparative Biology and Evolution of Aging', in Caleb E. Finch and Leonard Hayflick, eds, *Handbook of the Biology of Aging* (New York, 1977), p. 5.
3. A. de Moivre, *Annuities for Life* (London, 1725), pp. iv–v. See also M.D. Grmek, *On Ageing and Old Age: Basic Problems and Historical Aspects of Gerontology and Geriatrics* (The Hague, 1958), pp. 29–41.
4. Robert R. Kohn, 'Heart and Cardiovascular System', in Finch and Hayflick, eds, *Handbook of the Biology of Aging*, pp. 295–6, observes that, in the US female population of 1966, individuals who did not die from other causes died from cardiovascular disease, pneumonia, or accident at a modal age of 86 to 88 years. 'Which cause they will die from cannot be predicted, but the cause would appear to be fortuitous because deaths will occur at around the same age regardless of the terminal disease or injury.' Also James F. Fries and Lawrence M. Crapo, *Vitality and Aging: Implications of the Rectangular Curve* (San Francisco, CA, 1981), pp. 69–77.
5. E.A. Wrigley and R.S. Schofield, *The Population History of England, 1541–1871* (Cambridge, MA, 1981), p. 230.
6. Gy. Acsádi and J. Nemeskéri, *History of Human Life Span and Mortality*, trans. by K. Balás (Budapest, 1970); Mark Nathan Cohen, *Human Health and the Rise of Civilization* (New Haven, 1989) forthcoming; Jane E. Buikstra and Della C. Cook, 'Palaeopathology: An American Account', *Annual Review of Anthropology*, 9 (1980), pp. 433–70; Francis L. Black,' Modern Isolated Pre-agricultural Populations as a Source of Information on Prehistoric Epidemic Patterns', in N.F. Stanley and R.A. Joske, eds, *Changing Disease Patterns and Human Behaviour* (London,

1980), pp. 37–54; Keith Manchester, *The Archaeology of Disease* (Bradford, 1983).

7. Cohen, *Human Health*, Mark Nathan Cohen and George J. Armelagos, eds, *Paleopathology at the Origins of Agriculture* (New York, 1984), esp. pp. 585–601 explore the controversy. See also F. Macfarlane Burnet, *Virus as Organism* (Cambridge, MA, 1946); Ronald Hare, *Pomp and Pestilence: Infectious Disease, Its Origins and Conquest* (New York, 1955); Gerald D. Hart, ed., *Disease in Ancient Man: An International Symposium* (Toronto, 1983).

8. Alan H. Goodman *et al.*, 'Health Changes at Dickson Mounds, Illinois (A.D. 950–1300)', in Cohen and Armelagos, eds, *Paleopathology*, pp. 272–7.

9. Three of the curves (Alsónémedi, Late Woodland mixed, and Middle Mississippian) are based directly on excavations, and two (model A and the Maghreb-type) are model curves based on mixed experience. Notice also that the radix has been changed to 100 to signal how small the skeletal samples are. Goodman *et al.*, 'Health Changes', report from a total of 572 deaths, which is a particularly large population.

10. The model A population suggests 22.3 per cent. The best case, the Alsónémedi neolithic, indicates 34 per cent, but it is based on only 60 individuals. Age at death is particularly difficult to distinguish after 70, with the result that paleolithic and neolithic series may understate the ages achieved by the oldest individuals whose remains have been examined. This likelihood guides the notion that the maximum life span of paleolithic and neolithic humankind was quite similar to that of modern humans, the difference lying more in the proportion reaching advanced age.

11. For example, James C. Riley, *The Eighteenth-Century Campaign to Avoid Disease* (New York, 1987).

12. Acsádi and Nemeskéri, *Human Life Span*, p. 224. These observations take into account the likelihood that slaves will have entered observation at younger ages than people identified as free. On recent evidence of differentiation see Jacques Dupâquier, 'La contre-offensive de la mortalité dans le dernier quart du XXe siècle', *Histoire, économie et société*, 3, no. 3 (1984), pp. 477ff.

13. The Maghreb-type population represents especially North Africa; the Roman era is based on epitaphs at Intercisa and Brigetio (present-day Hungary) from the imperial period; the medieval on several series of Hungarian cemetery excavations from the tenth to the twelfth century; the mid-nineteenth century on males in England and Wales; and the early twentieth century from the US life table for 1910.

14. Acsádi and Nemeskéri, *Human Life Span*, pp. 182ff., estimate that female mortality in paleolithic and neolithic populations exceeded male by some 20 per cent.

15. It is important to notice that neither trend has been derived from age-specific data. R. Ted Steinbock, *Paleopathological Diagnosis and Interpretation: Bone Diseases in Ancient Human Populations* (Springfield, IL, 1976), p. 23; William Black, *A Comparative View of the Mortality of the Human Species* (London, 1788), the table between pp. 64 and 65 (reporting on cause of death from the London bills of mortality

from 1701–76); and any of a variety of vital statistics series for recent populations, such as the annual series from the US, National Center for Health Statistics, *Vital Statistics of the United States*. Considering violent deaths within Britain only, however, Hair infers a trend decline from the nineteenth century to the twentieth. P.E.H. Hair, 'Deaths from Violence in Britain: A Tentative Secular Survey', *Population Studies*, 25, no. 1 (Mar. 1971), pp. 5–24. War casualties are excluded.

16. This discussion is not intended to be exhaustive. Some other factors will be discussed below. Particularly useful summary treatments may be found in B[ernard] Benjamin, *Health and Vital Statistics* (London, 1968), which treats especially occupation and locale; Louis I. Dublin, Alfred J. Lotka, and Mortimer Spiegelman, *Length of Life: A Study of the Life Table* (rev. ed.; New York, 1949), esp. pp. 99–118 on genetic and environmental factors in the inheritance of a propensity to be long-lived.

2 Sickness, Aging and Death

1. Richard G. Cutler, 'Life-Span Extension', in James L. McGaugh and Sara B. Kiesler, eds, *Aging: Biology and Behavior* (New York, 1981), p. 66.
2. Alex Comfort, *The Biology of Senescence* (3rd edn; Edinburgh, 1979), p. 22, his italics. The elipses and brackets signal that I have changed the order of the sentence by shifting the qualifying phrase to the end. More extreme versions of this proposition may also be found. See, for example, Ralph Goldman, 'Aging and Geriatric Medicine', in James B. Wyngaarden and Lloyd H. Smith, eds, *Textbook of Medicine* (3rd edn; Philadelphia, 1982), p. 36.
3. Comfort, *Senescence*, p. 23. Also R.E. Beard, 'A Theory of Mortality based on Actuarial, Biological and Medical Considerations', *Proceedings of the International Population Conference* (New York, 1961), pp. 611–26.
4. Benjamin Gompertz, 'On the Nature of the Function Expressive of the Law of Human Mortality . . .', *Philosophical Transactions*, 115 (1825), pp. 513–85; William Siler, 'Parameters of Mortality in Human Populations with Widely Varying Life Spans', *Statistics in Medicine*, 2 (1983), pp. 373–80, gives a recent reinterpretation.
5. The literature on aging is vast. Some especially useful books and essays include: Comfort, *Senescence*; Caleb E. Finch and Edward L. Schneider, eds, *Handbook of the Biology of Aging* (2nd edn; New York, 1985); A.H. Bittles and K.J. Collins, eds, *The Biology of Human Ageing* (Cambridge, 1986); McGaugh and Kiesler, eds, *Aging: Biology and Behavior*; Nathan W. Shock *et al.*, *Normal Human Aging: The Baltimore Longitudinal Study of Aging* (Washington, 1984); Bernard L. Strehler, *Time, Cells, and Aging* (2nd edn; New York, 1977); Samuel H. Preston, ed., *Biological and Social Aspects of Mortality and the Length of Life* (Liege, 1982), pp. 223–9. Theodore J. Gordon, Herbert Gerjuoy, and Mark Anderson, eds, *Life-Extending Technologies: A Technology Assessment* (New York, 1979), attempts to foresee life span extending biomedical means likely to appear before the year 2000. On the specific

case of burns, see J.P. Bull and J.R. Squire, 'A Study of Mortality in a Burns Unit', *Annals of Surgery*, 130 (July-Dec. 1949), pp. 160–73.

6. Life tables are usually brought to a close at a lower age than the oldest survivors in a population. The most common method of closure is to apply a Makeham term, another curve named after a nineteenth-century actuary. Makeham closures turn the curve upward, and imply a catastrophic increase in the risk of death. Unretouched data, never plentiful for ages 100 + and usually troubled by age misreporting, suggest instead a tailing off toward closure. That is, in reality the rate of increase in the death rate slows and loses stability.

7. Kenneth G. Manton, 'Changing Concepts of Morbidity and Mortality in the Elderly Population', *Milbank Memorial Fund Quarterly/Health and Society*, 60, no. 2 (Spring 1982), pp. 183–244; Kenneth G. Manton and Beth J. Soldo, 'Dynamics of Health Changes in the Oldest Old: New Perspectives and Evidence', *Milbank Memorial Fund Quarterly/Health and Society*, 63, no. 2 (Spring 1985), pp. 224–6; Kenneth G. Manton and Eric Stallard, *Recent Trends in Mortality Analysis* (Orlando, 1984); Beard, 'A Theory of Mortality'. Matilda White Riley and Kathleen Bond, 'Beyond Ageism: Postponing the Onset of Disability', in Matilda White Riley, Beth Hess, and Kathleen Bond, eds, *Aging in Society: Selected Reviews of Recent Research* (Hillsdale, N.J., 1983), pp. 243–52, interpret the movement of individual variability toward higher ages as evidence of deferral of the onset of health problems. As will be shown below, it may more securely be seen as a deferral of the onset of terminal sickness rather than of sickness in general. On heterogeneity see Kenneth G. Manton and Eric Stallard, 'Heterogeneity and Its Effect on Mortality Measurement', in Preston, ed., *Aspects of Mortality*, pp. 265–99; George Alter and James C. Riley, 'Frailty, Sickness, and Death: Models of Morbidity and Mortality in Historical Populations', forthcoming. J.H. Sheldon, *The Social Medicine of Old Age: Report of an Inquiry in Wolverhampton* (London, 1948), gives an empirical demonstration.

8. In addition to the sources cited in n. 5 above, see Edward L. Schneider and John D. Reed, Jr., 'Life Extension', *New England Journal of Medicine*, 312, no. 18 (May 2, 1985), pp. 1159–68; Arthur Schatzkin, 'How Long Can We Live? A More Optimistic View of Potential Gains in Life Expectancy', *American Journal of Public Health*, 70, no. 11 (Nov. 1980), pp. 1199–1200.

9. Cutler, 'Life-Span Extension', pp. 40–2.

10. George Cheyne, *An Essay of Health and Long Life* (4th edn; London, 1725), p. 30 for the quote and pp. 30-42. To an historian, Cheyne's comments form part of a sustained discussion on health maintenance, of which a recent and often cited example is Nedra B. Belloc and Lester Breslow, 'Relationship of Physical Health Status and Health Practices', *Preventive Medicine*, I (1972), pp. 409–21. One significant difference between Cheyne and Belloc and Breslow is that Belloc and Breslow show no awareness of antecedents of their advice. The Belloc-Breslow case is developed further in Lisa F. Berkman and Lester Breslow, *Health and Ways of Living: The Alameda County Study* (New York, 1983).

11. Roy L. Walford, *Maximum Life Span* (New York, 1983), p. 99. On Cornaro see William F. Butler, ed., *The Art of Living Long* [by Luigi Cornaro], new ed. (Milwaukee, 1903); Henry E. Sigerist, *Landmarks in the History of Hygiene* (New York, 1956), pp. 36–46.

12. See below, pp. 38–9.

13. Cutler, 'Life-Span Extension', p. 53.

14. Strehler, *Time, Cells, and Aging*, p. 128; George A. Sacher, 'Life Table Modification and Life Prolongation', in Finch and Hayflick, eds, *Handbook of the Biology of Aging*, p. 601; Arthur C. Upton, 'Pathobiology,' in id., pp. 515–16. Cutler, 'Life-Span Extension', pp. 39–40, doubts that a useful distinction can be made at the population rather than the individual level, but also (p. 33) complicates the issue by suggesting comparatively low values for his equivalent of modal age of death (the point at which 90 per cent of a cohort has died) and potential life span. The latter he estimates at age 100, at which age as many as 1150 per 100 000 members of the US population of 1979-81 remained alive. The former, a variable term, appears at age 91-92 in the US population of 1979-81, still an age at which it seems unlikely that the aging term will approach 100 per cent. See also Manton, 'Changing Concepts', pp. 204–5; J. Grimley Evans, 'The Health of an Ageing Population', in Bittles and Collins, eds, *Biology of Human Ageing*, pp. 201–14; Angelos C. Economos, 'Rate of Aging, Rate of Dying and the Mechanism of Mortality', *Archives of Gerontology and Geriatrics*, 1 (1982), pp.3 –27. Riley and Bond, 'Ageism', point out the fatalism and age bias that may follow from stressing intrinsic causes, and suggest the malleability of some biological markers associated with aging.

15. That is, the death rate was higher even though its rate of increase followed the Gompertz function.

16. This is Sacher's point in 'Life Table Modification'; and Bernard L. Strehler's in 'Implications of Aging Research for Society', *Federation* [of American Societies for Experimental Biology] *Proceedings*, 34, no. 1 (Jan. 1975), pp. 5–8. It is developed further by John W. Rowe and Robert L. Kahn, 'Human Aging; Usual and Successful', *Science*, 237 (July 10, 1987), 143–9.

17. Abdel R. Omran, 'The Epidemiologic Transition: A Theory of the Epidemiology of Population Change', *Milbank Memorial Fund Quarterly*, 49, no. 4 (Oct. 1971), pp. 509–38. Also Arthur E. Imhof, 'From the Old Mortality Pattern to the New: Implications of a Radical Change from the Sixteenth Century to the Twentieth Century', *Bulletin of the History of Medicine*, 59 (1985), pp. 1–29.

18. E.g., Roy M. Acheson and Spencer Hagard, *Health, Society and Medicine: An Introduction to Community Medicine* (Oxford, 1984).

19. Stanley L. Robbins, Ramzi S. Cotran, and Vinay Kumar, *Pathologic Basis of Disease* (3rd edn; Philadelphia, 1984), p. 479; Acheson and Hagard, *Health, Society and Medicine*, p. 45. The historical trend of environmentally-influenced malformations is an important but neglected issue. Some environmental causes of malformations (e.g., dietary deficiency during pregnancy, rubella) were more prevalent in the past, but other causes (for example, cigarette smoking and chemotherapies with

unsuspected side-effects, such as thalidomide) were less prevalent.
20. Arthur C. Upton, 'Pathobiology', in Finch and Hayflick, *Biology of Aging*, p. 529, reviews recent evidence.
21. Acheson and Hagard, *Health, Society and Medicine*, p. 43.
22. Hardin B. Jones, 'The Relation of Human Health to Age, Place, and Time', in James E. Birren, ed., *Handbook of Aging and the Individual* (Chicago, 1959), p. 339.
23. The phrase 'new survivor' was coined by Lois M. Verbrugge, 'Longer Life but Worsening Health? Trends in Health and Mortality of Middle-aged and Older Persons', *Milbank Memorial Fund Quarterly/Health and Society*, 62, no. 3 (Summer 1984) pp. 475–519.
24. Lucinda McCray Beier, 'In Sickness and in Health: A Seventeenth Century Family's Experience', in Roy Porter, ed., *Patients and Practitioners: Lay Perceptions of Medicine in Pre-industrial Society* (Cambridge, 1985), pp. 101–28; Alan Macfarlane, ed., *The Diary of Ralph Josselin, 1616–1683* (London, 1976). Macfarlane points out (pp. xx and xxvi) that the period 1646–53 is especially well covered, claiming 40 per cent of total pages, and that entries become briefer from the mid-1660s.
25. Alain F. Corcos, 'Jean Astruc (1684–1766) on Old Age: A Man of his Time?', *Clio Medica*, 18, nos. 1–4 (1983), pp. 141–54.
26. See, for instance, Friedrich Hoffmann, *Fundamenta Medicinae*, trans. by Lester S. King (London, 1971), pp. 47 and 49. Also, Mirko D. Grmek, 'Préliminaires d'une étude historique des maladies', *Annales: économies, sociétés, civilisations*, 24, no. 6 Nov.-Dec. 1969)., pp. 1476–80.
27. Hardin B. Jones, 'A Special Consideration of the Aging Process, Disease, and Life Expectancy', in John H. Lawrence and Cornelius A. Tobias, eds, *Advances in Biological and Medical Physics*, vol. 4 (New York, 1956), pp. 281–337. This essay appeared initially in 1955 under the same title but in slightly different form in a series published by the University of California Radiation Laboratory, 3105 (Berkeley, 1955). The ideas are restated and developed further in Jones, 'Relation of Human Health'. R.A.M. Case, 'Cohort Analysis of Mortality Rates as an Historical or Narrative Technique', *British Journal of Preventive and Social Medicine*, 10 (1956), pp. 159–71, surveys some earlier versions of the cohort theory of mortality rate determination.
28. This distinction, in which physiologic age is often called 'functional' or 'biological' age, remains important but troubled. G.A. Borkan, 'Biological Age Assessment in Adulthood', in Bittles and Collins, eds, *Biology of Human Ageing*, pp. 81–3, reviews recent techniques and conclusions. Also William Regelson and F. Marott Sinex, *Intervention in the Aging Process* (2 vols; New York, 1982); Ian W. Webster and Alexander R. Logie, 'A Relationship between Age and Health Status in Female Subjects', *Journal of Gerontology*, 31, no. 5 (1976), pp. 546–50, who associate healthy females with lower biological ages but on the basis of small numbers (97 subjects) and a narrowly selected group. S. Jay Olshansky, 'Simultaneous/Multiple Cause-Delay (SIMCAD): An Epidemiological Approach to Projecting Mortality', *Journal of Gerontology*, 42, no. 4 (1987) pp. 358–65, considers this question in terms of

successive birth cohorts in which the progression of degenerative disease is delayed.

29. This suggestion was in keeping with earlier work regarding the importance of care from birth to age 15. W.O. Kermack, A.G. McKendrick, and P.L. McKinlay, 'Death-Rates in Great Britain and Sweden: Some General Regularities and Their Significance', *Lancet*, 1 (March 31, 1934), pp. 698–703.

30. Jones, 'A Special Consideration', pp. 298 and 304, respectively. The association, which can be stated also as an assertion that past health is a good predictor of future health, has been shown in clinical studies. Lawrence E. Hinkle, Norman Plummer, and L. Holland Whitney, 'The Continuity of Patterns of Illness and the Prediction of Future Health', *Journal of Occupational Medicine*, 3 (Sept. 1961), pp. 417–23; W. Dab, J. Rochon, and L. Bernard, 'L'absence au travail comme prédicteur de morbidité grave . . .', *Revue d'épidémiologie et de santé publique*, 34 (1986), pp. 252–60.

31. Mervyn W. Susser, *Causal Thinking in the Health Sciences: Concepts and Strategies of Epidemiology* (New York, 1973), is especially helpful in organizing thoughts on this issue.

32. See above pp. 250–1, n.15, and the discussion of war fatalities and casualties on pp. 204–5.

33. L.J. Rather, 'The "Six Things Non-Natural": A Note on the Origins and Fate of a Doctrine and a Phrase', *Clio Medica*, 3 (1968), pp. 337–47; and, for examples, Cheyne, *Essay of Health*, pp. 19–20, 176–80, and *passim*.

34. On stress, which I take to be the least familiar item in this list, see esp. Sheldon Cohen and S. Leonard Syme, eds, *Social Support and Health* (Orlando, FL, 1985); Lisa F. Berkman, 'Social Networks, Support, and Health: Taking the Next Step Forward', *American Journal of Epidemiology*, 123, no. 4 (Apr. 1986), pp. 559–62.

35. Sacher, 'Life Table Modification', pp. 604–5; Bernard Benjamin, 'Smoking and Mortality', in Preston, ed., *Biological and Social Aspects*, pp. 433–46; Kenneth G. Manton and Eric Stallard, 'Heterogeneity and Its Effect on Mortality Measurement', in Jacques Vallin, John H. Pollard and Larry Heligman, eds, *Methodologies for the Collection and Analysis of Mortality Data* (Liege, 1984), p. 288. Also below, pp. 205–6.

36. Iwao M. Moriyama, 'Mortality Effects of Physical and Chemical Contamination of the Environment', in Preston, *Biological and Social Aspects*, p. 69.

37. For instance, in England between 1661 and 1666, attributable to the last plague epidemic. E.A. Wrigley and R.S. Schofield, *The Population History of England, 1541–1871* (Cambridge, Mass., 1981), p. 230.

38. Sacher, 'Life Table Modification', p. 601; Upton, 'Pathobiology', pp. 513–17; Strehler, *Time, Cells, and Aging*, pp. 114–15. Sacher subdivides the vulnerability term to distinguish period and cohort effects.

39. T.B.L. Kirkwood and R. Holliday, 'Ageing as a Consequence of Natural Selection', in Bittles and Collins, eds, *Biology of Human Ageing*, 1–16; Kirkwood and Holliday, 'The Evolution of Ageing and Longevity', *Proceedings of the Royal Society of London*, B205, no. 1161 (Sept. 21,

1979), pp. 531–46; Thomas B.L. Kirkwood, 'Comparative and Evolutionary Aspects of Longevity', in Finch and Schneider, eds, *Biology of Aging*, pp. 27–44.

40. Strehler, *Time, Cells, and Aging*, pp. 113–15.

41. Trevor H. Howell, 'Multiple Pathology in Nonagenarians', *Geriatrics*, 18 (Dec. 1963) pp. 899–902.

42. See below, pp. 79–80. Also Samuel H. Preston, *Older Male Mortality and Cigarette Smoking: A Demographic Analysis* (Westport, Conn., 1976), pp. 38–9, shows the importance of health experience at adult ages in the case of cigarette smoking; and Richard H. Steckel, 'A Peculiar Population: The Nutrition, Health, and Mortality of American Slaves from Childhood to Maturity', *Journal of Economic History*, 46, no. 3 (Sept. 1986), pp. 721–41, considering nutrition and growth, suggests that developmental status in childhood is not decisive for later experience.

43. Jones, 'A Special Consideration', p. 291.

44. Alter and Riley, 'Frailty, Sickness, and Death'; James C. Riley, 'Ill Health during the English Mortality Decline: The Friendly Societies' Experience', *Bulletin of the History of Medicine*, 61, no. 4 (1987), pp. 563–88.

45. See below, p. 235.

3 Sickness Risk

1. George Cheyne, *An Essay of Health and Long Life* (4th edn; London, 1725), pp. 1–2.

2. For this section I have drawn on a variety of sources of which the most important are: B[ernard] Benjamin, 'The Measurement of Morbidity', *Journal of the Institute of Actuaries*, 83 (1957), pp. 225–67; J.N. Biraben, 'Morbidity and the Major Processes Culminating in Death', in Samuel H. Preston, ed., *Biological and Social Aspects of Mortality and the Length of Life* (Liege, 1982) pp. 385–92; E.J.M. Campbell, J.G. Scadding and R.S. Roberts, 'The Concept of Disease', *British Medical Journal*, 2 (Sept. 29, 1979), pp. 757–62; the essays in A.J. Culyer, ed., *Health Indicators* (Oxford, 1983), especially Ernest Schroeder, 'Concepts of Health and Illness', pp. 22–33; Arthur L. Caplan, H. Tristram Engelhardt, Jr. and James J. McCartney, eds, *Concepts of Health and Disease: Interdisciplinary Perspectives* (Reading, Mass., 1981); Edwin J. Faulkner, *Health Insurance* (New York, 1960); Harald Hanoluwka, 'Measuring the Health of Populations, Indicators and Interpretations', *Social Science and Medicine*, 20, no. 12 (1985), pp. 1207–24; R.M. Kaplan, J.W. Bush and C.C. Berry, 'Health Status: Types of Validity and the Index of Well-Being', *Health Services Research*, 11 (1976), pp. 478–507; Horacio Fabrega, Jr., *Disease and Social Behavior: An Interdisciplinary Perspective* (Cambridge, Mass., 1974); Henry E. Sigerist, 'The Special Position of the Sick', in Milton I. Roemer, ed., *On the Sociology of Medicine* (New York, 1960), pp. 9–22; Daniel F. Sullivan, 'Conceptual Problems in Developing an Index of Health', in US, Department of Health, Education, and Welfare, Public Health Service,

Vital and Health Statistics, National Center for Health Statistics, Series 2, no. 17 (Washington, 1966); Mervyn Susser, William Watson and Kim Hopper, *Sociology in Medicine* (3rd edn; New York, 1985). Sigerist's essay, published initially in 1929, is interesting also for its assertion of the doctrine of perfect repair, according to which most sickness episodes resolved in recovery have no lasting effect on the vitality of the individual.

3. In the collection of morbidity data there are also variations on the diagnostic model. The most important of these extracts information about self-reported cases of ill health, identified either as events (episodes) or as specific illnesses. The degree to which individuals know about their health problems, or can identify them accurately, is often uncertain.

4. E.g., Sidney Katz *et al.*, 'Active Life Expectancy', *New England Journal of Medicine*, 309, no. 20 (Nov. 17, 1983), pp. 1218–23, use certain 'activities of daily living' to distinguish active from restricted periods within remaining life expectancy. Martin K. Chen and Bertha E. Bryant, 'The Measurement of Health – A Critical and Selective Overview', *International Journal of Epidemiology*, 4, no. 4 (1975), p. 261, observe that the ADL index 'applies essentially to [the] home-bound or institutionalized chronically ill and aged'.

5. James C. Riley, 'Disease without Death: New Sources for a History of Sickness', *Journal of Interdisciplinary History*, 17, no. 3 (Winter 1987), pp. 537–63; id., 'Ill Health during the English Mortality Decline: The Friendly Societies' Experience', *Bulletin of the History of Medicine* 61, no. 4 (1987), pp. 563–88; id., 'Characteristics of Sick Funds and Their Members', unpublished. These sources, and an abundant literature which is referenced in them, consider such issues as rule variations among sick funds, changes in survey methodology, economic incentives and disincentives to enter claims, and the effects of introducing paid sickness absence. For present purposes the important point to note is that these potential and actual causes of distortion have been acknowledged in the selection and treatment of sickness rates which are reported here.

6. Lucinda McCray Beier, 'In Sickness and in Health: A Seventeenth Century Family's Experience', in Roy Porter, ed., *Patients and Practitioners: Lay Perceptions of Medicine in Pre-industrial Society* (Cambridge, 1985), pp. 111, 113, and 123.

7. The association is to ill health in general, but not to all diagnostic or functional measurements of health status. For example, Susan Reisine and Julia Miller, 'A Longitudinal Study of Work Loss Related to Dental Disease', *Social Science and Medicine*, 21, no. 12 (1985), pp. 1309–14, argue that age does not much affect work loss in dental disease. However, that lack of association may have more to do with professional repair or replacement of diseased teeth than with risk in the absence of treatment.

8. For example, US, Department of Health, Education, and Welfare, *Healthy People: The Surgeon General's Report on Health Promotion and Disease Prevention 1979* (Washington, 1979), p. 1.

9. During the survey period Foresters membership increased from 217 000 to 296 000. Whereas Watson dealt with 3 180 378.5 years at risk to death and 2 995 724 years at risk to sickness, Neison worked with a total of 1 302 166 years at risk to death. The men who were Foresters lived mostly in England and Wales and, like the Odd Fellows, followed a wide range of occupations.

10. Neison provides information about the number of members who experienced any sickness at each age, and the number who died. As calculated here, the risk of falling sick is the proportion entering claims or dying to member years at risk. Francis G.P. Neison, Jr., *The Rates of Mortality and Sickness According to the Experience for the Five Years, 1871–1875, of the Ancient Order of Foresters Friendly Society* . . . (London, 1882), p. 81, shows that members who died were sick for longer periods than those who recovered, as might be expected. This suggests that the number of people in the category of deaths without prior claims is small.

W[illiam] Sutton, *Special Report on Sickness and Mortality Experienced in Registered Friendly Societies* . . ., House of Commons, Sessional Papers 1896, LXXIX, 79, also furnishes information on the event rate for the period 1876–80. His data indicate a somewhat higher risk of falling sick at ages 30–34 and up, but they describe both a highly similar age curve and similar age-specific levels.

11. Sutton, *Special Report*. Sutton counted only people who had belonged to a society for at least three years, a simple device that eliminated most of the instances in which entrances or exits threatened to distort the denominator and most of the effect of rule variations among societies. This procedure may also have measured sickness in a population different in some respects from that belonging to a single society for any period. For example, longer-term members may have been more settled, an issue of potential significance for an interpretation in which attitude toward risk is one of the characteristics to be considered. Alfred Williams Watson, *Friendly Society Finance Considered in its Actuarial Aspect: A Course of Lectures* (London, 1912), p. 48, attributes high turnover at ages 17–19 to transfers from juvenile to adult branches, and remarks that entrants to adult societies were screened again for health status. Sutton seems to have counted sickness from the first day of eligibility for benefits, and it is not apparent whether the length of the waiting period varied among the societies he investigated.

12. Sutton, *Special Report*, pp. 4–7, 12–15, and 15a–15tt. The additional surveys, also reported by Sutton, deal with experience in some friendly societies in England during 1856–60 and 1861–70 and in Wales 1856–75. They report peaks in the risk of being sick at ages 18 to 20. The same sources indicate a corresponding mortality peak.

13. US, Bureau of the Census, *United States Life Tables, 1929 to 1931* . . . *1900 to 1902* (Washington, 1936); James F. Fries and Lawrence M. Crapo, *Vitality and Aging: Implications of the Rectangular Curve* (San Francisco, 1981), pp. 27–8.

14. Carl L. Erhardt and Joyce E. Berlin, eds, *Mortality and Morbidity in the United States* (Cambridge, Mass., 1974), pp. 28–30; J. Roswell Gal-

lagher, Felix P. Heald and Dale C. Garell, eds, *Medical Care of the Adolescent* (3rd edn; New York, 1976), pp. 11–14 and 697–9.

15. Thomas McKeown, *The Modern Rise of Population* (London, 1976), p. 58, reports rates.

16. W. Palin Elderton and Richard C. Fippard, *The Construction of Mortality and Sickness Tables* (London, 1914), p. 111.

17. Gallagher, Heald, and Garell, eds, *Medical Care of the Adolescent*.

18. N.S. Scrimshaw *et al.*, 'Nutrition and Infection Field Study in Guatemalan Villages, 1959–1964', *Archives of Environmental Health*, 16 (Feb. 1968), pp. 228–34; Leonardo J. Mata, *The Children of Santa María Cauqué: A Prospective Field Study of Health and Growth* (Cambridge, Mass., 1978), esp. pp. 254–92. Steven K. Clarke, 'Early Childhood Morbidity Trends in Prehistoric Populations', *Human Biology*, 52, no. 1 (Feb. 1980), pp. 79–85, also notes a peak at age 2 or 3 and relates that to weaning and its effects on nutrition and immunity.

19. For example, Beverly Winikoff, 'Weaning: Nutrition, Morbidity, and Mortality Consequences', in Samuel H. Preston, ed., *Biological and Social Aspects of Mortality and the Length of Life* (Liege, 1982), pp. 113–49; John H. Dingle, George F. Badger and William S. Jordan, *Illness in the Home: A Study of 25 000 Illnesses in a Group of Cleveland Families* (Cleveland, 1964, esp. pp. 22, 29, and 314–19; and Eduard J. Beck, *The Enigma of Aboriginal Health: Interaction between Biological, Social and Economic Factors in Alice Springs Town-camps* (Canberra, 1985), pp. 55–9. Cleveland families experienced 25 000 illnesses, but included only 85 different families. Winikoff campares mortality between breastfed and non-breastfed infants without considering other differences between the two populations and their environments.

20. For instance, Elisabeth Schach and Barbara Starfield, 'Acute Disability in Childhood: Examination of Agreement between Various Measures', *Medical Care*, 11 (July-Aug. 1973), pp. 297–309.

21. Robert D. Retherford, *The Changing Sex Differential in Mortality* (Westport, Conn., 1979). Also Alex Comfort, *The Biology of Senescence* (3rd edn; Edinburgh, 1979), pp. 163–7, regarding the sex differential among animals.

22. Samuel H. Preston, Nathan Keyfitz and Robert Schoen, *Causes of Death: Life Tables for National Populations* (New York, 1972), pp. 224 and 226; B.R. Mitchell and Phyllis Deane, *Abstract of British Historical Statistics* (Cambridge, 1971), pp. 38 and 40; and R.A.M. Case *et al.*, *The Chester Beatty Research Institute Serial Abridged Life Tables* (London, 1962), pp. 1–3 and 20–2.

23. For instance, Retherford, *Changing Sex Differential*, pp. 12–13. That is, environmental changes may have been responsible for most of the increasing sex mortality differential observed in the last 50 years, as Retherford argues, but a different mixture of biological and environmental factors obtained in earlier periods and that mixture changed over time.

24. Sutton, *Special Report*, pp. 8–11. It should be noticed that survey periods and membership durations do not overlap exactly. See also Francis G.P.

Neison, Sr., *Contributions to Vital Statistics: Being a Development of the Rate of Mortality and the Laws of Sickness* . . . (3rd edn; London, 1857), pp. 462–4, regarding 1836–40.

25. The inclusion of a few individuals at lower ages again signals that not all members of friendly societies held jobs. Francis G.P. Neison, Jr., *The Rates of Mortality and Sickness According to the Experience for the Ten Years 1878-1887, of the Independent Order of Rechabites* . . . (Manchester, 1889), pp. 92–3, provides data on female Rechabites at ages 13–62, but these include only 1441.5 years at risk.

26. US, Commissioner of Labor, Twenty-Fourth Annual Report, *Workmen's Insurance and Compensation Systems in Europe* (2 vols; Washington, 1911), I, pp. 364–8.

27. Lois M. Verbrugge, 'Gender and Health: An Update on Hypotheses and Evidence', *Journal of Health and Social Behavior*, 26, no. 3 (Sept. 1985), pp. 156–82. Also id., 'Sex Differentials in Morbidity and Mortality in the United States', *Social Biology*, 23, no. 4 (Winter 1976), pp. 275–96; id., 'From Sneezes to Adieux: Stages of Health for American Men and Women', *Social Science and Medicine*, 22, no. 11 (1986), pp. 1195-1212; Mary T. Westbrook and Linda L. Viney, 'Age and Sex Differences in Patients' Reactions to Illness', *Journal of Health and Social Behavior*, 24 (Dec. 1983), pp. 313–24; Constance Holden, 'Why Do Women Live Longer Than Men?' *Science*, 238 (Oct. 9, 1987), pp. 158–60. In the 1976 essay Verbrugge portrayed the NHIS as 'a social record of illness, not a purely epidemiological one' (pp. 294–5); in the 1985 essay her view was that the sex differential can be better related to actual differences in sickness risk than to differences in perceptions of illness.

28. Cheyne, *Essay of Health*, p. 173.

29. See the following chapter for more information about some representative diseases and their clinical courses. Information on clinical course is derived usually from late nineteenth- and early twentieth-century measures, and there may be instances in which it is inappropriate to assume that the diseases and treatments of that era may be transposed to interpret earlier disease experience.

30. Øivind Larsen, 'Eighteenth-Century Diseases, Diagnostic Trends, and Mortality', *The Fifth Scandinavian Demographic Symposium* (Hurdalssjøen, 1979) pp. 44 and 51; Ann G. Carmichael, 'Infection, Hidden Hunger, and History', *Journal of Interdisciplinary History*, 14, no. 2 (Autumn 1983), pp. 256–64, are especially helpful on this point.

31. E.g., Philip Cole, 'Morbidity in the United States', in Erhardt and Berlin, eds, *Mortality and Morbidity*, pp. 69 and 76. Cheyne, *Essay of Health*, p. 176, put the division at age 35 or 36, the 'meridian of life'.

32. The actuaries usually followed a society for five years, a period chosen in order to ensure that short-term events like epidemics did not distort findings. One of the advantages of five-year-long surveys is that they make it possible to follow long-term sicknesses.

33. Watson took sicknesses continuing into the survey period into account in locating claims weeks in each term, but did not count any claims preceding 1 January 1893. For this figure and some of the tables that follow, rates have been calculated from 52.18 weeks per year, that is, 365.25

days/7. Present-day actuarial methods are discussed in P[eter] Geddes and J[ohn] P. Holbrook, *Friendly Societies: A Text-Book for Actuarial Students* (Cambridge, 1963).

34. Watson's survey understates long-lasting sicknesses at ages at which entrances were numerous because fewer members had been in the society for more than two years. Sutton corrected most of this under-statement by considering only individuals who had belonged for at least three years, and who therefore had belonged long enough to be at risk to sickness lasting longer than two years. As a result Sutton's survey shows slightly higher proportions of sick time in weeks 105–260 in the age group 20–24, but the difference (4 per cent rather than 2 per cent) does not affect the broader argument presented here.

35. Sutton, *Special Report*, pp. 1134–51. Sutton labels these as weeks 0 to 4, 4 to 8, and 8 to 13, indicating that he counted the first week as week 0. He does not discuss how he located claims continuing into the survey period, and it is likely that his data include some episodes beginning before 1 January 1876. This probably helps explain why he found a higher risk of being sick in weeks 1–13 than did Watson.

36. The proportions do not sum to 100 per cent because of the omission of information about weeks 14–104.

37. Neison, *Rechabites*, pp. 11–12, divides members of this society into those who died after a sickness and those who died without an immediately preceding sickness. In the aggregate, concerning individuals aged 18 to 91, 152 died suddenly, and 833 after sickness. Neison (p. 20) regarded this as a high proportion of sudden deaths.

38. Neison, *Foresters*, p. 96, lists these as the leading causes of extended claims.

39. Neison, *Contributions*, pp. 162–3. On the general issue of outcomes see also Neison, *Rechabites*, pp. 55–6.

40. The number of years at risk declines sharply at age 75–79, but propor-tions in this and the following age group appear to be in line with what would be expected from the trend established at earlier ages. It is assumed that individuals compensated for part or all of a work week lost were sick for the entire week or portion thereof, and not just during working hours.

41. The figures given here slightly understate sick time because permanent disability is counted only through the five years of the survey, not through its actual duration.

42. However, Odd Fellows sickness rates show higher percentages of sick time especially in ages 60–64 and above. The average duration of sicknesses was increasing between 1870 and 1900. See Riley, 'Ill Health'.

43. Cheshire Record Office, Chester, DDX 186. Some episodes – during the first month after childbirth and those associated with pre-existing condi-tions or immoral behavior – were uncompensated. Male members were mostly agricultural laborers, and females mostly domestic servants.

44. Henry Ratcliffe, *Observations on the Rate of Mortality and Sickness Existing amongst Friendly Societies* . . . (Colchester, 1862) p. 84, ap-pears to recognize this possibility (' . . . it was seen that in many instances a large quantity of the lives extracted, presented no sickness,

and in other instances many cases arose together'). Some twentieth-century studies also suggest a bimodal distribution, but this issue awaits close scrutiny. See Johannes Due, 'Sygelighedsudvikling og sygdomsfordelinger blandt 1,791 smede', *Ugeskrift for Læger*, 138, no. 40 (Sept. 27, 1976), 2459–65; Lawrence E. Hinkle, Jr. *et al.*, 'The Distribution of Sickness Disability in a Homogeneous Group of "Healthy Adult Men"', *American Journal of Hygiene*, 64 (1956), pp. 220–42; and Barbara Starfield and I.B. Pless, 'Physical Health', in Orville G. Brim, Jr. and Jerome Kagan, eds, *Constancy and Change in Human Development* (Cambridge, Mass., 1980), pp. 277–79 and *passim*.

45. To the epidemiologist, incidence measures the number of new cases within a specific interval of time, and is distinguished from prevalence, which measures the number of cases of a disease in a population at a specific point in time. Period prevalence, another measure used by epidemiologists, is equivalent to duration or the risk of being sick.

4 Health and Sickness in Europe, 1600–1870

1. Alfred Perrenoud, *La population de Genève du seizième au début du dix-neuvième siècle: Etude démographique* (Geneva, 1979), p. 478.
2. Massimo Livi Bacci, *La société italienne devant les crises de mortalité* (Florence, 1978), pp. 41 and 58; L. Del Panta and M. Livi Bacci, 'Chronologie, intensité et diffusion des crises de mortalité en Italie: 1600–1850', *Population*, 32 (Sept. 1977, Special Number), pp. 401–46, esp. 432–6. The years at risk represent years under observation in various towns in the sample.
3. High prices for grain, the basic staple of most regions, signal crop shortfalls and dearth. In some regions and periods of the seventeenth century high prices preceded mortality spasms, often with a lag between the appearance of signs of dearth on grain markets and the rise of mortality rates. Jean Meuvret, 'Les crises de subsistances et la démographie de la France d'ancien régime', *Population*, 1, no. 4 (Oct.-Dec. 1946), pp. 643–50. But the relationship was not apparently as strong across Europe as it was in the areas of France where it was first detected. Even in adjacent areas with closely integrated markets – such as Brabant and Flanders in the seventeenth-century Spanish Netherlands – dearth did not regularly precede a mortality spasm, and many periods of high prices were not followed by higher than ordinary mortality. Claude Bruneel, *La mortalité dans les campagnes: Le duché de Brabant aux XVIIe et XVIIIe siècles* (2 vol.; Leuven, 1977), I, pp. 577–84; and Stefaan Lechat, *Mortaliteitscrisissen te Izegem van 1630 tot 1870* (unpublished *licentiaat* thesis, Katholieke Universiteit Leuven, 1986), I, pp. 134–6, summarizing results of studies of Flanders and reporting his own findings from the town of Izegem.) Most mortality peaks, and an increasing proportion of them, seem to have been either independent of harvest failures or to have been related to food shortages in a more complex way than appears from the simple comparison of wheat and rye

price series with deaths. See also Perrenoud, *Genève*, p. 446; Bruneel, *Brabant*, I. pp. 463–72 and 599–609.

4. E.A. Wrigley and R.S. Schofield, *The Population History of England, 1541–1871* (Cambridge, Mass., 1981), pp. 645–56, esp. p. 650. Also useful are George Alter, 'Plague and the Amsterdam Annuitant: A New Look at Life Annuities as a Source for Historical Demography', *Population Studies*, 37 (1983), pp. 23–41; and Hubert Charbonneau and André Larose, eds, *The Great Mortalities: Methodological Studies of Demographic Crises in the Past* (Liege, n.d.).

5. Perrenoud, *Genève*, pp. 421–9, data from 425 and 525–30.

6. [Jean] Razoux, *Tables nosologiques et météorologiques très-étendues dressées à l'hôtel-dieu de Nîmes . . . 1757 . . . [à] 1762* (Basle, 1767).

7. For a broader discussion see James C. Riley, 'Insects and the European Mortality Decline', *American Historical Review*, 91, no. 4 (Oct. 1986), pp. 833–58. Also Bruneel, *Brabant*, I, 463 and 473–537; Charles Creighton, *A History of Epidemics in Britain* (2 vols; Cambridge, 1891–94), I, pp. 463–578, 646–92, and II, pp. 4–132 and *passim*; Jean-Pierre Peter, 'Une enquête de la Société Royale de Médecine (1774–94): Malades et maladies à la fin du XVIIIe siècle', *Annales: économies, sociétés, civilisations*, 22 (1967), pp. 741–2.

8. Bernard Knight, *The Coroner's Autopsy: A Guide to Non-Criminal Autopsies for the General Pathologist* (Edinburgh, 1983), pp. 2 and 54.

9. Paul D. Hoeprich, ed., *Infectious Diseases: A Modern Treatise of Infectious Processes* (3rd edn; Philadelphia, 1983), pp. 665–6. Also Frederick P. Gay, *Typhoid Fever*, (New York, 1918). On the acute phase response see Irving Kushner, 'The Phenomenon of the Acute Phase Response', in Irving Kushner *et al.*, eds, *C-reactive Protein and the Plasma Protein Response to Tissue Injury*, Annals of the New York Academy of Sciences, 389 (1982), pp. 39–48.

10. For example, Donald G. Bates, 'Thomas Willis and the Epidemic Fever of 1661: A Commentary', *Bulletin of the History of Medicine*, 39, no. 5 (Sept.–Oct. 1965), pp. 393–414.

11. Ann G. Carmichael, 'Infection, Hidden Hunger, and History', *Journal of Interdisciplinary History*, 14, no. 2 (Autumn 1983), pp. 256–64; Jere Housworth and Alexander D. Langmuir, 'Excess Mortality from Epidemic Influenza, 1957–1966', *American Journal of Epidemiology*, 100 (July 1974), pp. 40–8; James C. Riley, *The Eighteenth-Century Campaign to Avoid Disease* (New York, 1987); J.L. Anderson and E.L. Jones, 'Natural Disasters and the Historical Response', *Australian Economic History Review*, (1988), forthcoming.

12. Raymond Pearl, 'Cancer and Tuberculosis', *American Journal of Hygiene*, 9 (1929), pp. 97–159; Mirko D. Grmek, 'Préliminaires d'une étude historique des maladies', *Annales: économies, sociétés, civilisations*, 24 (1969), pp. 1473–83; id., *Les maladies à l'aube de la civilisation occidentale* (Paris, 1983), esp. pp. 11–34; René Dubos, *Mirage of Health: Utopias, Progress, and Biological Change* (New York, 1959), pp. 66–74; id., *Men, Medicine, and Environment* (New York, 1968); Perrenoud, *Genève*, pp. 466 and 468; Thomas McKeown, *The Modern Rise of*

Population (London, 1976). Also Arthur E. Imhof, 'Statistiker und Historiker – und die andern: Ein Kapitel angewandter Berliner Bevölkerungsstatistik', in Wolfgang Ribbe (ed.), *Berlin-Forschungen* (Berlin, 1986) pp. 296–332.

13. Sporotrichosis is worldwide in incidence and is often diagnosed today in France. It occurs when the fungus, lying in soil or on vegetation, enters through a small wound, and is most common among agricultural workers. Death is rare and sporotrichosis seldom restricts ordinary activities but usually has a prolonged course and may produce pulmonary complications. Although not identifying sporotrichosis, Larsen notices the frequency of skin diseases in the eighteenth century. Øivind Larsen, 'Eighteenth-Century Diseases, Diagnostic Trends, and Mortality', *The Fifth Scandinavian Demography Symposium* (Hurdalssjøen, 1979), pp. 43 and 51. Round worm infection is common in temperate zones where sanitation is poor. It rarely causes death, especially with treatments now available, but is associated with pulmonary and intestinal complications, which may have been common or even prevalent in historical populations. It also has complex nutritional and immunologic implications. Robert E. Baldwin and Burton A. Weisbrod, 'Disease and Labor Productivity', *Economic Development and Cultural Change*, 22, no. 3 (Apr. 1974), pp. 414–35, assess the economic effect of ascariasis. Folke Henschen, *The History and Geography of Diseases*, trans. by Joan Tate (New York, 1966), p. 151, identifies ascariasis as rare in Sweden by the 1960s, but present in 63 per cent of First World War combatants.

14. Information on these diseases has been drawn from standard texts, James B. Wyngaarden and Lloyd H. Smith, Jr, eds, *Cecil Textbook of Medicine* (16th edn; Philadelphia, 1982); Hoeprich, ed., *Infectious Diseases*; Alfred S. Evans and Harry A. Feldman, eds, *Bacterial Infections of Humans: Epidemiology and Control* (New York, 1982). See also Wesley W. Spink, *Infectious Diseases: Prevention and Treatment in the Nineteenth and Twentieth Centuries* (Minneapolis, 1978); Perrenoud, *Genève*, pp. 450–2 and 458–66; Jean-Noël Biraben, *Les hommes et la peste en France et dans les pays européens et méditerranéens* (2 vols; Paris, 1976), I, 11 and 295–306; Gay, *Typhoid Fever*, esp. pp. 13–15; W.H. Mosley, 'Biological Contamination of the Environment by Man', in Samuel H. Preston, ed., *Biological and Social Aspects of Mortality and the Length of Life* (Liege, 1982), p. 49; R[obert] Pollitzer, *Plague* (Geneva, 1954), p. 418; K. David Patterson, *Pandemic Influenza, 1700–1900: A Study in Historical Epidemiology* (Totowa, NJ, 1986); and Zbigniew S. Pawlowski, 'Ascariasis: Host-pathogen Biology', *Reviews of Infectious Diseases*, 4, no. 4 (Aug., 1982), pp. 806–14.

15. Perrenoud, *Genève*, p. 468 (my translation).

16. Hoeprich, ed., *Infectious Diseases*, p. 653.

17. Detail about diseases not resolved in death may be found in physicians' case studies and in the investigation sponsored toward the end of the eighteenth century by the Société Royale de Médecine. For an example of the first, see Saul Jarcho, ed. and trans., *The Clinical Consultations of Giambattista Morgagni* (Boston, 1984); and on the second see Jean-Paul Desaive, *et al.* (eds), *Médecins, climat et épidémies à la fin du XVIII siècle*

(Paris, 1972), esp. the essay by Jean-Pierre Peter. Also the Josselin family's health record, on which see Lucinda McCray Beier, 'In Sickness and in Health: A Seventeenth Century Family's Experience', in Roy Porter, ed., *Patients and Practitioners: Lay Perceptions of Medicine in Pre-industrial Society* (Cambridge, 1985), pp. 101–28.

18. For instance, Satya Swaroop, 'Study of Morbidity in Underdeveloped Areas', in Louis Henry and Wilhelm Winkler, eds, *Proceedings of the International Population Conference* (Vienna, 1959), p. 544, regarding specifically lice and flea infestation in a village near Cairo.

19. Elborg Forster, 'From the Patient's Point of View: Illness and Health in the Letters of Liselotte von der Pfalz (1652–1722)', *Bulletin of the History of Medicine*, 60, no. 3 (Fall, 1986), pp. 297–320 (quote from 301, n. 11); Elborg Forster, ed., *A Woman's Life in the Court of the Sun King: Letters of Liselotte von der Pfalz, 1652–1722* (Baltimore, 1984), pp. xix, 11, and 83; Margaret Pelling, 'Appearance and Reality: Barber-Surgeons, the Body and Disease', in L. Beier and R. Finlay, eds, *London, 1500–1700: The Making of the Metropolis* (London, 1986), p. 91.

20. Wyngaarden and Smith, *Medicine*, pp. 326–7. Ann Carmichael called the frostbite case to my attention.

21. The following section relies on Milton Markowitz and Leon Gordis, *Rheumatic Fever* (2nd edn; Philadelphia, 1972); and William Ophüls, 'Arteriosclerosis, Cardiovascular Disease: Their Relation to Infectious Diseases', Stanford University Publications, *Medical Sciences*, I, no. 1 (1921), pp. 1–102. It exemplifies rather than exhausts possibilities of the insult accumulation model.

22. There are more than 50 types of group A streptococci which stimulate chiefly type-specific antibodies and thus immunity to that type alone. Rheumatic fever tends to recur, but the recurrence is linked to risk factors rather than to prior experience with the disease itself.

23. McKeown, *Modern Rise*, pp. 82–3; George Rosen, *A History of Public Health* (New York, 1958), pp. 90–1 and 279–80, who furnishes a chronology of changes in the virulence level of scarlet fever, based apparently on a survey of medical interest in the disease and cause of death data. He believes that scarlet fever was a leading cause of death in the last decades of the eighteenth century, of limited significance until the 1830s, and then severely virulent in Europe and North America from about 1840 to 1880.

24. Rosen, *Public Health*, p. 280.

25. William Ophüls, 'A Statistical Survey of Three Thousand Autopsies', Stanford University Publications, *Medical Sciences*, 1, no. 3 (1926), p. 131 and *passim*. See also W.S. Thayer, 'On the Late Effects of Typhoid Fever on the Heart and Vessels: A Clinical Study', *American Journal of the Medical Sciences*, 127 (1904), pp. 391–422.

26. Ophüls, 'Arteriosclerosis', pp. 9 (for the quote), 35, and 95. Predecessors had suspected a negative association between tuberculosis and arteriosclerosis. Ophüls could find no association, perhaps because so few people with active cases of tuberculosis lived to an age at which they might develop arterial disease. Recent work at the cellular level has

detected other vascular changes in infancy and childhood, but their origin remains unexplained. K.T. Lee, ed., *Atherosclerosis* (New York, 1985), esp. pp. 2–3 and 325.

27. Thomas Royle Dawber, *The Framingham Study: The Epidemiology of Atherosclerotic Disease* (Cambridge, Mass., 1980); Ancel Keys *et al.*, *Seven Countries: A Multivariate Analysis of Death and Coronary Heart Disease* (Cambridge, Mass., 1980); Wyngaarden and Smith, eds, *Medicine*, pp. 239–42.

28. Maurice Sandler and Geoffrey H. Bourne, eds, *Atherosclerosis and Its Origins* (New York, 1963), p. 41.

29. The post-mortem characteristics of disease are surveyed in Wiley D. Forbus, *Reaction to Injury: Pathology for Students of Disease Based on the Functional and Morphological Responses of Tissues to Injurious Agents* (2 vols; Baltimore, 1943–52). William B. Kannel and Thomas J. Thom, 'Declining Cardiovascular Mortality', *Circulation*, 70 (September 1984), pp. 333–4, notice autopsy results. Also Bernard Knight, *The Coroner's Autopsy: A Guide to Non-Criminal Autopsies for the General Pathologist* (Edinburgh, 1983), p. 56, points out that damages that might cause death cannot always be said to have caused death.
Some diseases of leading importance in causing lasting damage cannot be induced in laboratory animals in ways that satisfy the model. For example, typhoid fever cannot be introduced to animal models via the mouth. R.B. Hornick *et al.*, 'Typhoid Fever: Pathogenesis and Immunologic Control', *New England Journal of Medicine*, 283 (Sept. 24, 1970), pp. 686–91 and (Oct. 1, 1970), pp. 739–46. Ophüls' line of inquiry seems to have been given up at about the time the infectious diseases whose association with artery damage he studied ceased to be major causes of death, but some 40 to 60 years before effects from episodes suffered earlier would cease to be felt as cohorts bearing lesions died.

30. Henry E. Sigerist, *Landmarks in the History of Hygiene* (New York, 1956), pp. 41–2; and William F. Butler, ed., *The Art of Living Long* (Milwaukee, 1903), pp. 55 and *passim*.

31. See Figure 1.3.

32. Imhof, 'Statistiker, Historiker – und die andern', promises the first extensive demonstration of the possibilities of this approach, as applied to Berlin records.

33. George Alter and James C. Riley, 'Frailty, Sickness, and Death: Models of Morbidity and Mortality in Historical Populations', forthcoming.

5 The Experience of Sickness before 1870

1. John Brownlee, 'The Health of London in the Eighteenth Century', *Proceedings of the Royal Society of Medicine*, 17 (1925), p. 73.

2. William H. McNeill, *Plagues and Peoples* (Garden City, N.Y., 1976), esp. pp. 218–20. McNeill infers health levels from mortality rates and more directly still from diet, especially protein intake.

3. Marjorie Nicolson and G.S. Rousseau, *'This Long Disease, My Life': Alexander Pope and the Sciences* (Princeton, 1968), pp. 7–82; William B.

Ober, *Boswell's Clap and Other Essays* (Carbondale, Ill., 1979), pp. 1, 2, and 24; and Lucinda McCray Beier, 'In Sickness and in Health: A Seventeenth Century Family's Experience', in Roy Porter, ed., *Patients and Practitioners: Lay Perceptions of Medicine in Pre-industrial Society* (Cambridge, 1985), pp. 106–7. Beier counts events but not their duration.
4. William Paton, *Man and Mouse: Animals in Medical Research* (Oxford, 1984), p. 2.
5. Øivind Larsen, 'Eighteenth-Century Diseases, Diagnostic Trends, and Mortality', *Fifth Scandinavian Demographic Symposium* (Hurdalssjøen, 1979), p. 43.
6. Mireille Laget, 'Les livrets de santé pour les pauvres aux XVIIe et XVIIIe siècles', *Histoire, économie, société*, no. 4 (1984), pp. 567–82; and, for an example, William Buchan, *Domestic Medicine: Or, a Valuable Treatise on the Prevention and Cure of Diseases by Regimen and Simple Medicines . . .* (Leominster, 1804), which appeared in more than 20 editions between 1769 and 1804.
7. Thomas McKeown, *The Modern Rise of Population* (London, 1976), p. 4.
8. Simon Kuznets, *Modern Economic Growth* (New Haven, 1966), p. 58. Also H[ector] Correa, *The Economics of Human Resources* (Amsterdam, 1963), pp. 42–5; and Odin W. Anderson, 'Age-Specific Mortality in Selected Western Countries with Particular Emphasis on the Nineteenth Century: Observations and Implications', *Bulletin of the History of Medicine*, 29, no. 3 (May-June 1955), p. 239.
9. Imhof's introduction in Arthur E. Imhof, ed., *Biologie des Menschen in der Geschichte* (Stuttgart, 1978), p. 70.
10. Roy M. Acheson and Spencer Hagard, *Health, Society and Medicine: An Introduction to Community Medicine* (Oxford, 1984), p. 12.
11. Donald G. Bates, 'Thomas Willis and the Epidemic Fever of 1661: A Commentary', *Bulletin of the History of Medicine*, 39, no. 5 (Sept.–Oct. 1965), p. 400.
12. Mary Kilbourne Matossian, 'Death in London, 1750–1909', *Journal of Interdisciplinary History*, 10, no. 2 (Autumn 1985), p. 189.
13. Louis Torfs, *Fastes des calamités publiques survenues dans les Pays-Bas et particulièrement en Belgique . . .* (2 vols; Paris, 1859–62).
14. T.R. Edmonds, 'On the Laws of Sickness, According to Age, Exhibiting a Double Coincidence Between the Laws of Sickness and the Laws of Mortality', *Lancet*, no. 1 (1835–36), pp. 855–8.
15. Gilbert Blane, *Select Dissertations on Several Subjects of Medical Science* (London, 1833), pp. 149 and 207.
16. [Nicolas] G[ustave] Hubbard, *De l'organisation des sociétés de prévoyance ou de secours mutuels* (Paris, 1852), pp. liv–lv.
17. Edmonds, 'On the Laws of Sickness', 856; id., *Life Tables, Founded upon the Discovery of a Numerical Law Regulating the Existence of Every Human Being . . .* (London, 1832), p. xxxix; and [William Farr], 'Vital Statistics', in J[ohn] R[amsay] McCulloch, ed., *Statistical Account of the British Empire* (3rd edn; 2 vols; London, 1847), II, pt. 5, p. 577. Also L. Deboutteville, *Des sociétés de prévoyance ou de secours mutuels* (Rouen,

1844), p. 47; John M. Eyler, 'The Conceptual Origins of William Farr's Epidemiology: Numerical Methods and Social Thought in the 1830s', in Abraham M. Lilienfeld (ed.), *Times, Places, and Persons: Aspects of the History of Epidemiology* (Baltimore, 1980), pp. 1–21.

18. Arlette Farge, 'Les artisans malades de leur travail', *Annales: économies, sociétés, civilisations*, 32 (Sept.-Oct. 1977), p. 993. To the same effect Abel Poitrineau, *Remues d'hommes: Essai sur les migrations montagnardes en France aux XVIIe et XVIIIe siècles* (Paris, 1983), pp. 156–7 and 172–81, regarding migrant laborers.

19. [Farr], 'Vital Statistics', pp. 584, 589, and 591.

20. Respectively, James C. Riley, 'Sickness in an Early Modern Workplace', *Continuity and Change*, 2, no. 3 (1987), pp. 363–86; Jean-François Brière, 'L'armement français pour la pêche à Terre-Neuve au XVIIIe siècle' (York University, Ph.D. thesis, 1980), pp. 33–8 and *passim*; and Pierre Goubert, *The French Peasantry in the Seventeenth Century*, trans. by Ian Patterson (Cambridge, 1986), p. 105.

21. Philip Cole, 'Morbidity in the United States', in Erhardt and Berlin, eds, *Mortality and Morbidity in the United States* (1964), p. 65.

22. The same holds when the comparison involves earlier periods. Since 1960 it has begun to break down as the life expectancy of the old and the so-called old old has increased markedly in many developed countries.

23. Plantijnsch Archief, Antwerp, in the Museum Plantin-Moretus, 334, 432–433, 666, 697, 772, 781, and 1168. Riley, 'Sickness in an Early Modern Workplace', provides further detail.

24. The manuscript records of the fund seldom reveal age, date of birth, or place of birth. Since age is such an important force in shaping the morbidity risk, it is necessary either to track age-specific (or age-standardized) sickness rates, to follow a group with a stable age structure, or to find ways to compensate for the absence of age data. In the case of small sick funds, age-specific rates hold little value because the funds were too small to subdivide members into many age cells. By estimating age at first employment, charter members were aged between 29 and 61, with an average of 40.

25. Except briefly in 1681, benefits were paid for episodes lasting at least six days. Some shorter episodes are represented by deaths, which have been included in calculations of the rate of falling sick but not in the rate of being sick.

26. See n. 24 above.

27. Claims were paid only for full weeks but, on average, each claim can be assumed to represent additional sickness on both sides.

28. Both calculations include a half week for the week of death. Only 43 of 44 deaths can be considered, as one occurred on 1 March 1654, the first day of eligibility. Some sick fund members were sick intermittently. Deciding how to count the durations of their sicknesses requires that a convention be created. I decided to count as continuous all claims weeks not separated by at least four weeks without claims and, in the case of intermittent sickness, to count claims weeks but not intervening non-claims weeks.

29. That rate is expected because this population was skewed toward older

members. Thus while it omits the high mortality risk of infancy, it also omits the low risk of adolescence and early adulthood. More extensive information about Antwerp in this period, especially serial data about deaths, prices, or other economic variables, would permit further comment. But Antwerp is poorly served, having only a chronicle of city ordinances regarding pestilence. A.F.C. van Schevensteen, *Documents pour servir à l'étude des maladies pestilentielles dans le marquisat d'Anvers jusqu'à la chute de l'ancien régime* (2 vols; Brussels, 1931). Antwerp's population totalled some 57 000 in 1644 and 66 000 in 1698. R. Boumans, 'L'évolution démographique d'Anvers (XVe-XVIIIe siècle)', *Bulletin de statistique* (Belgium), 34, no. 11 (Nov. 1948), 1693.

30. Derbyshire Record Office, Matlock, D747A/PZ1/1.
31. Manchester Central Library, Archives Department, Bennett Street Sunday School Sick and Funeral Society, M103/10; Great Britain, Parliamentary Papers, vol. XIX, 1834, *Factories Inquiry Commission Supplementary Report*, pp. 276–7.
32. See Chapter 3.
33. All these characteristics determine the way in which the surviving record can be used. To simplify, a short period has been chosen because, on the basis of age at death information, the average age seems to have remained stable from 1816 through 1835 but to have increased thereafter. The denominators – the time at risk – have been reduced to account for turnover (estimated at 10 per cent a year) and changes from year to year in the time during which members were eligible for benefits.
34. See especially the annual reports for 1838 and 1860 in Manchester Central Library, Archives Department, M103/10/24/1–2.
35. Gloucester County Record Office, D4733/7/6. In this case, too, turnover has been estimated to adjust the denominator. Dursley is situated in southwestern England between Gloucester and Bristol.
36. *Factories Inquiry Commission Supplementary Report*, pp. 268–71.
37. [Farr], 'Vital Statistics', p. 589. However, Hawkins confused the age profile of the burial society (5 and up) with that of the sick society, and made no adjustment for the initiation period.
38. Committee of the Highland Society of Scotland, *Report on Friendly or Benefit Societies, Exhibiting the Law of Sickness* . . . (Edinburgh, 1824), esp. pp. 17, 58–9, 93, and 148–9; Francis G.P. Neison, Sr., *Contributions to Vital Statistics* . . . (3rd edn; London, 1857), esp. pp. 74–5 and 160–2.
39. At age 21 a member of these societies could, on average, expect to live 38.2 years, but only 35.5 years after eliminating survival after age 70.
40. Neison provides some information about the age groups 11–15 and 76–80 to 91–95, but the number of individuals is small.

6   Sickness in the Second Half of the Nineteenth Century

1. From an anonymous article called 'Registration of Sickness' in Charles Dickens's magazine *All the Year Round*, 4 (Dec. 15, 1860), p. 228.
2. Henry Ratcliffe, *Observations on the Rate of Mortality & Sickness Existing among Friendly Societies* (Manchester, 1850); id., *Observations on*

the Rate of Mortality and Sickness Existing amongst Friendly Societies . . . (Colchester, 1862); and [Henry Ratcliffe], *Independent Order of Odd-Fellows, Manchester Unity Friendly Society, Supplementary Report, July 1st, 1872* (n.p., 1872).

3. Francis G.P. Neison, Jr., *The Rates of Mortality and Sickness According to the Experience for the Five Years, 1871–1875, of the Ancient Order of Foresters Friendly Society* . . . (London, 1882).

4. W[illiam] Sutton, *Special Report on Sickness and Mortality Experienced in Registered Friendly Societies* . . ., House of Commons, Sessional Papers, 1896, LXXIX; F.G.P. Neison, Sr., *Contributions to Vital Statistics: being a Development of the Rate of Mortality and the Laws of Sickness* . . . (3rd edn; London, 1857), p. 465; Neison, Jr., *Foresters*, p. 43; and Alfred W. Watson, *An Account of an Investigation of the Sickness and Mortality Experience of the I.O.O.F. Manchester Unity . . . 1893–1897* (Manchester, 1903), p. 22.

5. Watson, *Manchester Unity*, p. 39.

6. Compare Neison, Jr., *Foresters*, p. 40; Watson, *Manchester Unity*, p. 65. Watson later suggested that a 10 per cent reduction in claims would satisfactorily adjust to the standard concept of claims. That may be so in the aggregate, but it will not have been so at each age because the risk of protracted sickness changed with age. Alfred William Watson, *Friendly Society Finance Considered in its Actuarial Aspect: A Course of Lectures* (London, 1912), p. 35.

7. James C. Riley, 'Ill Health during the English Mortality Decline: The Friendly Societies' Experience', *Bulletin of the History of Medicine*, 61, no. 4 (1987), tables 3 and 4. This essay also discusses other features of the actuarial reports.

8. George F. Hardy, 'Friendly Societies', *Journal of the Institute of Actuaries*, 27 (Oct. 1888), pp. 291–2.

9. E.J. Hobsbawm, *Labouring Men: Studies in the History of Labour* (London, 1964), pp. 272–5.

10. According to the standard interpretation, some combination of public health reforms, improvements in the standard of living, and improved medical therapies reduced the risk of dying from infectious diseases, allowing more youths to survive to ages at which they would die from chronic diseases. Abdel R. Omran, 'The Epidemiologic Transition: A Theory of the Epidemiology of Population Change', *Milbank Memorial Fund Quarterly*, 49, no. 4 (Oct. 1971), pp. 509–38; S. Jay Olshansky and A. Brian Ault, 'The Fourth Stage of the Epidemiologic Transition: The Age of Delayed Degenerative Diseases', *Milbank Quarterly*, 64, no. 3 (1986), pp. 355–7.

11. George Rosen, *A History of Public Health* (New York, 1958), pp. 90–1 and 279–80.

12. Neison, Jr., *Foresters*, p. 49.

13. The Hearts of Oak was not an affiliated but a centralized society, which means that members belonged directly to the central organization rather than through local units.

14. It is important to notice that the economic data do not represent Hearts of Oak members, who cannot be distinguished from the larger experience upon which the economic series are based. However, the geo-

graphical distribution of Hearts of Oak members and their numbers suggest that they will have shared in the national experience. In the Hearts of Oak the age-specific risk of being sick increased but the average duration of each episode decreased for some ages between 1884 and 1891. That is, the risk of falling sick (which is included in the risk of being sick) increased but sicknesses became less protracted. In the longer run, however, Hearts of Oak experience participated in the trend increase. See Hardy's comparison of 1884–91 with Odd Fellows experience during 1866–70. The Hearts of Oak included few men in hazardous occupations, and Hardy's comparison did not adjust for this difference.

15. Several other versions have been suggested for predicting an expectation of ill health (or health) time or episodes. See especially Monroe Lerner and Odin W. Anderson, *Health Progress in the United States, 1900–1960* (Chicago, 1963), pp. 337–47; Daniel F. Sullivan, 'Conceptual Problems in Developing an Index of Health', in US, Department of Health, Education, and Welfare, *Vital and Health Statistics*, National Center for Health Statistics, Series 2, no. 17 (Washington, 1966); Milton M. Chen and James W. Bush, 'Health Status Measures, Policy, and Biomedical Research', in Selma J. Mushkin and David W. Dunlop, eds, *Health: What is it Worth? Measures of Health Benefits* (New York, 1979), pp. 15–41; Sidney Katz *et al.*, 'Active Life Expectancy', *New England Journal of Medicine*, 309, no. 20 (1983), pp. 1218–23; and Eileen M. Crimmins and Yasuhiko Saito, 'Changes in Life Expectancy and Disability-free life Expectancy in the U.S.: 1970–1980' (unpublished).

16. Neison counted all episodes experienced by the same individual within one year as one episode, so these values understate somewhat the cumulative risk of falling sick.

17. That is, ill-health time not compensated under the Foresters' rules is included.

18. The estimates for ages 80+ have limited value because of the small number of members at those ages.

19. Michael Flinn *et al.*, *Scottish Population History from the 17th Century to the 1930s* (Cambridge, 1977), pp. 242, 246, 248–9, and 483–8.

20. The trend of the risk of falling sick among the Foresters escapes observation but shifts in disease and cause-of-death patterns – specifically the epidemiologic transition as conventionally understood – lead to the expectation that the risk of falling sick will have remained stable or declined.

21. Certain hazardous jobs, for instance, mining, are often held to be associated with markedly higher illness and injury risks, but the case about illness risk is disputed. See Bernard Knight, *The Coroner's Autopsy: A Guide to Non-Criminal Autopsies for the General Pathologist* (Edinburgh, 1983), pp. 163–4. In this connection it is important to remember that people change jobs, and that people whose health has been impaired by their jobs but who remain able to work may be especially likely to shift occupations. Also, higher risk occupations are in general more demanding in terms of physical fitness, which means that they impose a lower sickness threshold (that is, incapacity to work occurs earlier and more often).

22. Watson, *Manchester Unity*, pp. 180–2, 204–5, and 210–12. The risk of

Sickness, Recovery and Death

falling sick is inferred via Watson's method of counting claims, which inflates the number of claims. However, the error should be proportional for the different categories. The occupations listed are mostly those followed at joining; disabled miners, for example, continued to be listed as miners even at advanced ages.

23. Ibid., pp. 54 and 65.
24. It is worth noticing that this form of the injury risk may have been a recent innovation. As antiseptic and aseptic treatment spread in accident cases in the 1880s and thereafter, it is plausible to suppose a lower case fatality rate and longer average durations.
25. [William Farr], 'Vital Statistics', in J[ohn] R[amsey] McCulloch, ed., *Statistical Account of the British Empire* (2 vol; 3rd edn; London, 1847), II, pt. 5, pp. 572–3. The data include episodes lasting less than three days.
26. Walter Dickson, *On the Numerical Ratio of Disease in the Adult Male Community, deduced from the Sanitary Statistics of Her Majesty's Customs, for the Years 1857–74* (London, 1876), p. 8.
27. See the essays in Paul Weindling, ed., *The Social History of Occupational Health* (London, 1985), especially Karl Figlio, 'What is an Accident?' and Peter Bartrip, 'The Rise and Decline of Workmen's Compensation'.
28. Leslie Hannah, *Inventing Retirement: The Development of Occupational Pensions in Britain* (Cambridge, 1986).
29. Jill S. Quadagno, *Aging in Early Industrial Society: Work, Family, and Social Policy in Nineteenth-Century England* (New York, 1982), provides a particularly intelligent survey. Excepted were individuals earning more than £26 a year, and some others.
30. Great Britain, House of Commons Sessional Papers, *Report by the Government Actuary on an Examination of the Sickness and Disablement Experience of a Group of Approved Societies in the period 1921–27*, Cmd. 3548 (London, 1930), p. 9.
31. Independent Order of Odd Fellows Manchester Unity Friendly Society, *For Your Benefit . . .* ([Manchester], [c. 1967]), p. 3.
32. Some observers (see notes 33 and 34 below) asserted that those who joined because of the 1911 act held different attitudes, regarding the sickness coverage as an insurance contract without important implications about responsibility to fellow insureds rather than a contract supplied by a fraternal or friendly society with such implications. While that may be true, it is to be expected that the two putative attitudes would have converged after 1911.
33. See, for example, A.J. Fox and P.F. Collier, 'Low Mortality Rates in Industrial Cohort Studies Due to Selection for Work and Survival in the Industry', *British Journal of Preventive and Social Medicine*, 30 (1976), pp. 225–30. Chapter 7 provides an example of how the healthy worker effect influences the morbidity curve.
34. For example, see Alfred W. Watson, 'The Analysis of a Sickness Experience', *Journal of the Institute of Actuaries*, 62 (1931), pp. 26 and 28; E.C. Snow, 'Some Statistical Problems Suggested by the Sickness and Mortality Data of Certain of the Large Friendly Societies', *Journal of the*

Royal Statistical Society, 76, pt. 5 (April 1913), p. 513; W.T.C. Blake and J.M. Moore, *Friendly Societies* (Cambridge, 1951), p. 9; and P. Geddes and J.P. Holbrook, *Friendly Societies: A Text-Book for Actuarial Students* (Cambridge, 1963), pp. 87–9.
35. In addition to the sources cited in the previous note, see Alfred W. Watson, 'National Health Insurance: A Statistical Review', *Journal of the Royal Statistical Society* (London), 90 (1927), pp. 433–86; Victor Burrows, 'On Friendly Societies since the Advent of National Health Insurance', *Journal of the Institute of Actuaries*, 63 (1932), pp. 307–82; and Great Britain, House of Commons Sessional Papers 1964–65, XVIII, *Report of the Government Actuary on the Third Quinquennial Review* (London, 1964), p. 42; and Noel Whiteside, 'Counting the Cost: Sickness and Disability among Working People in an Era of Industrial Recession, 1920–39', *Economic History Review*, 2nd. ser., 40, no. 2 (1987), pp. 228–46. Copies of some valuation reports were generously supplied by the Independent Order of Odd Fellows Manchester Unity Friendly Society.
36. The number of members ranged from 113 to 156.
37. See Chapters 3 and 5.
38. See especially Thomas McKeown, *The Modern Rise of Population* (London, 1976); Robert Woods and John Woodward, eds, *Urban Disease and Mortality in Nineteenth-Century England* (London, 1984); F.B. Smith, *The People's Health, 1830–1910* (New York, 1979); F.B. Smith, 'Health', in John Benson, ed., *The Working Classes in England, 1875–1914* (London, 1985), pp. 36–62.

7   **Sickness and Death in the Twentieth Century**

1. See below, p. 22.
2. Edward Meeker, 'The Improving Health of the United States, 1850–1915', *Explorations in Economic History*, 9 (Summer 1972), p. 353.
3. US, Bureau of the Census, *Population and Housing Inquiries in US Decennial Censuses, 1790–1970*, Working Paper no. 39 (Washington, 1973), pp. 57–67, shows the questions put (answers to which appear in the manuscript census but were not reported in US, Department of the Interior, Census Office, *Compendium of the Tenth Census* (June 1, 1880) [rev. ed.; Washington, 1885–88]); William Franklin Willoughby, *Workingmen's Insurance* (New York, 1898); H.J. Messenger, 'The Rate of Sickness with Special Reference to the Experience of the Travelers Insurance Company of Hartford on Their Health Policies', *Transactions of the Actuarial Society of America*, 10 (1908), pp. 371–82; Irving Fisher, *Economic Aspect of Lengthening Human Life* (n.p., 1909); and, for example, Lee K. Frankel and Louis I. Dublin, *A Sickness Survey of Boston, Mass.* (New York, 1916).
4. US, Department of Commerce, *Historical Statistics of the United States: Colonial Times to 1970* (Washington, 1975), I, p. 61; US, Department of Health and Human Services, *Vital Statistics of the United States: 1981* (Hyattsville, MD. 1986), II, part A, p. 3; and US, National Center for

Health Statistics, *Monthly Vital Statistics Report*, vol. 34, no. 13 (Sept. 19, 1986), p. 15. Figures for 1984 and 1985 are estimates. In 1900 the death registration area included only ten states and 26 per cent of the US population.

5. Deaths reported are those occurring in the ten (ultimately 50) states and the District of Columbia, and include military personnel dying in that area.

6. See also Eileen M. Crimmins, 'The Changing Pattern of American Mortality Decline, 1940–1977, and Its Implications for the Future', *Population and Development Review*, 7, no. 2 (June 1981), pp. 229–54; Carl L. Erhardt and Joyce E. Berlin, eds, *Mortality and Morbidity in the United States* (Cambridge, Mass., 1974); Paul H. Jacobsen, 'Cohort Survival for Generations since 1840', *Milbank Memorial Fund Quarterly*, 42, no. 3 (1964), pp. 36–53; John B. McKinlay and Sonja M. McKinlay, 'The Questionable Contribution of Medical Measures to the Decline of Mortality in the United States in the Twentieth Century', *Milbank Memorial Fund Quarterly/Health and Society*, 55, no. 3 (Summer 1977), pp. 405–28; John B. McKinlay, Sonja M. McKinlay, Susan Jennings and Karen Grant, 'Mortality, Morbidity, and the Inverse Care Law', in Ann Lennarson and Scott Greer, eds, *Cities and Sickness: Health Care in Urban America* (Beverly Hills, 1983), pp. 99–138; Solomon Schneyer, J. Steven Landenfeld and Frank H. Sanifer, 'Biomedical Research and Illness: 1900–1979', *Milbank Memorial Fund Quarterly/Health and Society*, 59, no. 1 (Winter 1981), pp. 44–58; Clifford C. Clogg, 'The Effect of Personal Health Care Services on Longevity in an Economically Advanced Population', *Health Services Research*, 14 (1979), pp. 5–32; US, National Center for Health Statistics, Iwao M. Moriyama and Susan O. Gustavus, 'Cohort Mortality and Survivorship: United States Death-Registration States, 1900–1968', *Vital and Health Statistics*, Ser. 3, no. 16 (Washington, 1972); L.A. Fingerhut, R.W. Wilson and J.J. Feldman, 'Health and Disease in the United States', *Annual Review of Public Health*, I (1980), pp. 1–36; S.L.N. Rao, 'On Long-Term Mortality Trends in the United States, 1850–1968', *Demography*, 10 (Aug. 1973), p. 405; George C. Myers, 'Mortality Decline, Life Extension and Population Aging', *Proceedings of the International Population Conference* (held in Manila, 1981), 5 (1983), pp. 691–703; Robert W. Fogel, 'Nutrition and the Decline in Mortality since 1700: Some Preliminary Findings', in Stanley L. Engerman and Robert E. Gallman (eds), *Long-term Factors in American Economic Growth* (Chicago, 1986), pp. 439–555; Louis I. Dublin, Alfred J. Lotka and Mortimer Spiegelman, *Length of Life: A Study of the Life Table*, rev. edn (New York, 1949).

7. Harry F. Dowling, *Fighting Infection: Conquests of the Twentieth Century* (Cambridge, MA, 1977); Wesley W. Spink, *Infectious Diseases: Prevention and Treatment in the Nineteenth and Twentieth Centuries* (Minneapolis, 1978), pp. 61–130 and *passim*; and C.C. Dauer, 'A Demographic Analysis of Recent Changes in Mortality, Morbidity, and Age Group Distribution in Our Population', in Iago Galdston (ed.), *The Impact of the Antibiotics on Medicine and Society* (New York, 1958), pp. 98–120. McKinlay and McKinlay, 'Questionable Contributions of Medi-

cal Measures', 405–28, observe that very little of the overall mortality decline can be attributed to medical innovations. In most specific diseases the largest quantities of decline in death rates preceded the widespread use of new therapies. However, new therapies often did increase the rate of decline in specific age groups.

8. Paul B. Beeson, 'Changes in Medical Therapy during the Past Half Century', *Medicine*, 59, no. 2 (1980), pp. 79–99.

9. US, Department of Health, Education and Welfare, *Healthy People: The Surgeon General's Report on Health Promotion and Disease Prevention 1979* (Washington, 1979), p. 1.

10. S. Jay Olshansky, 'Simultaneous/Multiple Cause-Delay (SIMCAD): An Epidemiological Approach to Projecting Mortality', *Journal of Gerontology*, 42, no. 4 (1987), pp. 358–65, observes that the removal of a single risk factor may lead to a reduced risk of death from several degenerative diseases at the same time (that is, a delay in death). However, when risk factors (or morbidities) are multiple, as they are for middle-aged and older Americans, deferral of death adds to the prevalence of morbidity.

11. Alan S. Morrison, *Screening in Chronic Diseases* (New York, 1985), discusses health screening and its effect on measuring ill health. By detecting episodes earlier in their course, screening has the effect of making episodes appear longer. Prominent and effective in some diseases, screening has had limited effect on the broad range of illnesses in the US population.

12. Jones's theory therefore forecasts a quite different effect than Spiegelman's hypothesis of impaired lives, according to which the postponement of death at lower ages was expected to lead eventually to higher mortality rates at higher ages. Mortimer Spiegelman, 'Mortality in the United States: A Review and Evaluation of Special Reports of the National Center for Health Statistics', *Demography*, 5 (1968), pp. 525–33. See also W.O. Kermack, A.G. McKendrick and P.L. McKinlay, 'Death-Rates in Great Britain and Sweden: Some General Regularities and Their Significance', *Lancet*, I (1934), pp. 698–703. This effect has not been observed in the US, although it seems plausible to suppose that, if the new survivors could be distinguished within each cohort, observed mortality rates would be higher than those obtaining among 'old' survivors (that is, all survivors less new survivors) only.

13. On cohort analysis and US population experience see Jacobson, 'Cohort Survival', pp. 36–53; James J. Collins, 'The Contribution of Medical Measures to the Decline of Mortality from Respiratory Tuberculosis: An Age-Period-Cohort Model', *Demography*, 19, no. 3 (August 1982), pp. 409–27.

14. The 1918 influenza epidemic intensified the mortality risk toward the end of the First World War. It was not caused by the war, but its transmission and focus on young men were assisted by war mobilization. See Alfred W. Crosby, *Epidemic and Peace, 1918* (Westport, Conn., 1976). Vietnam War casualties are cited for years in which annual deaths (mostly occurring in Vietnam) surpassed 1000.

15. US, Bureau of the Census, *Historical Statistics of the United States: Colonial Times to 1970* (Washington, 1975), pt 2, p. 1140; and US,

Bureau of the Census, *Statistical Abstract of the United States: 1986* (Washington, 1985), p. 342. The Vietnam War data concern 1959–84.

16. US, Department of Health, Education and Welfare, *Smoking and Health: A Report of the Surgeon General* (Washington, 1979); George A. Sacher, 'Life Table Modification and Life Prolongation', in Caleb E. Finch and Leonard Hayflick (eds), *Handbook of the Biology of Aging* (New York, 1977), pp. 604–5; US, National Center for Health Statistics, *Mortality from Diseases Associated with Smoking: United States, 1960–77*, National Vital Statistics System, Series 20, no. 17 (Washington, 1982); Samuel H. Preston, *Older Male Mortality and Cigarette Smoking: A Demographic Analysis* (Westport, Conn., 1976).

17. Otto von Mering and Frederick L. Weniger, 'Social-Cultural Background of the Aging Individual', in James E. Birren (ed.), *Handbook of Aging and the Individual* (Chicago, 1959), p. 311.

18. Lisa F. Berkman and S. Leonard Syme, 'Social Networks, Host Resistance, and Mortality: A Nine-Year Follow-Up Study of Alameda County Residents', *American Journal of Epidemiology*, 109, no. 2 (1979), p. 188.

19. G. Anthony Ryan, 'The Automobile and Human Health', in N.F. Stanley and R.A. Joske, eds, *Changing Disease Patterns and Human Behaviour* (London, 1980), pp. 467–90.

20. René Dubos, 'The Evolution of Microbial Diseases', in R. Dubos and J.G. Hirsch (eds), *Bacterial and Mycotic Infections of Man* (4th edn; Philadelphia, 1965), pp. 20–1.

21. Louis Weinstein, 'Infectious Disease: Retrospect and Reminiscence', *Journal of Infectious Diseases*, 129, no. 4 (Apr. 1974), pp. 480–92. Also Ivan Illich, *Medical Nemesis: The Expropriation of Health* (New York, 1976), pp. 3 and *passim*.

22. Ingrid Waldron and Joseph Eyer, 'Socioeconomic Causes of the Recent Rise in Death Rates for 15–24-Yr-Olds', *Social Science and Medicine*, 9, no. 7 (July 1975), pp. 383–96; Darnell F. Hawkins, ed., *Homicide among Black Americans* (Lanham, MD, 1986).

23. Edwin J. Faulkner, *Health Insurance* (New York, 1960), considers the problem of definition and measurement from the perspective of twentieth-century US health insurers.

24. Figure 7.3 does not attempt to compare levels of ill health, only the shape of the age curve derived from different surveys.

25. For example, the NHIS reference period is two weeks and the Foresters five years, and this range affects the average duration of episodes.

26. William Graebner, *A History of Retirement: The Meaning and Function of an American Institution, 1885–1978* (New Haven, 1980), p. 12; Harold L. Sheppard, 'Work and Retirement', in Robert H. Binstock and Ethel Shanas, eds, *Handbook of Aging and the Social Sciences* (New York, 1976), pp. 286–309.

27. Kenneth G. Manton, 'Changing Concepts of Morbidity and Mortality in the Elderly Population', *Milbank Memorial Fund Quarterly/Health and Society*, 60, no. 2 (Spring 1982), pp. 183–244; Ronald W. Wilson, 'Trends in Illness and Disability', *Proceedings of the American Statistical Association: Social Statistics Section* (1983), pp. 93–96; James W. Vaupel, Kenneth G. Manton and Eric Stallard, 'The Impact of Heterogeneity in Individual Frailty on the Dynamics of Mortality', *Demogra-*

phy, 16, no. 3 (Aug. 1979), pp. 439–54; McKinlay, McKinlay, Jennings and Grant, 'Mortality', pp. 116–22; George Alter and James C. Riley, 'Frailty, Sickness, and Death: Models of Morbidity and Mortality in Historical Populations', forthcoming. See also the sources cited in the following note, and in n. 12, Chapter 8. Earlier commentators (for example, Philip Cole, 'Morbidity in the United States', in Erhardt and Berlin, eds, *Mortality and Morbidity*, esp. pp. 80–1) tended to doubt evidence of a trend rise and suspected measurement errors.

28. P.J. Taylor, 'Some International Trends in Sickness Absence 1950–68', *British Medical Journal*, 4, no. 5684 (Prac. obs. ed.) (Dec. 20, 1969), pp. 705–7; T. Lecomte, 'La morbidité déclarée, description et évolution: France 1970–1980', *Solidarité Santé: Etudes statistiques* (1984), pp. 41–56; United Nations, Economic and Social Commission for Asia and the Pacific, Country Monograph Series no. 11, *Population of Japan* (New York, 1984).

29. Eileen M. Crimmins and Yasuhiko Saito, 'Changes in Life Expectancy and Disability-free Life Expectancy in the U.S.; 1970–80', (unpublished).

30. Thomas N. Chirikos, 'Accounting for the Historical Rise in Work-disability Prevalence', *Milbank Quarterly*, 64, no. 2 (1986), pp. 271–301; Lois M. Verbrugge, 'Longer Life but Worsening Health? Trends in Health and Mortality of Middle-aged and Older Persons', *Milbank Memorial Fund Quarterly/Health and Society*, 62, no. 3 (Summer 1984), pp. 475–519; Dorothy P. Rice and Mitchell P. LaPlante, 'Chronic Illness, Disability, and Increasing Longevity', forthcoming. Rice and LaPlante show a trend increase in restricted activity and explain that hospital statistics (hence bed disability measurements) are unlikely to capture this trend because the length of hospital stays has been curtailed. See also Martin Neil Baily, 'Aging and the Ability to Work: Policy Issues and Recent Trends', and James M. Poterba and Lawrence H. Summers, 'Public Policy Implications of Declining Old-Age Mortality', in Gary Burtless, ed., *Work, Health and Income among the Elderly* (Washington, 1987), respectively, pp. 59–102 and 19–58.

31. Chirikos also employs factor analysis to estimate the degree to which changes in measured health experience may be influenced by measurement error and economic incentives. He finds that those factors account for no more than a third of the trend growth.

32. Verbrugge, 'Longer Life', p. 477, notes that the NHIS is a 'social record of health' in that respondents underreport and overreport conditions when responses are compared to medical records. On the whole respondents underreport conditions.

33. Ibid., p. 479.

34. Ibid., p. 509.

35. US, National Center for Health Statistics, *Health – United States: 1985* (Washington, 1985), p. 128.

8 Sickness and Death in the Twenty-First Century

1. See below, p. 248.

2. In effect, forecasts given below assume that predictors related to sex, income, residence, occupation, and some other population characteristics will retain constant values, and that age-specific period mortality and morbidity rates will accurately reflect future experience at each age. Those assumptions are unlikely to prove accurate. Adopting them simplifies the task of forecasting, but more complex predictive models are called for.

3. See below, p. 235.

4. James F. Fries and Lawrence M. Crapo, *Vitality and Aging: Implications of the Rectangular Curve* (San Francisco, CA, 1981), p. 82. Also James F. Fries, 'Aging, Natural Death, and the Compression of Morbidity', *New England Journal of Medicine*, 303, no. 3 (July 17, 1980), pp. 130–5; id., 'The Compression of Morbidity', *Milbank Memorial Fund Quarterly/Health and Society*, 61, no. 3 (Summer 1983), pp. 397–419; S. Jay Olshansky and A. Brian Ault, 'The Fourth Stage of the Epidemiologic Transition: The Age of Delayed Degenerative Diseases', *Milbank Quarterly*, 64, no. 3 (1986), pp. 374–8; Beth J. Soldo and Kenneth G. Manton, 'Health Status and Service Needs of the Oldest Old: Current Patterns and Future Trends', *Milbank Memorial Fund Quarterly/Health and Society*, 63, no. 2 (Spring 1985), pp. 286–319; Erdman D. Palmore, 'Trends in the Health of the Aged', *Gerontologist*, 26, no. 3 (June 1986), pp. 298–302; Tom Hickey, *Health and Aging* (Monterey, CA, 1980), pp. 169–71.

5. Fries, 'Compression', p. 406.

6. Fries and Crapo, *Vitality*, p. 107. Some commentators object to the Fries-Crapo model on grounds that it seems arbitrary to suggest that health policy should be based on the assumption that age 85 is a fair representation of the maximum average life span (or modal age at death) that should be expected or aimed for. If aging is plastic, as Fries and Crapo argue, and the exhaustion of organ reserve can be deferred, why not attempt to put it off to some higher age? The essential point of the Fries-Crapo case, however, is that there is a boundary; the evidence that the human life span is more or less fixed by characteristics peculiar to the species is more compelling than suggestions that the span itself can be manipulated. Once that point has been made, it becomes clear that the boundary will fall between 70 and 100 and that, for purposes of illustration, age 85 is a reasonable choice. For criticism of Fries, see G.C. Myers and K.G. Manton, 'Compression of Mortality: Myth or Reality?', *Gerontologist*, 24, no. 4 (August 1984), pp. 346–53; Edward L. Schneider and Jacob A. Brody, 'Aging, Natural Death, and the Compression of Morbidity: Another View', *New England Journal of Medicine*, 309, no. 14 (October 6, 1983), pp. 854–6; J. Grimley Evans, 'The Health of an Ageing Population', in A.H. Bittles and K.J. Collins, eds, *The Biology of Human Ageing* (Cambridge, 1986), p. 205; *Gerontologica Perspecta*, 1 (1987).

7. Fries and Crapo, *Vitality*, pp. 3–4, 89–90 and *passim*.

8. Ibid., pp. 86–9 and 100–5. Also Richard G. Cutler, 'Life-Span Extension', in James L. McGaugh and Sara B. Kiesler, eds, *Aging: Biology and Behavior* (New York, 1981), pp. 31–76.

9. George Alter and James C. Riley, 'How to Bet on Lives: A Guide to Life Contingent Contracts in Early Modern Europe', *Research in Economic History*, 10 (1986), pp. 29–31.
10. Kenneth G. Manton, 'Changing Concepts of Morbidity and Mortality in the Elderly Population', *Milbank Memorial Fund Quarterly/Health and Society*, 60, no. 2 (Spring 1982), pp. 183–244; Kenneth G. Manton and Beth J. Soldo, 'Dynamics of Health Changes in the Oldest Old: New Perspectives and Evidence', *Milbank Memorial Fund Quarterly/ Health and Society*, 63, no. 2 (Spring 1985), pp. 206–85; Kenneth G. Manton, 'Past and Future Life Expectancy Increases at Later Ages: Their Implications for the Linkage of Chronic Morbidity, Disability, and Mortality', *Journal of Gerontology*, 41, no. 5 (1986), pp. 672–81; and id., 'The Population Implications of Breakthroughs in Biomedical Technologies for Controlling Mortality and Fertility', in Thomas J. Espenshade and George J. Stolnitz, eds, *Technological Prospects and Population Trends* (Washington, 1987), pp. 147–93. James W. Vaupel, Kenneth G. Manton and Eric Stallard, 'The Impact of Heterogeneity in Individual Frailty and the Dynamics of Mortality', *Demography*, 16, no. 3 (Aug. 1979), p. 447, argue that the increase in life expectancy among the aged may be rapid. Also R.W. Wilson and T.F. Drury, 'Interpreting Trends in Illness and Disability: Health Statistics and Health Status', *Annual Review of Public Health*, 5 (1984), pp. 83–106, who seem unable to decide on the likely morbidity trend.
11. Manton, 'Changing Concepts', p. 233.
12. Thomas N. Chirikos, 'Accounting for the Historical Rise in Work-disability Prevalence', *Milbank Quarterly*, 64, no. 2 (1986), p. 289; Lois M. Verbrugge, 'Longer Life but Worsening Health? Trends in Health and Mortality of Middle-aged and Older Persons', *Milbank Memorial Fund Quarterly/Health and Society*, 62, no. 3 (Summer 1984), pp. 475–519; Jacob J. Feldman, 'Work Ability of the Aged under Conditions of Improving Mortality', *Milbank Memorial Fund Quarterly/ Health and Society*, 61, no. 3 (Fall 1983), pp. 430–44; A. Colvez and M. Blanchet, 'Disability Trends in the United States Population 1966–1976: Analysis of Reported Causes', *American Journal of Public Health*, 71, no. 5 (May 1981), pp. 464–71; Schneider and Brody, 'Another View', p. 855; Jerome L. Avorn, 'Medicine: The Life and Death of Oliver Shay', in Alan Pifer and Lydia Bronte, eds, *Our Aging Society: Paradox and Promise* (New York, 1986), pp. 283–97.
13. Ernest M. Gruenberg, 'The Failures of Success', *Milbank Memorial Fund Quarterly/Health and Society*, 55, no. 1 (Winter 1977), pp. 3–24. See also Manton, 'Changing Concepts', esp. pp. 200ff.; Emily Grundy, 'Mortality and Morbidity among the Old', *British Medical Journal*, 288, no. 6418 (Prac. Obs. ed.) (Mar. 3, 1984), pp. 663–4; Mervyn Susser, 'Environment and Biology in Aging: Some Epidemiological Notions', in James L. McGaugh and Sara B. Kiesler, *Aging: Biology and Behavior* (New York, 1981), pp. 77–96; Donald S. Shepard and Richard J. Zeckhauser, 'Long-term Effects of Interventions to Improve Survival in Mixed Populations', *Journal of Chronic Diseases*, 33 (1980), pp. 413–33, for discussion of some long-run effects of selection in survival rates.

14. J.F. Faber and A.H. Wade, *Life Tables for the United States, 1900–2050*, Social Security Administration Pub. no. 11–11536 (Washington, 1983), pp. 62–4. See also Eileen M. Crimmins, 'The Changing Pattern of American Mortality Decline, 1940–1977, and Its Implications for the Future', *Population and Development Review*, 7, no. 2 (June 1981), pp. 229–54. Other particularly useful previews of experience in a society in which the aged will become more numerous include the essays in Pifer and Bronte, eds, *Our Aging Society*, esp. Jacob S. Siegel and Cynthia M. Taeuber, 'Demographic Dimensions of an Aging Population', pp. 79–110, esp. pp. 94–6.

   If Figure 8.2 were complete, the survival curves would show some people living to age 110 or longer.

15. The ill-health rate in the first year of life will probably exceed the rate inferred by interpolation, but the difference will not be large enough to affect results. Interpolated values were derived by using Waring's formula for a fifth degree polynomial. The technique is explained in US, Bureau of the Census, *The Methods and Materials of Demography*, Henry S. Shryock, Jacob S. Siegel, and others, 2nd printing revised (Washington, 1973), II, pp. 683–4.

16. This effect will show up before age 64 because the labor participation rate declines from an earlier age. Dividing projections at age 64 implies that the labor force participation rate of people aged less than 64 will remain stable after 1985. That is a convenient assumption that simplifies the task at hand, but it is probably inaccurate. Sickness rates may tend to increase more rapidly, or diminish less rapidly, to the degree that labor participation rates decline below 1982–5 levels.

17. People remember ill-health episodes more reliably when asked about the last fourteen days than about periods more distant from the present, but the projection of experience within a short reference period into annual averages understates the actual average of sickness through the year. Protracted or permanent incapacity weighs much less heavily in a reference period of fourteen days than in a longer period, such as a year.

18. Given only five point estimates, it is not possible to discover whether ill-health rates in the US population increase temporarily at or around age 20, as mortality risks do especially for the male population. Thus the age curve is U- rather than W-shaped.

19. US, Bureau of the Census, *Statistical Abstract of the United States 1985* (Washington, 1984), p. 71; and US, National Center for Health Statistics, *Health – United States: 1982* (Washington, 1983), pp. 80–1. The age-adjusted proportion of the population whose activity is limited by health problems remained stable, but the two most widely cited measures of time lost to ill health – restricted activity and bed disability – increased by 5.7 and 4.6 per cent, respectively.

20. The projection varies by age because the predicted change of mortality rates varies by age. Thus the difference between curves A and B is not the same at each age.

21. Since the 1985 population is not stationary, there is a difference between the aggregate sickness time calculated from the life table and the sum that would be derived if the actual distribution of the population were

used to make the calculation. The chief difference is caused by the bulge of baby boomers, aged 21–39 in 1985. Because of this bulge and the lower sickness risk of those ages, the aggregate sickness time in Table 8.1 is somewhat overstated. In the long run a stationary population is usually projected, although the projection is a matter of convenience arising from the difficulty of foreseeing future birth rates. Another way to project aggregate health needs is followed in US, National Center for Health Statistics, D.P. Rice *et al.*, 'Changing Mortality Patterns, Health Services Utilization, and Health Care Expenditures, United States, 1978–2003', *Vital and Health Statistics*, Series 3, no. 23 (Washington, 1983), which forecasts health care utilization under an assumption of fixed age-specific ill-health rates and changing mortality rates.

22. US, National Center for Health Statistics, Aging in the Eighties, Preliminary Data from the Supplement on Aging to the National Health Interview Survey, United States, January-June 1984, *Advance Data from Vital and Health Statistics*, No. 115 (Hyattsville, MD, 1986), p. 4. Also Ira Rosenwaike, *The Extreme Aged in America: A Portrait of an Expanding Population* (Westport, Conn., 1985).

23. US, National Center for Health Statistics, The National Nursing Home Survey: 1977 Summary for the United States, *Vital and Health Statistics*, Series 13, no. 43 (Washington, 1979), pp. 28–9.

24. Compare rates for the closest age groups from the survey used as a basis for Figure 8.4 (US, National Center for Health Services Research, National Health Care Expenditures Study, Marc L. Berk, Gail Lee Cafferata and Michael M. Hagan, *Persons with Limitations of Activity: Health Insurance, Expenditures and Use of Services*, Data Preview 19 [Washington, 1984] p. 2) with those in US, Bureau of the Census, *Persons with Work Disability, Census of Population: 1970*, Subjects Report PC (2)-6C (Washington, 1973), p. 1 (regarding partial or complete work disabilities in the non-institutionalized population). The 1977 NMCES survey also provides a rate for ages 75 and over, but it has been discarded because it applies only to the non-institutionalized population. See further Joan C. Cornoni-Huntley, *et al.*, 'Epidemiology of Disability in the Oldest Old: Methodologic Issues and Preliminary Findings', *Milbank Memorial Fund Quarterly/Health and Society*, 63, no. 2 (Spring 1985). pp. 350–76; Manton and Soldo, 'Dynamics of Health Changes', 206–85.

25. The rate at age 65 has been interpolated from rates at lower ages plus that at ages 65–74, assigned to 69.5. Rates at ages 70 and above follow the same interpolation curve. See n. 21 above on method.

26. Kenneth L. Minaker and John Rowe, 'Health and Disease among the Oldest Old: A Clinical Perspective', *Milbank Memorial Fund Quarterly/ Health and Society*, 63, no. 2 (Spring 1985), pp. 334–5.

27. Ibid., pp. 324–5.

28. Manton and Soldo, 'Dynamics of Health Changes', pp. 247–8, observe that 29 per cent of the non-institutionalized population aged over 90 in one study remained capable of performing basic functions.

In the absence of reliable measurements, estimating the shape of the curve at age 85 and above depends on resolution of a debate recently joined about the way selection operates in this segment of the age spectrum. Manton argues that people 85 + are more robust and represent a population selected for its ability to survive life threatening events at all earlier ages. That is, he hypothesizes that the selection effect shifts around 85 so that only more rather than predominantly less robust people survive. He adopts this view to explain why the life expectancy of disadvantaged populations (all US versus all Swedish, US blacks versus US whites) appears to exceed that of advantaged populations at age 85 and above. But A.J. Coale and Ellen Kisker, 'Mortality Crossovers: Reality or Bad Data?', *Population Studies*, 40, no. 3 (November 1986), pp. 389–402, attribute the effect to measurement error.

29. Manton and Soldo, 'Dynamics', pp. 256 and 262. Also Laurence J. Kotlikoff, 'Some Economic Implications of Life-Span Extension', in McGaugh and Kiesler, eds, *Aging*, pp. 97–114, projecting on the basis of an extended life and work span.
30. Current Estimates from the National Health Interview Survey, 1985, pp. 82–3, adding up columns of conditions reported for selected problems ranging from acne to heart disease. The age-related increase may be understated also because of the selection of conditions. For comparison, see Ethel Shanas, *et al.*, *Old People in Three Industrial Societies* (New York, 1968), pp. 36–44.

Select Bibliography

Acheson, Roy M. and Spencer Hagard, *Health, Society and Medicine: An Introduction to Community Medicine* (Oxford, 1984).

Acsádi, Gy. and J. Nemeskéri, *History of Human Life Span and Mortality*, trans. by K. Balás (Budapest, 1970).

Alter, George and James C. Riley, 'Frailty, Sickness, and Death: Models of Morbidity and Mortality in Historical Populations', forthcoming *Population Studies* (1989).

Ansell, Charles, *A Treatise on Friendly Societies . . .* (London, 1835).

Beeson, Paul B., 'Changes in Medical Therapy during the Past Half Century', *Medicine*, 39 (1980), pp. 79–99.

Beier, Lucinda McCray, 'In Sickness and in Health: A Seventeenth Century Family's Experience', in Roy Porter, ed., *Patients and Practitioners: Lay Perceptions of Medicine in Pre-industrial Society* (Cambridge, 1985).

Benjamin, Bernard, 'The Measurement of Morbidity', *Journal of the Institute of Actuaries*, 83 (1957), pp. 225–67.

Binstock, Robert H. and Ethel Shanas, eds, *Handbook of Aging and the Social Sciences* (New York, 1976).

Birren, James E., ed., *Handbook of Aging and the Individual* (Chicago, 1959).

Bittles, A.H. and K.J. Collins, eds, *The Biology of Human Ageing* (Cambridge, 1986).

Bruneel, Claude, *La mortalité dans les campagnes: Le duché de Brabant aux XVIIe et XVIIIe siècles*, 2 vols (Leuven, 1977).

Burnet, F. Macfarlane and David O. White, *Natural History of Infectious Disease*, 4th edn (Cambridge, 1972).

Caplan, Arthur L., H. Tristram Engelhardt, Jr, and James J. McCartney, eds, *Concepts of Health and Disease: Interdisciplinary Perspectives* (Reading, Mass., 1981).

Carmichael, Ann G., 'Infection, Hidden Hunger, and History', *Journal of Interdisciplinary History*, 14 (1983), pp. 249–64.

Charbonneau, Hubert and André Larose, eds, *The Great Mortalities: Methodological Studies of Demographic Crises in the Past* (Liege, n.d.).

Cheyne, George, *An Essay of Health and Long Life*, 4th edn (London, 1725).

Chirikos, Thomas N., 'Accounting for the Historical Rise in Work-disability Prevalence', *Milbank Quarterly*, 64 (1986), pp. 271–301.

Cohen, Mark Nathan and George J. Armelagos, eds, *Paleopathology at the Origins of Agriculture* (New York, 1984).

Cohen, Sheldon and S. Leonard Syme, eds, *Social Support and Health* (Orlando, 1985).

Colvez, A. and M. Blanchet, 'Disability Trends in the United States Population 1966–1976: Analysis of Reported Causes', *American Journal of Public Health*, 71 (1981), pp. 464–71.

Comfort, Alex, *The Biology of Senescence*, 3rd edn (Edinburgh, 1979).

Committee of the Highland Society of Scotland, *Report on Friendly or*

Benefit Societies, Exhibiting the Law of Sickness . . . (Edinburgh, 1824).

Crimmins, Eileen M., 'The Changing Pattern of American Mortality Decline, 1940–1977, and Its Implications for the Future', *Population and Development Review*, 7 (1981), pp. 229–54.

Culyer, A.J., ed., *Health Indicators* (Oxford, 1983).

Dab, W., J. Rochon and L. Bernard, 'L'absence au travail comme prédicteur de morbidité grave . . .', *Revue d'épidémiologie et de santé publique*, 34 (1986), pp. 252–60.

Del Panta, L. and M. Livi Bacci, 'Chronologie, intensité et diffusion des crises de mortalité en Italie: 1600–1850', *Population*, 32 (1977), pp. 401–46.

Desaive, Jean-Paul *et al.*, *Médecins, climat et épidémies à la fin du XVIII siècle* (Paris, 1972).

Dowling, Harry F., *Fighting Infection: Conquests of the Twentieth Century* (Cambridge, Mass., 1977).

Dubos, René, *Man, Medicine, and Environment* (New York, 1968).

——, *Mirage of Health* (New York, 1959).

Economos, Angelos C., 'Rate of Aging, Rate of Dying and the Mechanism of Mortality', *Archives of Gerontology and Geriatrics*, 1 (1982), pp. 3–27.

Edmonds, T.R., *Life Tables, Founded upon the Discovery of a Numerical Law Regulating the Existence of Every Human Being* . . . (London, 1832).

——, 'On the Laws of Sickness, According to Age, Exhibiting a Double Coincidence Between the Laws of Sickness and the Laws of Mortality', *Lancet*, no. 1 (1835–6), pp. 855–8.

Erhardt, Carl L. and Joyce E. Berlin, eds, *Mortality and Morbidity in the United States* (Cambridge, 1974).

Espenshade, Thomas J. and George J. Stolnitz, eds, *Technological Prospects and Population Trends* (Washington, 1987).

Faber, J.F. and A.H. Wade, *Life Tables for the United States, 1900–2050* Social Security Administration Pub. no. 11–11536 (Washington, 1983).

Farge, Arlette, 'Les artisans malades de leur travail', *Annales: économies, sociétés, civilisations*, 32 (1977), pp. 993–1006.

[Farr, William], 'Vital Statistics', in J.R. McCulloch, ed., *Statistical Account of the British Empire*, 3rd edn, 2 vols (London, 1847).

Feldman, Jacob J., 'Work Ability of the Aged under Conditions of Improving Mortality', *Milbank Memorial Fund Quarterly/Health and Society*, 61 (1983), pp. 430–44.

Finch, Caleb E. and Leonard Hayflick, eds, *Handbook of the Biology of Aging* (New York, 1977).

—— and Edward L. Schneider, eds, *Handbook of the Biology of Aging*, 2nd edn (New York, 1985).

Fogel, Robert W., 'Nutrition and the Decline in Mortality since 1700: Some Preliminary Findings', in Stanley L. Engerman and Robert E. Gallman, eds, *Long-term Factors in American Economic Growth* (Chicago, 1986).

Forster, Elborg, 'From the Patient's Point of View: Illness and Health in the Letters of Liselotte von der Pfalz (1652–1722)', *Bulletin of the History of Medicine*, 60 (1986), pp. 279–320.

Fries, James F., 'Aging, Natural Death, and the Compression of Morbidity',

New England Journal of Medicine, 303 (1980), pp. 130–5.

_____ and Lawrence M. Crapo, *Vitality and Aging: Implications of the Rectangular Curve* (San Francisco, 1981).

Gompertz, Benjamin, 'On the Nature of the Function Expressive of the Law of Human Mortality . . .', *Philosophical Transactions*, 115 (1825), pp. 513–85.

Grmek, Mirko D., 'Préliminaires d'une étude historique des maladies', *Annales: économies, sociétés, civilisations*, 24 (1969), pp. 1473–83.

Gruenberg, Ernest M., 'The Failures of Success', *Milbank Memorial Fund Quarterly/Health and Society*, 55 (1977), pp. 3–24.

Hannah, Leslie, *Inventing Retirement: The Development of Occupational Pensions in Britain* (Cambridge, 1986).

Hinkle, Lawrence E., Jr, *et al.*, 'The Distribution of Sickness Disability in a Homogeneous Group of "Healthy Adult men"', *American Journal of Hygiene*, 64 (1956), pp. 220–42.

Howell, Trevor H., 'Multiple Pathology in Nonagenarians', *Geriatrics*, 18 (1963), pp. 899–902.

Imhof, Arthur Erwin, 'From the Old Mortality Pattern to the New: Implications of a Radical Change from the Sixteenth Century to the Twentieth Century', *Bulletin of the History of Medicine*, 59 (1985), pp. 1–29.

_____, *Die gewonnenen Jahre: Von der Zunahme unserer Lebensspanne seit dreihundert Jahren oder von der Notwendigkeit einer neuen Einstellung zu Leben und Sterben* (Munich, 1981).

_____ and Øivind Larsen, *Sozialgeschichte und Medizin: Probleme der quantifizierenden Quellenbearbeitung in der Sozial- und Medizingeschichte* (Oslo, 1976).

Jones, Hardin B., 'A Special Consideration of the Aging Process, Disease, and Life Expectancy', in John H. Lawrence and Cornelius A. Tobias, eds, *Advances in Biological and Medical Physics*. vol. IV (New York, 1956).

Katz, Sidney *et al.*, 'Active Life Expectancy', *New England Journal of Medicine*, 309 (1983), pp. 1218–23.

Kermack, W.O., A.G. McKendrick and P.L. McKinlay, 'Death-Rates in Great Britain and Sweden: Some General Regularities and Their Significance', *Lancet*, no. 1 (1934), pp. 698–703.

Kirkwood, T.B.L. and R. Holliday, 'The Evolution of Ageing and Longevity', *Proceedings of the Royal Society of London*, B205 (1979), pp. 531–46.

Knight, Bernard, *The Coroner's Autopsy: A Guide to Non-Criminal Autopsies for the General Pathologist* (Edinburgh, 1983).

Larsen, Øivind, 'Eighteenth-Century Diseases, Diagnostic Trends, and Mortality', *The Fifth Scandinavian Demographic Symposium* (Hurdalssjøen, 1979).

Livi Bacci, Massimo, *La société italienne devant les crises de mortalité* (Florence, 1978).

McGaugh, James L. and Sara B. Kiesler, eds, *Aging: Biology and Behavior* (New York, 1981).

McKeown, Thomas, *The Modern Rise of Population* (London, 1976).

McKinlay, John B. and Sonja M. McKinlay, 'The Questionable Contribution of Medical Measures to the Decline of Mortality in the United States in the Twentieth Century', *Milbank Memorial Fund Quarterly/Health and Society*, 55 (1977), pp. 405–28.

McNeill, William H., *Plagues and Peoples* (Garden City, N.Y., 1976).

Manton, Kenneth B., 'Changing Concepts of Morbidity and Mortality in the Elderly Population', *Milbank Memorial Fund Quarterly/Health and Society*, 60 (1982), pp. 183–244.

—— and Beth J. Soldo, 'Dynamics of Health Changes in the Oldest Old: New Perspectives and Evidence', *Milbank Memorial Fund Quarterly/ Health and Society*, 63, (1985), pp. 206–85.

Meeker, Edward, 'The Improving Health of the United States, 1850–1915', *Explorations in Economic History*, 9 (1972), pp. 353–73.

Minaker, Kenneth L. and John Rowe, 'Health and Disease among the Oldest Old: A Clinical Perspective', *Milbank Memorial Fund Quarterly/ Health and Society*, 63 (1985), pp. 324–49.

Morrison, Alan S., *Screening in Chronic Diseases* (New York, 1985).

Myers, George C. and Kenneth G. Manton, 'Compression of Mortality: Myth or Reality?', *Gerontologist*, 24 (1984), pp. 346–53.

Neison, Francis G.P., Sr., *Contributions to Vital Statistics: Being a Development of the Rate of Mortality and the Laws of Sickness . . .*, 3rd edn (London, 1857).

Neison, Francis G.P., Jr., *The Rates of Mortality and Sickness According to the Experience for the Five Years, 1871–1875, of the Ancient Order of Foresters Friendly Society . . .* (London, 1882).

——, *The Rates of Mortality and Sickness According to the Experience for the Ten Years 1878–1887, of the Independent Order of Rechabites . . .* (Manchester, 1889).

Neugarten, Bernice L. and Robert J. Havighurst, eds, *Extending the Human Life Span* (Chicago, 1977).

Oddy, Derek [J.] and Derek [S.] Miller, eds, *Diet and Health in Modern Britain* (London, 1985).

Olshansky, S. Jay and A. Brian Ault, 'The Fourth Stage of the Epidemiologic Transition: The Age of Delayed Degenerative Diseases', *Milbank Quarterly*, 64 (1986), pp. 355–91.

Omran, Abdel R., 'The Epidemiologic Transition: A Theory of the Epidemiology of Population Change', *Milbank Memorial Fund Quarterly*, 49 (1971), pp. 509–38.

Ophüls, William, 'Arteriosclerosis, Cardiovascular Disease; Their Relation to Infectious Diseases', Standford University Publications, *Medical Sciences*, vol. I, no. 1 (1921).

——, 'A Statistical Survey of Three Thousand Autopsies', Standford University Publications, *Medical Sciences*, vol. I (1926) no. 3.

Pelling, Margaret, 'Healing the Sick Poor: Social Policy and Disability in Norwich, 1550–1640', *Medical History*, 29 (1985), pp. 115–37.

Perrenoud, Alfred, 'Le biologique et l'humain dans le déclin séculaire de la mortalité', *Annales: économies, sociétés, civilisations*, 40 (1985), pp. 113–35.

——, *La population de Genève du seizième au début du dix-neuvième siècle: Etude démographique* (Geneva, 1979).

Pifer, Alan and Lydia Bronte, eds, *Our Aging Society: Paradox and Promise* (New York, 1986).

Preston, Samuel H., ed., *Biological and Social Aspects of Mortality and the Length of Life* (Liege, 1982).

____, Nathan Keyfitz and Robert Schoen, *Causes of Death: Life Tables for National Populations* (New York, 1972).

Quadagno, Jill S., *Aging in Early Industrial Society* (New York, 1982).

Ratcliffe, Henry, *Observations on the Rate of Mortality and Sickness Existing amongst Friendly Societies . . .* (Colchester, 1862).

Retherford, Robert D., *The Changing Sex Differential in Mortality* (Westport, Conn., 1979).

Riley, James C., *The Eighteenth-Century Campaign to Avoid Disease* (New York, 1987).

____, 'Disease without Death: New Sources for a History of Sickness', *Journal of Interdisciplinary History*, 17 (1987), pp. 537–63.

____, 'Ill Health during the English Mortality Decline: The Friendly Societies' Experience', *Bulletin of the History of Medicine*, 61 (1987), pp. 563–88.

____, 'Sickness in an Early Modern Workplace', *Continuity and Change*, 2 (1987), pp. 363–85.

Riley, Mathilda White, Beth B. Hess and Kathleen Bond, eds, *Aging in Society: Selected Reviews of Recent Research* (Hillsdale, N.J., 1983).

Rosen, George, *A History of Public Health* (New York, 1958).

Schneider, Edward L. and Jacob A. Brody, 'Aging, Natural Death, and the Compression of Morbidity: Another View', *New England Journal of Medicine*, 309 (1983), pp. 854–6.

____ and John D. Reed, Jr., 'Life Extension', *New England Journal of Medicine*, 312 (1985), pp. 1159–68.

Shock, Nathan W. *et al.*, *Normal Human Aging: The Baltimore Longitudinal Study of Aging* (Washington, 1984).

Siegel, Jacob S. and Cynthia M. Taeuber, 'Demographic Perspectives on the Long-Lived Society', *Daedalus*, 115 (1986), pp. 77–117.

Smith, F.B., 'Health', in John Benson, ed., *The Working Class in England, 1875–1914* (London, 1985).

____, *The People's Health, 1830–1910* (New York, 1979).

Soldo, Beth J. and Kenneth G. Manton, 'Health Status and Service Needs of the Oldest Old: Current Patterns and Future Trends', *Milbank Memorial Fund Quarterly/Health and Society*, 63 (1985), pp. 286–319.

Spink, Wesley W., *Infectious Diseases: Prevention and Treatment in the Nineteenth and Twentieth Centuries* (Minneapolis, 1978).

Stanley, N.F. and R.A. Joske, eds, *Changing Disease Patterns and Human Behaviour* (London, 1980).

Strehler, Bernard L., *Times, Cells, and Aging*, 2nd edn (New York, 1977).

Sutton, W[illiam], *Special Report on Sickness and Mortality Experienced in Registered Friendly Societies . . .*, House of Commons, Sessional Papers, 1896, LXXIX, 1.

Taylor, P.J., 'Some International Trends in Sickness Absence 1950–68', *British Medical Journal*, no. 4 (1969), pp. 705–7.

United States, National Center for Health Statistics, *Mortality from Diseases*

Associated with Smoking: United States, 1960–77, National Vital Statistics System, Series 20, no. 17 (Washington, 1982).

Vallin, Jacques, John H. Pollard and Larry Heligman, eds, *Methodologies for the Collection and Analysis of Mortality Data* (Liege, 1984).

Vaupel, James W. and Anatoli I. Yashin, 'Heterogeneity's Ruses: Some Surprising Effects of Selection on Population Dynamics', *The American Statistician*, 39 (1985), pp. 176–85.

Verbrugge, Lois M., 'Gender and Health: An Update on Hypotheses and Evidence', *Journal of Health and Social Behavior*, 26 (1985), pp. 156–82.

——, 'Longer Life but Worsening Health? Trends in Health and Mortality of Middle-Aged and Older Persons', *Milbank Memorial Fund Quarterly/ Health and Society*, 62 (1984), pp. 475–519.

Walford, Roy L., *Maximum Life Span* (New York, 1983).

Watson, Alfred W., *An Account of an Investigation of the Sickness and Mortality Experience of the I.O.O.F. Manchester Unity . . . 1893–1897* (Manchester, 1903).

Weindling, Paul, ed., *The Social History of Occupational Health* (London, 1985).

Weinstein, Louis, 'Infectious Disease: Retrospect and Reminiscence', *Journal of Infectious Diseases*, 129 (1974), pp 480–92.

Wilson, Ronald W. and Thomas F. Drury, 'Interpreting Trends in Illness and Disability: Health Statistics and Health Status', *Annual Review of Public Health*, 5 (1984), pp. 83–106.

Woods, Robert and John Woodward, eds, *Urban Disease and Mortality in Nineteenth-Century England* (London, 1984).

Wrigley, E.A. and R.S. Schofield, *The Population History of England, 1541–1871* (Cambridge, Mass., 1981).

Wunsch, Guillaume, 'Malades et maladies: La mesure de la morbidité et de la durée de la maladie', in *Morbidité et mortalité aux âges adultes dans les pays développés* (Louvain-la-neuve, 1983).

Index